Medicinal Chemistry: Principles and Practice

Medicinal Chemistry: Principles and Practice

Edited by

Frank D. King
SmithKline Beecham Pharmaceuticals, Harlow, UK

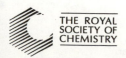

THE ROYAL
SOCIETY OF
CHEMISTRY

A catalogue record for this book is available from the British Library.

ISBN 0–85186–494–5

© The Royal Society of Chemistry 1994

Reprinted 1995

Published by The Royal Society of Chemistry,
Thomas Graham House, The Science Park, Cambridge CB4 4WF

Typeset by Computape (Pickering) Ltd, North Yorkshire
Printed in Great Britain by Athenaeum Press Ltd., Gateshead, Tyne & Wear.

Foreword

The excitement and challenges in Biochemical Research have never been greater. The breathtaking speed and diversity of scientific advance, coupled with the range and complexity of technology, can easily leave the scientist bemused, as well as exhausted. For medicinal chemists in many parts of the world, both aspiring and experienced, the RSC Medicinal Chemistry School has become a valuable means of acquiring new knowledge and recharging the cerebral batteries. It is a pleasure to have participated and a privilege to introduce this book, which gathers the formal inputs to lectures and workshops, but, of course, cannot reproduce the many hours of informal, but animated discussion.

Huge strides were taken in controlling infectious disease with the introduction of antibiotics, which resulted from the application of chemistry and microbiology to the search for new medicines. Equally, the efforts of pharmacologists and chemists led to significant advances in the treatment of the mentally ill. These are merely two examples of early success in the search for new medical products. The appearance of AIDS and the reemergence of tuberculosis, the inadequacy of neuroleptic drugs and the absence of therapy for neurodegenerative diseases, together with countless other diseases which have no cure or are inadequately treated, serve to remind us that we have only just begun the quest to alleviate human suffering.

Happily, we are better equipped than ever before. Molecular biology is having a profound impact on biomedical research. Pathological processes can now be understood at the molecular level and can quickly lead to the establishment of discerning tests to facilitate the early evaluation of compounds. Link these with the ability of computers to process enormous amounts of data and several thousand compounds can be put through such screens each week. Positive leads can be rapidly followed by the scanning through large collections of compounds seeking 3-D structural relationships. The structure of enzymes or receptors to be blocked can often be established by gene cloning, expression and X-ray or NMR analysis. Structural models are no longer cumbersome bits of engineering to be handled delicately, but 3-D graphics which only a few years ago would have been regarded as science fiction. Chemical libraries can now be created to allow rapid access to a wider range of structural diversity than ever before. Advances in molecular genetics permit rapid identification of genes 'associated with' particular human diseases. It will soon be possible to go from identifying a gene through understanding its function and creating high-throughput screens to candidate drugs in very short order.

It is paradoxical that just as this scientific momentum is opening the door to striking advances in disease therapy, society is questioning what it wants, or more precisely how much it can afford. Typically, developed countries spend about ten percent of Gross Domestic Product on health care, with about one tenth of this being spent of medicines, *i.e.* one percent of GDP. Rocketing overall health care costs are forcing governments everywhere to act and the small component put on medicines has become the focus of much attention. It is politically more acceptable to attack this target than to close hospitals or reduce local care. Pressure is being imposed on the pricing of medicines everywhere, just at a time when the costs of bringing a new product to the market have reached worryingly high levels; for instance, the US Pharmaceutical Manufacturers' Association has recently estimated an average figure of 260 million dollars.

It is inevitable that much biomedical research and many companies will not be adequately rewarded for their efforts by the introduction of successful new medicines. Indeed, there will be many losers. What is clear is that winners will bring forward new products which meet real medical needs and will be able to show an economic justification for the use of their products. In conducting their research, scientists need to be aware of this social and economic climate if their work is to be of more than academic interest. Today's medicinal chemists must add to their professional mastery of chemistry a great diversity of cognate science and a sharp politico-economic awareness – quite a challenge, but one made easier and more fun by activities such as the RSC Summer School.

Dr. T.F.W. McKillop
Zeneca Pharmaceuticals

Preface

This book is essentially a collation of the lectures presented at the 7th RSC Medicinal Chemistry School held between 28th June and 3rd July in 1993 at the University of Kent, Canterbury, UK (the 8th is due to be held in 1995). This residential course consists of a series of 1 hour lectures and three afternoon tutorials and is intended to provide an introduction to Medicinal Chemistry, primarily for synthetic chemists who have recently joined the industry. The teaching staff are taken from both pharmaceutical companies and academia to give as broad a perspective as possible. An integral and important part of the course is the informal discussions between the teaching staff and students. The course is intended to introduce most of the Principles of Medicinal Chemistry, given the time constraints, and includes a selection of Case Histories, examples of drug discovery which illustrate how these principles have been put into practice.

The main aim of the medicinal chemist is to identify a drug candidate from an initial lead compound which possesses all of the properties required for successful development. This compound should possess not only the desired level of biological activity in suitable disease models, but also satisfy other criteria such as being overtly non-toxic, stable, be preferably water soluble, have suitable pharmacokinetics and dynamics and have good bioavailability. The process by which this is accomplished can be viewed as a cyclic process, spiralling to the desired end with each turn of the cycle.

Initially a target compound would be identified from the lead compound. This would then be synthesised and tested to see whether an improvement in the desired properties has been achieved. The result would then be analysed and compared with results obtained from other compounds and a hypothesis or hypotheses produced. These hypotheses are then tested by identification of more target compounds and the cycle is repeated until a compound is identified which satisfies all of the criteria set for a development candidate. A good medicinal chemist must therefore be not just a good synthetic organic chemist, but also, amongst other things, have an understanding of intermolecular interactions which give molecules the desired biological activity.

The pharmaceutical industry is highly competitive and therefore it is essential to complete the spiral to success as quickly as possible. This relies not only on the **quality** of interpretation and understanding (mainly on the left hand side of the cycle) but also on the **quantity** (number) of compounds prepared and the **speed** with which each cycle is completed (mainly dependent on the right hand side). In

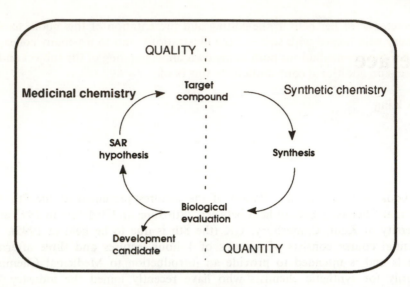

order to achieve results quickly, a research team will often be concurrently investigating a large number of different, interactive cycles. (It is becoming increasingly rare that the medicinal chemist has the luxury of being the only investigator working on an approach to a disease, where the competitive pressure to being first to the market is not so apparent.) The speed with which the cycle is completed is dependent upon a combination of the size and efficiency of the research team and the ease of synthesis and testing. However, the main aim of the course and of this book is to address the **quality of interpretation and understanding** which determines how far the research advances with each turn of the cycle.

Over the years the Medicinal Chemistry course has been highly successful and this has been due both to the high quality and enthusiasm of past organisers (two of whom, Prof. Robin Ganellin and Dr. Colin Greengrass are still involved) and that of the participants. (During the last 20 years the pharmaceutical industry has been one of the major industrial successes in the UK and the training of the scientists has played no small part in this success.) A special thanks is given to the teaching staff of the 1993 course, especially to those tutors whose contributions do not appear in this book. They include Dr. Ken Richardson, Dr. Nigel Cussans and Dr. Paul Finn (all from Pfizer), Dr. Colin Edge (SB), Dr. Howard Broughton (MS&D) and Dr. Peter Daley-Yates (Upjohn). I would also like to thank a number of pharmaceutical companies who sponsored the recent course, to enable a number of postgraduate students to attend. These include Boots Pharmaceuticals, Fisons Pharmaceuticals, Glaxo Group Research, Lilly Research Centre, Merck Sharp and Dohme Research Laboratories, Parke-Davis Research Unit, Pfizer Central Research, Roche Products, SmithKline Beecham Pharmaceuticals, Wellcome Research Laboratories, Wyeth Research UK and Zeneca Pharmaceuticals. Finally the course would not have been such a success without the organisational efficiency of Lorraine Hart from the RSC Education Department, to whom I give many thanks. Acknowledgement is also due to Kris Phillipson, my secretary, for her help in the editing and presentation of this book, to Sally Bradbury who helped with some of the illustrations, and to my many colleagues at SB for their contributions both to my own understanding of the subject and for their help on additional contributions to this book.

Frank King

GENERAL REFERENCES

Reference Books

'Comprehensive Medicinal Chemistry', ed. C. Hansch, J.C. Emmett, P.D. Kennewell, C.A. Ramsden, P.G. Sammes and J.B. Taylor, 1990, Vols 1–6. Pergamon, Oxford. 'Burger's Medicinal Chemistry', ed. M.E. Wolff, 1979–81, 4th Edn. Wiley, New York. 'The Merck Index', ed. S. Budavari, 1989, 11th Edn. Merck & Co., Rahway, New Jersey.

Journals

Annual Reports in Medicinal Chemistry
Bioorganic and Medicinal Chemistry Letters
Chemical and Pharmaceutical Bulletins
Drugs of the Future
Drug Design and Delivery
Drug News and Perspectives
European Journal of Medicinal Chemistry
Journal of Medicinal Chemistry
Medicinal Chemistry Research
Medicinal Research Review
Trends in Pharmacological Sciences

A very useful 'Pocket Guide to Pharmacology' is available from Glaxo by writing to: Dr. Michael J. Sheehan, Glaxo Group Research Ltd., Park Road, Ware, Herts., SG12 0DP, UK.

Contents

Chapter 8   **Quantitative Structure–Activity Relationships**
Andrew M. Davis

Contents xix

Contributors

J. Carey, *SmithKline Beecham Pharmaceuticals, Coldharbour Road, The Pinnacles, Harlow, Essex CM19 5AD, UK*

R.A. Coleman, *Glaxo Group Research Ltd., Park Road, Ware, Hertfordshire SG12 0DP, UK*

A. Davies, *Fisons Pharmaceuticals Bakewell Road, Loughborough, Leicestershire LE11 0RH, UK*

T. J. Franklin, *Zeneca Pharmaceuticals, Mereside, Alderley Park, Macclesfield, Cheshire SK10 4TG, UK*

C.R. Ganellin FRS, *Department of Chemistry, University College London, 20 Gordon Street, London WC1H 0AJ, UK*

N. Gensmantel, *Fisons Pharmaceuticals, Bakewell Road, Loughborough, Leicestershire LE11 0RK, UK*

C. W. Greengrass, *Discovery Chemistry, Pfizer Central, Sandwich, Kent CT13 9NJ, UK*

M. Hann, *Glaxo Group Research, Greenford, Middlesex UB6 9HE, UK*

C. Hill, *Roche Research Centre, P.O. Box 8, Welwyn Garden City, Hertfordshire AL7 3AY, UK*

S. T. Hodgson, *Wellcome Research Laboratories, Langley Court, South Eden Park Road, Beckenham, Kent BR3 3BS, UK*

D. C. Horwell, *Parke-Davis Neuroscience Research Unit, Addenbrookes Hospital Site, Hills Road, Cambridge CB2 2QB, UK*

B. Hunt, *School of Natural Science, University of Hertfordshire, College Lane, Hatfield, Hertfordshire, AL10 9AB UK*

R.M. Ings, *Upjohn Limited, Fleming Way, Crawley, West Sussex RH10 2LZ, UK*

F. D. King, *SmithKline Beecham Pharmaceuticals, Coldharbour Road, The Pinnacles, Harlow, Essex CM19 5AD, UK*

P. North, *Glaxo Group Research Limited, Ware, Hertordshire SG12 0DP, UK*

J. Ormerod, *Clinical Research and Project Management, SmithKline Beecham Pharmaceuticals, Yew Tree Bottom Road, Epsom, Surrey KT18 5XQ, UK*

D. A. Roberts, *Zenecca Pharmaceuticals, Mereside, Alderley Park, Macclesfield, Cheshire SK10 4TG, UK*

A.W. Tyrrell, *SmithKline Beecham Pharmaceuticals, Yew Tree Bottom Road, Epsom, Surrey KT18 5XQ, UK*

C. Vose, *Hoechst Pharmaceutical Research Laboratories, Walton Manor, Milton Keynes, Buckinghamshire MK7 7AJ, UK*

CHAPTER 1

An Introduction to Drug–Receptor Interactions

BARRY HUNT

1 INTRODUCTION

Many pharmacologically active substances exert their maximum effect on physiological function when they are present at their site of action in the body in minute quantities; some of these highly potent molecules have significant effects at tissue concentrations in the nanomolar range and are thus capable of inducing maximum cellular responses at concentrations far less than would be necessary to provide even a monomolecular coat. Additionally, their effects are usually biologically highly selective so that an effect of the agent in one type of tissue may be profound whereas the response of an apparently similar tissue may be either non-existent or opposite. For example the effect of the administration of histamine in different smooth muscle preparations illustrates this phenomenon, the substance producing a contraction of bronchiolar and a relaxation of vascular smooth muscle. Furthermore, even small manipulations to the structure of an active molecule may seriously affect its pharmacological activity.

For example, Figure 1 shows the effect on activity of introducing a methyl group into different parts of the histamine molecule. Substitution on either the α or the β carbon atom leads to a significant loss of pharmacological activity in both the isolated ileum and atrium preparations, whereas ring methylation in the 4 position causes a selective loss of effect in the ileum, explained by sub-types

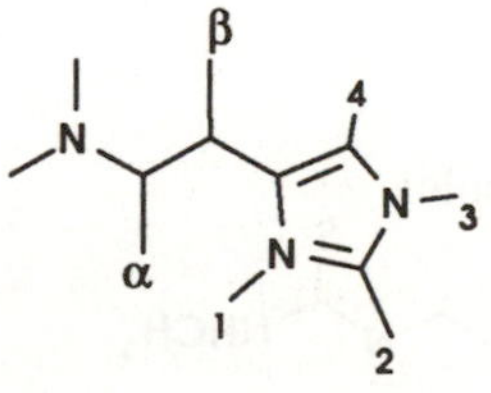

Substituent	Ileum*	Atrium*
N-methyl	70%	70%
N,N-dimethyl	45%	50%
α-methyl	<5%	<5%
β-methyl	<5%	<5%
1-methyl	<5%	<5%
2-methyl	25%	10%
3-methyl	<5%	<5%
4-methyl	<5%	50%

* Activity relative to histamine

Figure 1: *Effect of methyl substituent in histamine*

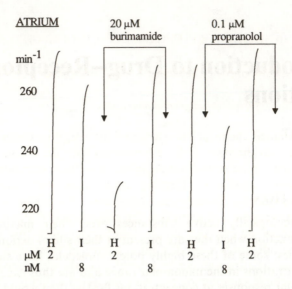

Figure 2:   *Action of histamine (H) and isoprenaline (I) on isolated atrium*

of histamine receptor. In many cases these specific biological responses to an active molecule (agonist) can be selectively disrupted by a substance (antagonist) that bears a structural resemblance. For example the action of both histamine (H) and isoprenaline (I) on the atrium of the heart is to increase its rate of beat and Figure 2 illustrates an experiment where these actions of histamine and isoprenaline were selectively blocked by burimamide and propranolol respectively; the structural similarity of each agonist/antagonist pair is shown in Figure 3.

Observations such as the above of high potency, biological selectivity, definite structural requirement for activity, and selective disruption of activity with other compounds can easily be explained in terms of drugs requiring only to interact with a specialised portion (receptors) of the target cell in order to produce their effects.

This notion of receptors that is central to our understanding of drug action

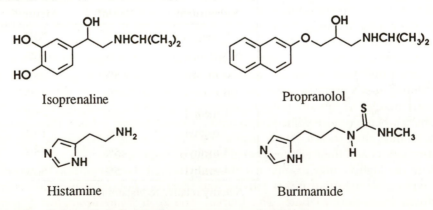

Figure 3:   *Structural similarities between agonists and antagonists*

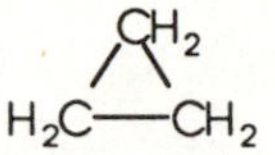

H_2C——CH_2 / CH_2 cyclopropane

$(C_2H_5)_2O$ diethyl ether

$CF_3CHClBr$ halothane

$CF_3CH_2OCH=CH_2$ fluoroxene

$CHCl_2CF_2OCH_3$ methoxyflurane

Figure 4: *Structures of a number of general anaesthetics*

predates any detailed chemical knowledge of the receptive material. In the 19th century Langley, on the basis of his experiments with the mutually antagonistic actions of the drugs pilocarpine and atropine on salivary secretion, assumed that both drugs were capable of forming compounds with some endogenous substance. Subsequently Ehrlich also considered the antagonistic actions of atropine and pilocarpine and expressed the classic view '*Corpora non agunt nisi fixata*'; (substances do not act unless fixed: in context this means bound). Nevertheless not all drugs show the same degree of structural specificity. For example the stucture of a number of general anaesthetics is shown in Figure 4; they are lipid soluble compounds but with unrelated structure. Therefore, non-receptor based mechanisms are required alongside drug-receptor concepts as part of the theoretical explanations of pharmacodynamics offered by pharmacologists.

Overall the concept that a majority of drugs work through specific receptors is highly acceptable. However, the notion that these receptors are present to render the effects of an ingested foreign chemical more potent is not tenable: more sensible is the idea that the drug utilises mechanisms evolved to receive signals from endogenous mediators. For example the characterisation of specific receptors for opiate drugs in the brain led to the search for and identification of natural agonists in brain extracts termed collectively endorphins. Furthermore, for an individual endogenous mediator a number of receptor sub-types may exist (also refer back to Figure 1).

To illustrate further the point the neurotransmitter acetylcholine has been shown to act through receptors designated both nicotinic and muscarinic; by a variety of pharmacological and molecular biology techniques the muscarinic receptor has been further sub-divided into M_1 to M_5 sub-types. In general, receptors for neurotransmitter substances have often proved to be valuable targets for drug action and Figure 5 depicts the classical features of a chemical synapse revealing both pre- and post-junctional receptors for the transmitter.

To take the example of the sympathetic nervous system noradrenaline acts as the transmitter and in blood vessels its action is to cause constriction by stimulating α-receptors (a sub-class of adrenaline receptors) on the innervated smooth muscle. At this site pre-junctional α-receptors are involved with negative feedback where noradrenaline acts to inhibit its own further release. Pharmacological studies have shown that a distinction can be made between the pre- and post-receptors and these are designated α_2 and α_1 respectively.

With the high volume of pharmacological research the recognition of receptor sub-types is an area that is fast moving and therefore nomenclature can become confused from time to time. The journal *Trends in Pharmacological Sciences* publishes a useful review of receptor classification on a yearly basis.

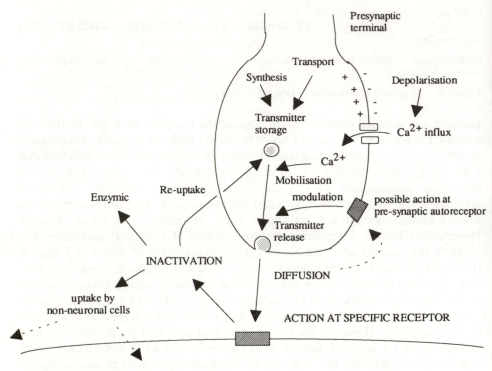

Figure 5:   *Features of a chemical synapse*

2 DRUG AGONISTS: DOSE–RESPONSE RELATIONSHIPS

To obtain an appreciation of the quantitative nature of drug–receptor interaction the use of isolated tissue (such as the guinea pig ileum in an organ-bath situation) is invaluable: with whole animal studies pharmacokinetic factors will impinge on the analysis of the effects of an administered drug. Table 1 indicates examples of the individual receptor system that can be explored using a particular isolated preparation. For example the guinea pig ileum set up in an isolated organ bath situation can be used to explore the action of the neurotransmitter acetylcholine and structurally related molecules. Typically increasing the concentration of the agonist leads to an increasingly larger response until a maximum response is achieved. See Figure 6 where a diagramatic representation of a response (r) trace to sequential application of increasing concentrations (D) of an agonist is provided; graphically this relationship is often presented as a log dose–response curve.

The dose–response relationships obtained can be explained in terms of the occupancy theory of Clark which states that the response to a drug is proportional to the number of receptors occupied at equilibrium and that a maximum response occurs when all the receptors are occupied. Thus:

Drug (D) + Receptor (R) $\leftrightarrow$ Drug Receptor complex (DR) $\Rightarrow$ Response

Table 1: *Common isolated tissue preparations*

Preparation	Receptors commonly studied
Guinea-pig ileum	ACh (muscarinic), histamine H_1 neurokinin NK_1, bradykinin B_2, 5-HT_3, CCKa
Guinea-pig ileum (field stimulated)	μ- and κ-opioid, α_2-adrenoceptors
Rabbit jejunum	α_2-adrenoceptors
Rat phrenic nerve/diaphragm	ACh (nicotinic)
Frog rectus abdominus	ACh (nicotinic)
Rat uterus	ACh (muscarinic), β_2-adrenoceptors, histamine H_2
Mouse vas deferens (field stimulated)	μ-, κ- and δ-opioid, DA_2
Rat vas deferens (field stimulated)	α_2-adrenoceptors, μ-opioid, prostanoid EP_3
Rabbit heart (Langendorff)	β_1-adrenoceptors
Rat or rabbit aorta	α_1-adrenoceptors, 5-HT_2, NK_1
Guinea-pig ascending colon	5-HT_4
Rat anococcygeus	α_1-adrenoceptors, GABAB
Rat atrium	β_1-adrenoceptors, ACh (muscarinic)
Guinea-pig tracheal muscle	β_2-adrenoceptors

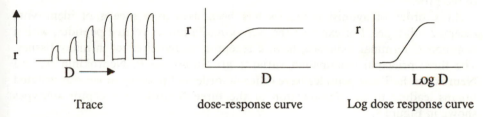

Trace	dose-response curve	Log dose response curve

Figure 6: *Diagramatic representation of a response (r) to sequential application of increasing concentration (D) of an agonist*

By applying the law of mass action the equilibrium constant (K_A) can be expressed as:

$$K_A = \frac{D.R}{DR}$$

If we assume that the proportion of receptors occupied at equilibrium is equal to y then the proportion of free receptors equals $1 - y$ thus:

$$K_A = \frac{D(1-y)}{y} \quad \text{or} \quad y = \frac{D}{D + K_A}$$

and the response is proportional to y. Then for a half maximal response, half the receptors would be occupied (*i.e.* $y = \frac{1}{2}$); therefore the concentration required (EC_{50}) would equal the equilibrium constant K_A or the reciprocal of the affinity constant. Comparisons of the affinity of agonists for receptors (and therefore potency) can be made on the basis of such estimations. See Figure 7 for comparisons for acetylcholine and propionylcholine acting at muscarinic

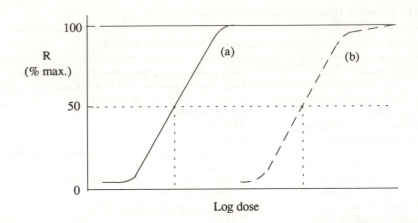

Figure 7: *Log dose–response curves for* (a) *ACh and* (b) *propionyl choline on guinea pig ileum*

receptors showing an apparently higher affinity of acetylcholine for this subclass of receptor.

Rank order of agonist potencies has been used as a means of identifying receptor sub-types. For example the tachykinin family of related peptides, with a common *C* terminal sequence, have a receptor mediated effect in many tissues. The three principal mammalian variants are Substance P, Neurokinin A, and Neurokinin B. These peptides have differing orders of potency in various isolated organs leading to the classification of the three Neurokinin receptor subtypes shown in Figure 8.

Primary structures of the Neurokinins
SP: Arg-Pro-Lys-Pro-Gln-Gln-Phe-Phe-Gly-Leu-MetNH$_2$
NK$_A$:   His-Lys-Thr-Asp-Ser-Phe-Val-Gly-Leu-MetNH$_2$
NK$_B$ Asp-Met-His-Asp-Phe-Phe-Val-Gly-Leu-MetNH$_2$

Potency order for Neurokinin receptor subtypes
NK$_1$ SP > NK$_A$ > NK$_B$ *e.g.* Dog carotid artery
NK$_2$ NK$_A$ > NK$_B$ > SP   *e.g.* Rabbit pulmonary artery
NK$_3$ NK$_B$ > NK$_A$ > SP   *e.g.* Rat portal vein

All three receptor subtypes are found in guinea pig ileum

Figure 8: *Neurokinin receptor subtypes*

3 DRUG ANTAGONISM

In contrast to an agonist a competitive antagonist can effectively bind to the receptor region without directly evoking a physiologal response. However *in vivo*, or in the presence of the agonist, the antagonist will hinder the access of the agonist to the receptors and thus completely or partially block the response. The establishment of agonist concentration response curves in the presence of

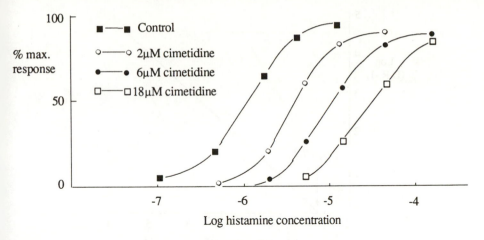

Figure 9: *Histamine concentration response curves in the presence of cimetidine in guinea pig atrium preparation*

increasing concentrations of the specific antagonist leads to a rightward shift in these curves as shown for the antagonism of histamine by cimetidine on the atrium in Figure 9.

Such interaction can also be considered quantitatively using the Occupancy Theory. Suppose a concentration of the agonist D' produces the same response in the presence of the antagonist (concentration B) that a concentration D of the agonist would alone; then applying the law of mass action the following relationship may be derived:

$$\frac{D'}{D} \text{ (Dose ratio)} = 1 + \frac{B}{K_B} \text{ or Dose ratio} - 1 = \frac{B}{K_B}$$

Where K_B is the equilibrium constant for antagonist–receptor reaction.

The pA scale provides a convenient measure for the potency of an antagonist drug at a particular receptor. An often quoted value for a competitive antagonist is the pA_2, which is the negative logarithm of the antagonist concentration required to halve the potency of the agonist; thus the dose ratio, defined above would equal two and therefore this antagonist concentration would reflect the equilibrium constant for antagonist receptor reaction. The value may be derived from a Schild Plot and an example is shown for acetylcholine and atropine competing for muscarinic receptors (see Figure 10).

The pA_2 value for atropine of 9.2 demonstrates a potent antagonist and the measurement of the rank order of this value for a series of antagonists in different tissues provides a further means of confirming receptor sub-types. Sometimes conflicting data may be obtained from the agonist and antagonist approach, as can be seen with the study of antagonists at neurokinin receptors. On the basis of such antagonist studies there appear to be differences in both the NK_1 and NK_2 receptor between various species whereas selective agonists show no species selectivity.

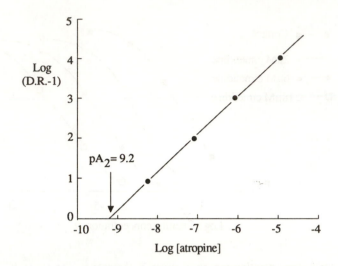

Figure 10: *Antagonism of ACh by atropine in a guinea pig ileum preparation*

Other types of antagonist include irreversible antagonists that bind covalently (see later) and non-competitive antagonists that bind at a different receptor site to reduce the effect of the agonist. Physiological antagonism is where two drugs produce physiologically opposite effects; *e.g.* acetylcholine's ability to cause a contraction of the ileum is reduced in the presence of adrenaline because of the latter's relaxant action in this tissue.

4 PARTIAL AGONISM

Thus an agonist is defined as an agent that can evoke a maximal response and an antagonist, while it is capable of combining with the receptor, produces no response. However, there is an intermediate position between these two extremes: an agent that will occupy the receptors but that will produce a response somewhat less than the maximum possible. The effect of trimethylammonium compounds on the guinea pig ileum illustrates this: as can be seen from Figure 11 the compounds have comparable affinities (compare EC_{50}'s) but differing abilities to generate the physiological response.

The terms Efficacy, Intrinsic Activity or Intrinsic Efficacy have been variously used to descibe this ability to activate transduction mechanisms. A partial agonist will act as a competitive antagonist in the presence of a full agonist. Oxprenolol, for example, is used clinically as a β-adrenoceptor blocker but in situations of low sympathetic tone will mimic the action of sympathetic nerve stimulation. Figure 12 provides a further example of the effect of a partial agonist on agonist activity from the *in vitro* pharmacology of histamine H_2 receptors; increasing the concentration of partial agonist in the presence of a fixed maximal concentration of the agonist leads to a reduction in the size of the response.

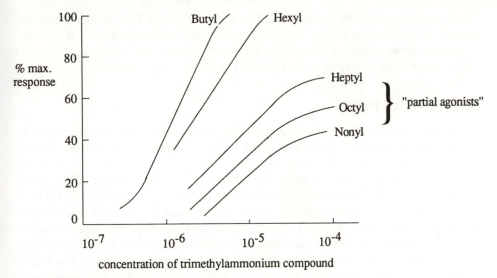

Figure 11: *Response of guinea pig ileum to trimethylammonium compounds*

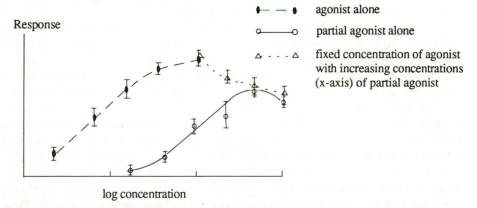

Figure 12: *Interaction of agonist and partial agonist*

5 RELATIONSHIP BETWEEN AFFINITY AND EFFICACY FACTORS

Overall the response to an agonist drug is dependent on the interplay of affinity and efficacy factors in a way that may vary with the receptor mechanisms involved. Occupation of the receptor by the drug requires affinity and the amount of response per drug–receptor complex reflects efficacy. However, whether the drug–receptor complex retains efficacy throughout its existence may depend on the particular receptor involved. If activity is maintained then increasing affinity would increase potency. On the other hand if the cell needs to recover between chemical stimuli the reformation of free receptors will be essential for a continued response; in this case high affinity would lead to a loss of effect. These two possibilities have been termed Type 1 (includes β-adrenoreceptor agonism) and Type 2 agonism (acetylcholine on nicotinic receptors) by Jack. An earlier view that contrasted with the Occupation Theory was Paton's Rate theory where the process of occupation rather than occupation itself was suggested to trigger the response: an analogy of the piano keyboard versus the organ keyboard as receptors evoking a 'response' mirrors the two contrasting theories

6 SPARE RECEPTORS

Observations of the effects of antagonists that bind irreversibly to receptors on the corresponding agonist responses have led to the concept of spare receptors. Thus, contrary to Clark's theory, some agonists can generate a maximum response without total receptor occupancy. For example, returning to the use of the guinea pig ileum with low doses of the irreversible histamine antagonist, GD 121, a parallel shift in log dose–response curve to histamine is observed while higher doses of the antagonist lead to the expected depression of the maximum response as shown in Figure 13. The observation of a maximum response to histamine being achieved without all the receptors needing to be occupied (as in graph B of Figure 13) means that some of the receptors can be considered as 'spare': it is important to recognise that these spare receptors are in no way different from the ones that had been occupied in producing the maximum response.

In general, therefore, the overall response is a function of efficacy and occupancy. Thus, full agonists have high efficacy and therefore operate at lower receptor occupancy and there is a bigger receptor reserve: this is the case for many natural agonists, neurotransmitters, and hormones. For a drug of lower efficacy the maximum response it can produce will depend on the extent of the receptor reserve and this may vary from tissue to tissue. In a tissue with a large receptor reserve where a high efficacy drug will produce a maximum response by occupying a small fraction of the receptors then a lower efficacy drug may still appear as a full agonist as a consequence of full receptor occupancy. For example from *in vitro* experiments prostaglandin PGD_2 inhibits platelet aggregation and promotes vasodilatation with a higher receptor reserve for the former. A PGD_2 partial agonist may thus inhibit platelets without an effect on blood vessels. Thus variability in receptor reserve may be exploited when attempting to obtain a selective effect. Additionally it means that the equilibrium dissociation constant K_A (the concentration of an agonist occupying 50% of the receptors) does not necessarily equal the concentration which produces the half maximal response.

7 TWO STATE THEORY

A further problem associated with the application of the occupancy theory as based on the Langmuir adsorption isotherm (derived to describe the adsorption of gases by metal surfaces) is that simple 1:1 binding would lead to an hyperbolic binding curve. However, in some circumstances, receptor activation follows a sigmoidal relationship, indicating co-operativity. Figure 14 shows the predicted and actual responses of the crustacean neuromuscular junction, measured as a fractional conductance change across the membrane to γ-aminobutyric acid (GABA).

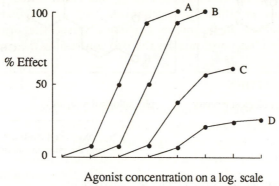

Agonist concentration on a log. scale

Figure 13: *Depression of maximum response to histamine by high concentrations of antagonist. B, C, and D are agonist response curves in the presence of increasing concentrations of GD 121*

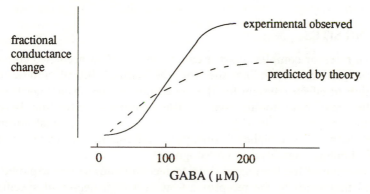

Figure 14: *Response of crustacean neuromuscular junction to GABA*

This notion of co-operative binding can be accommodated by introducing the concept that a receptor may exist in two states, an active (R*) and an inactive form (R), which are in equilibrium with one another; the equilibrium constant is referred to as the allosteric constant. Agonists have a higher affinity for R* in a quantitative way that reflects the efficacy of the agonist receptor complex; on the other hand, antagonists are non-selective in their binding to either form of the receptor thus not disturbing the normal equilibrium between the two receptor forms. The concept also introduces the possibility of a third type of drug that binds preferentially to R thus having negative efficacy and termed an inverse agonist.

This situation is illustrated by drug binding at the benzodiazepine receptor; benzodiazepine agonists are believed to bind to sites associated with the GABA receptor, an ion-channel linked receptor. The conformational form of the receptor complex that binds benzodiazepine agonists (*e.g.* diazepam) has a high affinity for GABA at its associated site. In equilibrium is a conformational form of the receptor complex that binds benzodiazepine inverse agonists (*e.g.* β-adrenaline and the physiological receptor   physiological receptor   exoreceptor

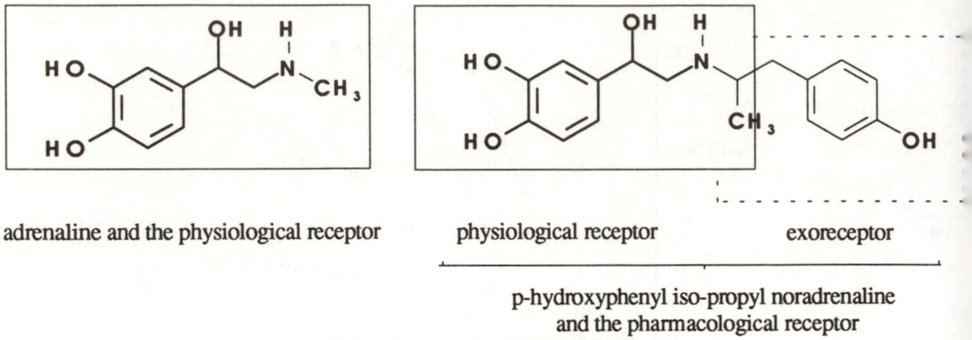

p-hydroxyphenyl iso-propyl noradrenaline
and the pharmacological receptor

Figure 15: *Concept of physiological receptor and exoreceptor*

carbolines), has a low affinity for GABA and thus is not associated with the opening of the associated ion channel. Antagonist drugs at the benzodiazepine receptor will prevent the binding of either agonists or inverse agonists.

8 BINDING SITES

Taking the receptor complex apart it can be reasoned to need two components, first a recognition or binding site for the natural ligand and secondly a transduction or effector system for the generation of the physiological response. Xenobiotics may bind to an area of the membrane extending beyond the physiological receptor as in Figure 15 where the natural agonist adrenaline is compared with *p*-hydroxyphenylisopropylnoradrenaline: separate agonist and antagonist binding domains may be recognised.

An assessment of the binding of drug to receptor sites can be explored using a compound that binds to the receptor site with a high degree of specificity and affinity (ligand). As this compound will need to be detected in minute quantities it should not be metabolised in the tissues and will be radiolabelled and have high specific activity. Thus, membrane fragments from homogenates of tissue under test are incubated with radiolabelled ligand and separated by filtration. After correction for non-specific binding, label bound to receptors can be determined. Assessment of affinity of ligand for binding sites and number of binding sites can be made using a Scatchard plot: a typical plot is shown in Figure 16 and deviations from the linear Scatchard plot shown may occur either because the tissue possesses two or more binding sites having different affinities for the ligand, or because binding does not obey the simple mass action equation and shows positive or negative co-operativity.

Assessment of the number of binding sites may provide useful information on the pathogenesis of disease and a means to explore the possible pharmacological mechanisms of action of therapeutically important drugs such as the antipsychotic drugs used in the treatment of schizophrenia: the inhibition of labelled spiperone binding to a class of dopamine receptor (D_2) parallels therapeutic potency as shown in Figure 17. However, assessment of antagonists

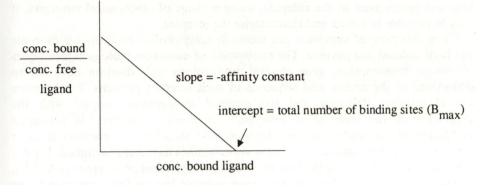

Figure 16: *Scatchard plot*

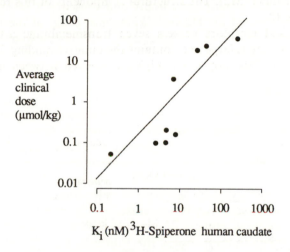

Figure 17: *Relationship of clinical potency of antipsychotics to potency in inhibiting ^{3}H-spiperone binding to human caudate membranes*

on the basis of radioligand binding assays where no response is measured may differ from activity assessed in functional assays.

Autoradiography has been used to explore the distribution of receptors in various organs. Furthermore using the technique of Positron Emission Tomography (PET scan) the distribution of receptors *in vivo* can be studied. For example using short-lived positron emitting isotopes such as [^{11}C]raclopride it has been possible to explore the distribution of D_2 receptors in schizophrenics.

9 RECEPTOR CHARACTERISATION

Approaches have been made to attempt to characterise the nature of the receptive material involved in the above interactions. Examination of the chemical structure of drugs that interact with specific receptors may allow some prediction of the complementary structure of the latter. Alternatively, if a label is available that will tightly bind to the receptor, using a range of biochemical strategies, it may be possible to isolate and characterise the receptor.

Using this type of approach the nicotinic acetylcholine receptor for example has been isolated and purified. The application of molecular biological techniques of reverse transcription, gene cloning, and colony hybridisation have led to deductions of the amino acid sequence of such receptor proteins. Furthermore use of selective deletions and site directed mutagenesis coupled with the expression of the receptor in cells such as *Xenopus oocytes* has permitted evaluation of the relationship of the molecular structure of receptors to their function. Overall a number of receptor superfamilies have been identified. Ligand gated ion channels are typified by the nicotinic acetylcholine receptor (nAChR), which is composed of five subunits, each subunit having four transmembrane domains crossing their cell membrane with one of the transmembrane domains lining the ion channel (M2). The structural components of this receptor type are shown in Figure 18.

G-Protein linked receptors possess seven transmembrane α-helices and the third cytoplasmic loop is large and contains the putative binding domain for a G-protein (see later). This loop is not highly conserved between members of the

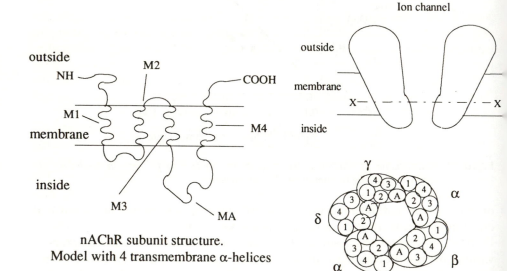

nAChR subunit structure.
Model with 4 transmembrane α-helices

$\alpha_2 \beta \gamma \delta$ stoichiometry of five subunits

Structure of the nAChR
M_{1-4} = hydrophobic, membrane spanning α-helical portions (approx. 20 amino acids each)
N-terminal glycosylated: in α-subunits the large N terminal sequence includes the binding site.
M_2 regions have clusters of negatively charged amino acids which may contribute to lining of ion channel

Figure 18: *Ligand-gated ion channel receptor superfamily*

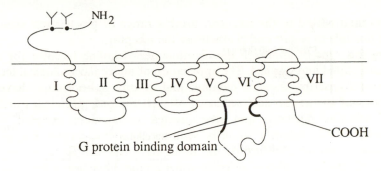

Main features:

Single polypeptide chain
Seven hydrophobic membrane-spanning α-helices
N-terminal extracellular and glycosylated
Third long cytoplasmic loop (between TM_5 and TM_6) may control G protein coupling
Ligand binding domains appear to reside in TM components (TM_2, TM_3 and TM_7?)

Figure 19: *G-Protein linked receptor superfamily*

superfamily reflecting the variety of distinct G-proteins involved in mediating responses. The location of the ligand binding region appears to be within the transmembrane components. The muscarinic acetylcholine and β-adrenaline receptor belong to this superfamily and the general structure is shown in Figure 19.

Tyrosine kinase linked receptors mediate the actions of growth factors and insulin and consist of large extra- and intra-cellular domains, the latter being rich in tyrosine residues where autophosphorylation occurs (see Figure 20).

The tyrosine kinase receptor is characterised by ligand stimulated intrinsic tyrosine domains which lie on the cytosolic side of these transmembrane proteins. The extracellular side contains regions rich in cysteine residues which probably contribute the secondary structure required of the ligand binding site. The extracellular region is also glycosylated; several receptors in this superfamily exist in at least two different glycosylation states. Ligand occupation results in activation of the intrinsic tyrosine kinase and autophosphorylation. This is thought to trigger kinase cascades which activate a number of serine protein kinases within the cell which mediate some of insulin's effects. Certain growth factors also have tyrosine kinase activity with a similar structure for their receptors.

A steroid receptor superfamily is located within the cell: thus the agonist molecule needs to cross the cell membrane to occupy the receptor. A schematic diagram of this set up is shown in Figure 21.

10 TRANSDUCTION LINKAGES

When a receptor is in its natural environment within the cell, occupation by an agonist drug leads to a specific biological response. As seen in the discussion of

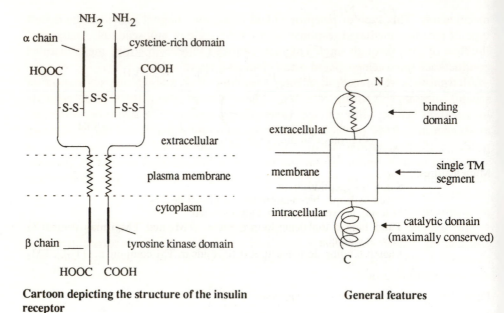

Cartoon depicting the structure of the insulin
receptor   General features

Figure 20: *Tyrosine kinase receptor superfamily*

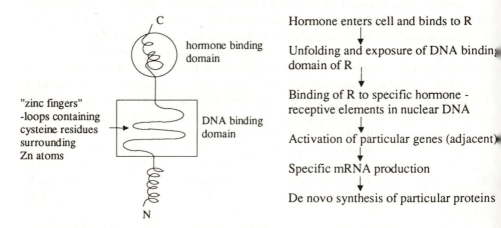

Hormone enters cell and binds to R

Unfolding and exposure of DNA binding
domain of R

Binding of R to specific hormone -
receptive elements in nuclear DNA

Activation of particular genes (adjacent)

Specific mRNA production

De novo synthesis of particular proteins

Figure 21: *Steroid receptors – intracellular*

receptor isolation, one possibility is that the receptors are linked directly to ion
channels. Thus, for example, at the voluntary neuromuscular junction postjunc-
tional nicotinic acetylcholine receptors bind the neurotransmitter inducing a
conformational change that opens the ion channels. Passage of cations through
the channel depolarises the muscle cell leading to an initiation of contractile

mechanisms. This type of receptor linked to an ion channel provides the fastest type of receptor-mediated response with a time-scale of milliseconds. Analysis of the flow of ions through single channels can lead to assessment of mean channel conductance (picosiemens) and mean channel open time (ms).

Alternatively the receptor effector coupling may involve the formation of second messengers within the cell. These second messengers then regulate intracellular activity with a longer timescale of response. The two types of second messenger are cAMP (cyclic 3',5'-adenosine monophosphate) and the breakdown products of phosphatidyl inositol. Activation of the second messenger systems as a result of drug–receptor interaction involves a link through regulatory proteins that are internally-facing and membrane-bound (G-proteins). The biochemical mechanisms involved with these processes are discussed elsewhere in this publication.

The scheme used earlier to describe receptor activation therefore could be adapted to reflect the effector mechanism. For receptors incorporating ion channels a two step process, the isomerisation mechanism, may provide one appropriate description:

$$D + R \overset{K_A}{\rightleftharpoons} DR \overset{E}{\rightleftharpoons} DR^* \Rightarrow \text{response}$$

DR* represents the state of the occupied receptor associated with the open ion channel and E determines the susceptibility of the receptor complex to isomerise to this state and therefore reflects efficacy. On the other hand, for the other group of receptors with slower response times and coupled to G-proteins the following ternary complex mechanism follows the process:

$$D + R \overset{K_A}{\rightleftharpoons} DR \overset{K_{DR}}{\rightleftharpoons} DRG^* \Rightarrow \text{response}$$

DRG* represents the state associated with the activated G-protein.

In both considerations the formation of the active state of the receptor complex cannot be achieved without depleting DR thus shifting the equilibrium of drug and receptor interaction to the right. The drug would therefore appear in response-based assays to have greater affinity for the receptor; the greater the efficacy of DR the greater this effect. However a general feature of receptor systems that have a number of coupling steps between activated receptor and response of the tissue is that of amplification through the steps. Thus only a small amount of activated receptor (DR* or DRG) may be required for a full response and this could be obtained without substantial effect on the initial equilibrium and affinity assessment.

11 RECEPTOR CONSTANCY

Finally, it is apparent that the consequences of a drug–receptor interaction may not be constant with time. Continued exposure to an agonist drug may lead to a loss of sensitivity (one mechanism producing tolerance). The receptor may become uncoupled from the second messenger system as a result of phosphorylation of the intracellular domain of the receptor adjacent to the site of G-protein binding; alternatively, the number of agonist binding sites might fall. Changes in receptor number may occur as a result of sequestration, where the receptors are transiently internalised within the cell or more long-term through adaptive change in receptor synthesis and degradation.

Such adaptive changes in receptors could even explain the time lag observed between pharmacological effect and therapeutic benefit seen with some medication (*e.g.* use of antidepressant drugs). Conversely, it is well known that to deprive a cell of its functional agonist will lead to an adaptive increase in sensitivity (up-regulation). This phenomenon might partially explain physical withdrawal symptoms in those dependent on opiates. It should be noted that changes in sensitivity to a drug may sometimes occur by other mechanisms. For example the loss of effect of tyramine in isolated organ-bath preparations may well be due to the depletion of noradrenaline in the tissue through repeated exposure to tyramine: this drug acts by releasing noradrenaline from nerve terminals.

As well as agonist exposure, disease processes may also alter receptor function. Endogenous antibodies to various receptors may lead to reduced function. Endogenous antibodies are found to nicotinic acetylcholine receptors in Myasthesia Gravis, insulin receptors in some patients with diabetes and thyroid receptors in Graves' disease.

12 CONCLUSION

Overall an understanding of the mechanisms involved with drug–receptor interaction is one of the central concepts of pharmacology and is essential to the development of rationally designed therapies for the treatment of disease.

13 BIBLIOGRAPHY

1. H.P. Rang and M.M. Dale, 'Pharmacology', 2nd Edn., Churchill, 1991.
2. W.B. Pratt and P. Taylor, 'Principles of Drug Action, The Basis of Pharmacology', 3rd Edn., Churchill Livingstone, 1990.
3. R.B. Barlow, 'Quantitative Aspects of Chemical Pharmacology', Crook-Helm, 1980.
4. T.P. Kenakin, 'Pharmacologic Analysis of Drug-Receptor Interaction', Raven, NY, 1987.
5. D. Jack, 'A Way of Looking at Agonism and Antagonists: Lessons from Salbutamol, Salmeterol and Other β-Adrenoreceptor Agonists', *Br. J. Clin. Pharm.*, 1991, **31**, 501.
6. T.P. Kenakin, R.A. Bond, and T.I. Bonner, 'Definition of Pharmacological Receptors', *Pharm. Rev.*, 1992, **44**, 351.

7. D. Hoyer, and H.W.G.M. Boddeke, 'Partial Agonists, Full Agonists, Antagonists: Dilemmas of Definition', *TiPS*, 1993, **167**, 270.
8. J.M. Hall, M.P. Caulfield, S.P. Watson and S. Guard, 'Receptor Subtypes or Species Homologues: Relevance to Drug Discovery', *TiPS*, 1993, **170**, 376.
9. *TiPS* Receptor Nomenclature Supplement (1993) 4th Edn., 1993.

CHAPTER 2

Signal Transduction and Second Messengers

TREVOR J. FRANKLIN

1 INTRODUCTION

The proper functioning of multicellular organisms is critically dependent upon the correct orchestration of the activities of the billions of constituent cells. Intercellular communication and response are essential to the maintenance of effective control over the cellular community. The communication process involves an extensive array of chemical messengers which are released from cells, including hormones, growth factors, and neuro-endocrine substances. In addition, the cells interact with the many macromolecular substances in their immediate environment which make up the extracellular matrix. These external stimuli are detected by the interaction of the ligands with specific proteinaceous receptor molecules on the cell surface. The purpose of this chapter is to provide an introduction to the many and complex biochemical changes within cells which result from the binding of the external ligands to their receptors and which culminate in specific biological end responses.

In many instances the ligand–receptor interaction leads to a rapid change in the intracellular concentration of a small molecular weight compound or ion referred to as a 'second messenger' which in turn initiates a cascade of biochemical events leading to the end response. The second messengers include adenosine 3',5'-cyclic monophosphate (cyclic AMP), guanosine 3',5'-cyclic monophosphate (cyclic GMP), products of membrane phospholipid hydrolysis (Figure 1), and the calcium ion (Ca^{2+}).

The other major mechanism of signal transduction does not involve second messengers directly but depends upon ligand–receptor interactions which activate specific protein phosphorylating enzymes associated with the receptor, known as tyrosine kinases. This second mechanism of signal transduction is especially typical of many cytokines and cellular growth factors, including insulin.

A notable feature of most signal transduction systems is the remarkable degree of amplification of the original ligand–receptor interaction that can be achieved. This is responsible for the classical observation in pharmacology of 'spare receptors', that is the ability of many agonists to elicit a maximum biological end response even though only a small fraction of the total receptor population is occupied by agonist molecules.

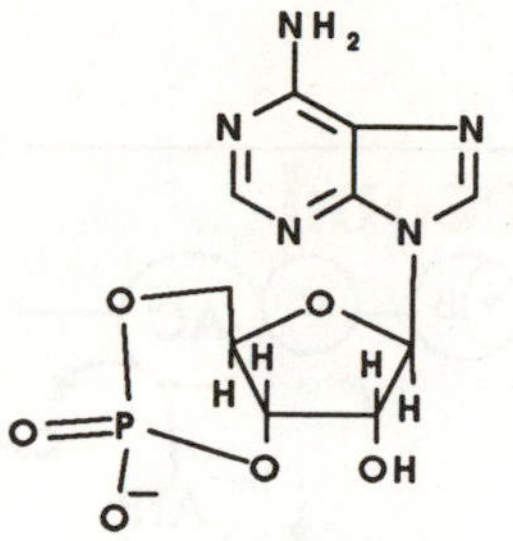

Cyclic AMP

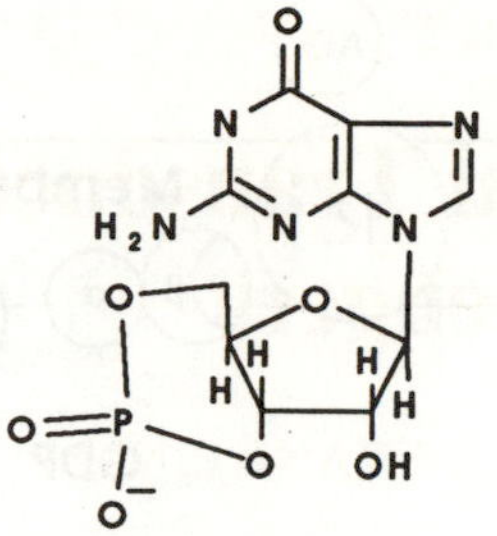

Cyclic GMP

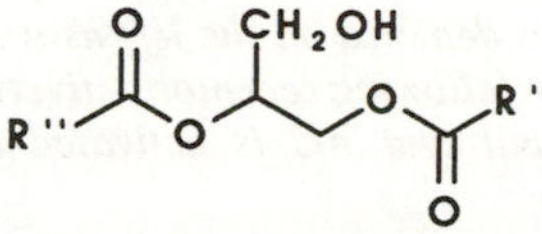

Diacylglycerol (DAG)
(R', R'': acyl residues)

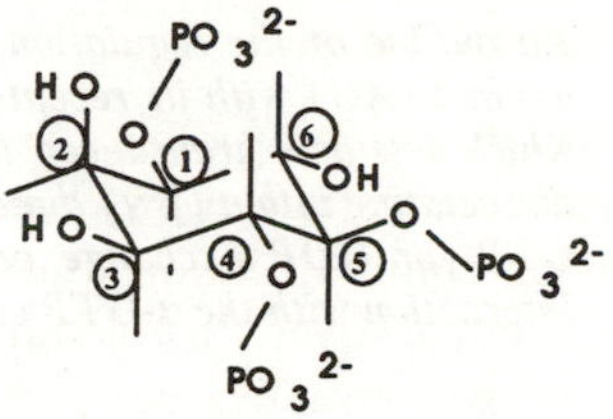

Inositol-1,4,5-triphosphate (IP$_3$)

Figure 1: *Four of the most important second messenger molecules. Not shown is the calcium ion, which is also an major second messenger*

2 SECOND MESSENGERS

Cyclic AMP

Cyclic AMP (cAMP) was the first of the second messenger molecules to be discovered. Over thirty years ago it was found to be the second messenger between the activation of the β-adrenergic receptors in liver cells and the initiation of glycogenolysis, *i.e.* the liberation of glucose from glycogen. Since then, cAMP has proved to be the second messenger for a host of hormonal and neuro-endocrine effectors. Some agonists, for example β-adrenergic and hista- mine-H$_2$ agonists, induce a rapid rise in the intracellular concentration of cAMP, whilst other agonists cause cAMP levels to fall (Table 1).

Table 1: *Stimulatory and inhibitory agonists of adenlylyl cyclase*

Stimulators	Inhibitors
β-Adrenergic agonists	α2-Adrenergic agonists
Dopamine (D$_1$)	Dopamine (D$_2$)
Histamine (H$_2$)	Adenosine (A$_2$)
Vasopressin (V$_2$)	Angiotensin II
Follicle Stimulating Hormone	Acetylcholine (muscarinic)
Luteinising Hormone	Somatostatin
Glucagon	

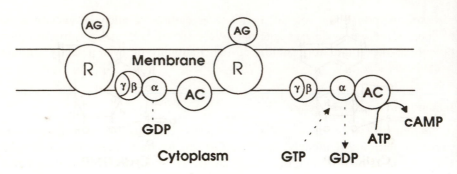

Figure 2: *An outline of the regulation of adenylyl cyclase (AC) via the interaction of an agonist (AG) with its receptor (R) in the cytoplasmic membrane. The G-protein, which acts as a 'transducer' between R and AC, is depicted on the left as a trimer dissociating into a (β γ) dimer and an α monomer following receptor activation. A GTP for GDP exchange occurs on the α-subunit and AC is activated by its interaction with the α-GTP complex*

How are these changes in the intracellular concentration of cAMP brought about? Figure 2 illustrates in an extremely simplified form the general nature of the interactions between the receptor, a 'transducing' protein, called a G-protein (with α, β, and γ subunits) and the enzyme, adenylyl cyclase, which catalyses the formation of cAMP from ATP. Interposed between the receptor protein and adenylyl cyclase is a specific member of the extensive family of G-proteins which determines whether receptor activation stimulates (G_s) or inhibits (G_i) adenylyl cyclase. The assembly of receptor–G-protein–adenylyl cyclase is associated with the cytoplasmic membrane, with the G-proteins and adenylyl cyclase being located on the inner face of the membrane.

Activation of Adenylyl Cyclase

Let us first look at the action of agonists which increase intracellular cAMP. In the 'resting' or unstimulated cells the activity of adenylyl cyclase and the concentration of cAMP are both low. In this state the G_s protein is bound to guanosine diphosphate (GDP). The α-subunit of the G protein has a single high affinity site for GDP or GTP. The α-GDP complex binds tightly to a (βγ) dimer and in this form the assembly is inactive. When a cAMP-enhancing agonist binds to its specific receptor on the outer surface of the cell, a conformational change (whose nature is unknown) in the receptor results in an increase in the off-rate of GDP from the α-subunit allowing the binding site to become occupied by GTP. The affinity of the α-subunit for the (βγ) dimer now declines sharply causing dissociation of the G-protein trimer into α-GTP and (βγ) components. Finally, the liberated α-GTP complex binds to adenylyl cyclase and activates the enzyme by an unknown molecular mechanism, However this activation of adenylyl cyclase is only transient. The α-subunit has a low level GTPase activity ($k_{cat} \sim 15$ m^{-1}). The ensuing cleavage of GTP to GDP leads to a reversal of the activation process which can be reinitiated if agonist remains available to interact with the receptor. Although the role of α_s in the activation of adenylyl cyclase is well established, recent evidence suggests that the ($\beta\gamma$) dimer can, in some situations, potentiate the stimulatory action of the α-subunit or even directly stimulate adenyl cyclase.

Inhibition of Adenylyl Cyclase

A different type of G-protein is involved in the transduction of receptors which cause inhibition of adenylyl cyclase. G-Proteins have been identified which contain a form of α-subunit (α_i) which, in its GTP-complexed state, may directly inhibit adenylyl cyclase. However, adenylyl cyclase is indirectly inhibited if the ($\beta\gamma$) dimer released from G_i competes with adenylyl cyclase for α_s-subunits liberated from stimulatory G_s trimers. At present the precise roles of the G-protein subunits in the control of adenylyl cyclase are not completely worked out.

Heterogeneity of G-Proteins and Adenylyl Cyclases

Trimeric G-proteins constitute a family of bewildering diversity, some of which, as we shall see later, regulate the activity of enzymes other than adenylyl cyclase. cDNA cloning reveals that there are several different forms of the α-, β-, and γ-subunits associated with the regulation of adenylyl cyclase, giving many possible different oligomeric combinations. With six types of mammalian adenylyl cyclase also having been identified, it will be a major task to work out their individual interactions with the physiologically significant G-protein trimeric combinations. Recent work suggests that there is considerable specificity in the regulation of the different types of adenylyl cyclase by G-protein isoforms. For example, whilst all forms of mammalian adenylyl cyclase are stimulated by $G_{\alpha s}$, the stimulation brought about by the $G_{(\beta\gamma)}$ dimer may be limited to types II and IV.

Intracellular Receptors for cAMP: cAMP-dependent Protein Kinases

Changes in the intracellular concentration of cAMP represent the first phase in the transduction of receptor activation. Cells respond to the altered concentration of cAMP through the participation of enzymes whose activity is regulated by cAMP. The cAMP-dependent protein kinases phosphorylate sequence-specific serine and threonine residues in target proteins, some of which are also protein kinases. Phosphorylation profoundly alters the activity of the target proteins and is essential to the extension and amplification of the signalling cascade culminating in the biological end response. A typical cAMP-dependent cascade, which leads to agonist-induced glycogenolysis, is illustrated in Figure 3.

In the absence of the nucleotide, the cAMP-dependent protein kinases are tetrameric in form comprising two catalytic and two regulatory subunits and are catalytically inactive. Two major types of regulatory (R) subunit have been identified for each of which there are several isoforms. The various types and subtypes of R may be functionally distinct since they are found in characteristic tissue distributions: types R_α^I and R_χ^{II} occur in most cells whereas R_β^{II} is found

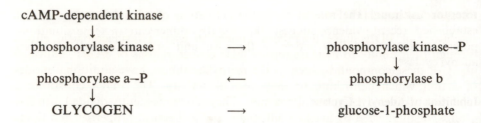

Figure 3: *The cyclic AMP-initiated cascade of protein phosphorylation which leads to the release of glucose-1-phosphate from glycogen in the liver*

mainly in neuronal tissues, granulosa cells, and adrenal tissue. All forms of R have two (A and B) high-affinity binding sites for cAMP at the carboxyl terminus. A and B sites show strong positive co-operativity for cAMP binding: the initial binding of cAMP to site B promotes binding to site A. Another characteristic domain of the R-subunit, which is located between residues 90 and 100, binds to a complementary site in the catalytic subunit and blocks its kinase activity.

There are two highly homologous forms of the catalytic subunit (C), C_α and C_β, which show considerable differences in tissue distribution, again hinting at functional specialisation. As the cytoplasmic concentration of cAMP increases both binding sites on R become occupied by cAMP, inducing a conformational change which decreases the affinity between R and C subunits by 10^4. The subsequent dissociation is followed by the binding of the C-subunits, via a specific peptide binding site, to target proteins to ensure their phosphorylation.

Termination of the cAMP Signalling Process

There is a considerable metabolic cost to the cell in the activation of the cAMP signalling system, both in the signalling cascade itself and more especially in the metabolic and physical responses evoked by the cascade, *e.g.* glycogenolysis, lipolysis, biosynthesis, muscular contraction, or relaxation. It is essential, therefore, that cells are able to shut down the signalling process as soon as its purpose is achieved. This can be accomplished in several ways:

1. Removal of the agonist from the receptor environment.
2. Degradation of GTP on the G_α–GTP complex by the intrinsic GTPase activity of the α-subunit.
3. Degradation of cAMP by phosphodiesterases.
4. Dephosphorylation of activated proteins by phosphoprotein phosphatases.
5. Desensitisation of the receptor–G-protein–adenylyl cyclase complex to continued agonist stimulation.

Mechanisms (3), (4), and (5) will be reviewed in more detail below. Mechanism (1) is outside the scope of this chapter and the GTPase involved in mechanism (2) has already been described.

Phosphodiesterases (PDEs)

Inhibitors of PDEs have long been known to exert pharmacological effects through their ability to increase intracellular concentrations of cAMP, although many of these compounds, such as the methylxanthines, have additional modes of action which contribute to their overall activity. The PDEs constitute a remarkably diverse assembly of enzymes. They are conveniently divided into five groups, distinguished by marked differences in biochemical properties and tissue distribution, differences which are strongly suggestive of specialised functions. A varied collection of inhibitors is available although inhibitors selective for individual subtypes of enzyme have been hard to come by. Such is the complexity of the PDE scene that it would be virtually impossible to predict all of the pharmacological effects of a novel selective inhibitor. Despite this, the indications of functional specificity amongst the PDEs provide encouragement for the continued search for such inhibitors.

Phosphoprotein Phosphatases

Relatively few serine-threonine specific protein phosphatases are involved in the reversal of the cAMP-activation process – for example only three phosphatases appear to be required for the dephosphorylation of some thirteen enzymes which regulate the major biodegradative and biosynthetic pathways in the liver. The question of how the activities of the phosphatases themselves are regulated is a subject which is attracting increasing attention, especially in view of the recently recognised role of insulin in promoting the activity of the key phosphatase, protein phosphatase I (see later).

Desensitisation of the Receptor–G-Protein–Adenylyl Cyclase Complex to Agonist Stimulation

Receptor-activated adenylyl cyclases are rapidly desensitised with a consequent loss of the cAMP response when the stimulation by agonist is continued for more than a few minutes. The mechanisms involved have largely been unravelled in the case of the β-adrenergic receptor and may well have general relevance for other receptors which evoke increases in cAMP. A rapidly developing, agonist-specific desensitisation results from the activation of a unique, β-receptor protein-specific protein kinase (cAMP-independent) which only phosphorylates the receptor when it is occupied by an agonist. Another protein, β-arrestin, prevents the coupling of the phosphorylated receptor to the G-protein and the subsequent activation of adenylyl cyclase. Desensitisation also results from the inactivation of the receptor by a cAMP-dependent protein kinase and does not require the receptor to be occupied by agonist for phosphorylation to occur. Yet another mode of desensitisation involves the internalisation of receptors from the cell surface and their subsequent proteolytic destruction within the cell. Unlike the other modes of desensitisation, which are readily reversible, recovery from the loss of surface receptors is a lengthy process requiring the synthesis of new receptors. All forms of desensitisation of the cAMP response serve to limit the metabolic cost to the cell of prolonged stimulation.

Cyclic Guanosine 3′,5′-monophosphate (cGMP)

Although cGMP was discovered soon after cAMP, success in identifying its role as a second messenger proved much more elusive. Nevertheless, its participation in the transduction of two important mammalian signalling systems has now been firmly established: those involving natriuretic peptides (NPs) and nitric oxide.

Guanylyl Cyclase

In contrast with adenylyl cyclase, which is confined to the inner leaflet of the cytoplasmic membrane, guanylyl cyclase occurs in both membrane-bound (particulate) and soluble forms, each serving different functions. Particulate guanylyl cyclase combines an enzymic function with that of receptor for the NPs. The extracellular domain, which contains a peptide-binding region, is connected to the intracellular, enzymic domain by a single trans-membrane region. Binding of the agonists to the receptor region induces a conformational change in the protein which activates the guanylyl cyclase. GTP and G-proteins are not involved in the activation process, although there appears to be a requirement for ATP.

The soluble, or cytoplasmic guanylyl cyclase presents a very different picture. It has two subunits, α and β, both of which contain sequences resembling those in the catalytic region of the particulate enzyme. However, the most striking feature of soluble guanylyl cyclase is a tightly associated haem entity which is the target for nitric oxide, the principal activator of the soluble enzyme. Nitric oxide is generated from arginine by either of two different forms of nitric oxide synthase. A Ca^{2+}-dependent enzyme, which is constitutively produced, is important in blood pressure regulation and in neuro-transmission in the central nervous sytem, whilst an inducible form, which is largely Ca^{2+} independent, has a major role in the host defence capability of macrophages. There is strong evidence that in its role as a relaxant of smooth muscle, nitric oxide operates through cyclic GMP as a second messenger. Nitric oxide reacts with the haem prosthetic group of soluble guanylyl cyclase to form nitro-haem which induces a marked increase in the rate of cGMP synthesis. No other physiologically significant activator of soluble guanylyl cyclase has yet been identified.

Intracellular Receptors for cGMP

It might be expected that cGMP would initiate its downstream effects by binding to cGMP-dependent protein kinases in a manner analogous to cAMP. Many cells do indeed contain a serine-threonine protein kinase which can be activated by cGMP. Two main forms of the enzyme exist. Type I, which is fairly widely distributed in the tissues, is a dimer, each subunit containing a cGMP-binding site and a catalytic region. Binding of cGMP activates the enzyme without provoking dissociation of the subunits. The Type II enzyme, which has only been identified in the epithelial cells of the intestines, is a monomer associated with the cytoplasmic membrane. Many proteins act as substrates for cGMP-dependent protein kinase *in vitro* although the functional significance of this is uncertain. Some biological activities of cGMP are known not to involve cGMP-dependent kinases. For example, cGMP has a key role in the functioning of the photosensitive rod cells of the retina. In resting cells the intracellular concentration of cGMP is high (~ 50 µM). The cGMP maintains Na^+/Ca^{2+} ion channels in the cell membrane in the open state by binding directly to specific cGMP sites in the channels. Photostimulation of the rod cells lowers the concentration of cGMP through the activation of cGMP phosphodiesterase. The consequent closure of the ion channels leads to neurotransmitter release at local synapses and the initiation of a nervous impulse.

Much work remains to be done in defining the range of functions of cGMP and simple analogies with cAMP can be misleading.

Products of Phospholipid Metabolism as Second Messengers

Over the last decade or so a remarkable series of biochemical investigations has revealed a complex signal transduction–second messenger system which relies upon agonist-induced hydrolysis of specific phospholipid components of the cytoplasmic membrane. For example, the receptors for a range of agonists (Table 2) are linked, through trimeric G-proteins (belonging to the Gq subfamily) to a phospholipid-specific phosphodiesterase called phospholipase C (PLC). Occupation of the receptor site by a specific agonist results in the activation of PLC and the hydrolysis of a minor component of the inner leaflet of the cytoplasmic membrane, phosphoinositol 4,5-bisphosphate (PIP_2), to release diacylglycerol (DAG) and inositol (1,4,5)-trisphosphate (IP_3) (Figure 1). As we shall see, both DAG and IP_3 act as second messengers.

Table 2: *Some important agonists which activate phospholipase C*

Acetylcholine (muscarinic)	Substance P
5-Hydroxytryptamine (5-HT_2)	Bombesin
α_1-Adrenergic agonists	Bradykinin
Histamine (H_1)	Angiotensin II
Adenosine (A_2)	Thyrotropin releasing hormone
Vasopressin (V_1)	

Numerous subtypes of both the Gq-protein and the PLC have been identified although their relationships to specific receptors remain to be clarified. The involvement of the Gq-protein subunits, α and ($\beta\gamma$), in the activation of PLC is analogous to that of adenylyl cyclase (Figure 4): the α subunit–GTP complex activates PLC and the addition of the ($\beta\gamma$) dimer reverses the activation by sequestering the α subunit. However, one form of PLC isolated from a line of leukemic cells, HL60, is stimulated by ($\beta\gamma$), suggesting that regulation by both α and ($\beta\gamma$) subunits is possible, as is the case with adenylyl cyclase.

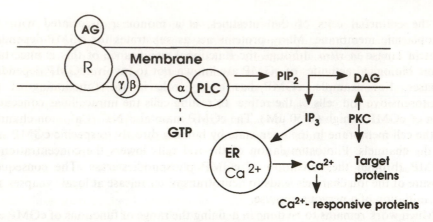

Figure 4: *An outline of the release of the second messengers inositol trisphophate (IP₃) and diacylglycerol (DAG) from the membrane phospholipid phosphoinositol 4,5-bisphosphate (PIP₂). The interaction of an agonist (AG) with its receptor (R) provokes the dissociation of the G-protein into a (βγ) dimer and an α-subunit complexed with GTP which activates PLC. The interaction of IP₃ with the endoplasmic reticulum (ER) releases Ca²⁺ ions into the cytoplasm. DAG promotes the activation of protein kinase C (PKC) by its association with the cytoplasmic membrane*

Diacylglycerol (DAG) and Protein Kinase C (PKC)

DAG is one of the two primary products generated by the action of PLC on the membrane phospholipid PIP_2. DAG is also generated by the hydrolysis of phosphatidic acid generated by the action of phospholipase D (PLD) on phosphatidylcholine. A broad range of agonists which activate PLC also activate PLD, apparently through a G-protein-dependent mechanism. However, it seems likely that DAG formation via PLD only becomes significant after sustained stimulation in contrast with the rapid (<1 second) but transient appearance of DAG after the stimulation of PLC.

The formation of DAG by phospholipid hydrolysis assumed major imprtance when it was discovered that DAG activates members of a family of enzymes collectively known as protein kinase C (PKC). In mammalian tissues there are numerous isoforms of PKC which phosphorylate sequence-specific serine and threonine residues in a wide range of target proteins. The various isoforms of PKC exhibit marked differences in tissue distribution, suggesting that functional specialisation is likely. Whilst all the isoforms depend on phospholipid for enzymic activity, some isoforms also require Ca^{2+} ions whereas others do not. Interaction with DAG increases the affinity for Ca^{2+} of the Ca^{2+}-dependent forms of PKC thus facilitating enzymic activity at micromolar concentrations of Ca^{2+}. The activation is potentiated by *cis*-unsaturated fatty acids. Overall, the various forms of PKC show considerable difference in biochemical properties although the relevance of of these differences to *in vivo* function is uncertain.

The activation of PKC in cells is associated with translocation of the enzyme to the inner face of the cytoplasmic membrane where it catalyses the phosphorylation of target proteins. Indications of the physiological functions of PKC have been obtained through the use of metabolically stable phorbol esters which diffuse into cells and activate the enzyme through the DAG binding site. The effects of phorbol esters indicate that PKC is involved in many cellular functions including secretion and exocytosis, gene expression, cell proliferation, modulation of ion channel conductance and smooth muscle contraction. PKC is also probably a major contributor to the 'cross talk' between the various signal transduction pathways since it is suspected that its ability to phosphorylate membranous regions of receptors, G-proteins, adenylyl cyclase, and cAMP phosphodiesterases and to activate Ca^{2+} channels and pumps may modulate the intensities of a variety of signals. A widely distributed enzyme, DAG kinase, converts DAG into phosphatidic acid. There are at least two isoforms of DAG kinase, which may regulate the availability of DAG in the signalling pathway.

Inositol 1,4,5,-Triphosphate (IP_3) and Intracellular Calcium

In contrast with DAG, which remains associated with the cell membrane because of its lipophilic character, the other product of PIP_2 hydrolysis, IP_3, is water-soluble and is released into the cytoplasm. IP_3 binds to specific receptors on the membrane of the endoplasmic reticulum (ER), otherwise called the sarcoplasmic reticulum in muscle cells. The ER is a complex intracellular network of membranous vesicles which provide numerous storage sites for Ca^{2+} ions in addition to accomodating enzymes of the P_{450} family and, in some regions of the network, the organelles for protein biosynthesis.

Before describing the activities of IP_3 a brief account of the significance of Ca^{2+} ions in cellular physiology is necessary. The requirement for Ca^{2+} in muscular contraction was discovered over a century ago and since then there has been an ever-increasing awareness of its involvement in many other cellular processes, including cell division, secretion, metabolic control, and changes in gene expression. The intracellular concentration of free Ca^{2+} in the cytoplasm of 'resting' cells is between 0.1 and 0.01 μM whereas its concentration in the extracellular space is maintained at approximately 1mM. Many cellular activities, including muscular contraction, are only activated when the cytoplasmic concentration of free Ca^{2+} ions reaches approximately 1 μM. An increase in the Ca^{2+} concentration is achieved partly by its rapid entry through voltage-gated Ca^{2+} channels in the cytoplasmic membrane and partly by its release from intracellular storage sites, mainly in the ER. The relative contributions of external and internal Ca^{2+} to muscle contractility depend to some extent on the type of muscle cell. Smooth muscle cells, for example, have only a sparse ER, in comparison with the abundant ER of skeletal and cardiac muscle cells. Ca^{2+} is released from its intracellular storage sites in the ER largely as a result of the interaction of IP_3 with its receptors on the surface of ER. These receptors act as specific ion channels for Ca^{2+}, which are closed down in the absence of IP_3. The binding of IP_3 to its receptor converts the channel to the open form and the Ca^{2+}

flux reaches a maximum within 140 ms. Cloning studies have revealed that there is a family of IP_3 receptor proteins although the specialised functions of the individual members are unknown. Their shared features include an N-terminal cytoplasmic domain which carries the IP_3 binding site, and a channel-forming region at the *C*-terminus.

Ryanodine Receptors

An added complication to the Ca^{2+} channel picture emerged with the discovery of a distinct, but related family of Ca^{2+} channels in the ER membrane which act as receptors for the plant alkaloid ryanodine. At nanomolar concentrations the alkaloid opens these channels but closes them at higher concentrations. The physiological significance of the ryanodine receptors was uncertain until the very recent discovery that the cellular metabolite, cyclic adenosine diphosphate ribose (cADPR), which is formed by the action of ADP ribose cyclase on nicotinamide adenine dinucleotide (NAD), binds to the ryanodine receptors and releases Ca^{2+} from within the ER. cADPR may therefore be a physiological ligand for the ryanodine receptor. External Ca^{2+} entering the cell through the voltage-dependent channels also activates the ryanodine receptors to release Ca^{2+} from the ER thereby augmenting the total Ca^{2+} signal. Recent interest in Ca^{2+} signalling has focused on the observation that there is not a uniform rise in internal Ca^{2+} but rather a series of waves or oscillations across the cell although the mechanism of propagation is controversial. It may be that cells can respond specifically to the amplitude and/or frequency of these Ca^{2+} oscillations.

Intracellular Receptors for Calcium

Ca^{2+} continues the activation cascade by binding to specific sites on several proteins thereby inducing changes in their conformation and function. Most of these Ca^{2+}-responsive proteins have a characteristic helix–loop–helix domain of 29 residues, often referred to as the E-F bend. The actual Ca^{2+}-binding site is a highly conserved, contiguous 12 residue sequence within the E–F bend which provides for seven-fold co-ordination of Ca^{2+} in a pentagonal pyramid. Despite the conserved structure of the binding site, the affinities of the different proteins for Ca^{2+} vary widely.

One of the most remarkable Ca^{2+}-responsive proteins is calmodulin, a protein which is highly conserved from *Paramecium* to man. Apart from its Ca^{2+}-binding function (served by two domains, each of which binds two Ca^{2+} ions), calmodulin has the ability, when complexed with Ca^{2+}, to bind to many different proteins, including phosphodiesterases, brain adenylyl cyclase, NAD kinase, Ca^{2+}-dependent nitric oxide synthase and protein kinases, including a multi-functional Ca^{2+}/calmodulin-dependent kinase which regulates many cellular activities. High affinity of calmodulin for its target proteins combined with low specificity is provided by two hydrophobic domains, flanked by regions of highly negative electrostatic potential, which are exposed in Ca^{2+}-activated-calmodulin. These are thought to bind strongly, probably as a single unit, to amphiphilic domains of varied structure in the target proteins. The interaction of the target proteins with calmodulin results in a marked increase in their functional activity. In 'resting' cells the cytoplasmic concentration of Ca^{2+} is too low to promote the occupation of the Ca^{2+} sites in calmodulin. However, the sites are all filled when the Ca^{2+} concentration increases to ~ 1 µM in stimulated cells. Conformational changes are induced in calmodulin and the protein activates a wide range of target proteins.

A component protein of the myofibrillar complex of muscle cells, troponin C, has about 70% sequence homology with calmodulin. Binding of Ca^{2+} to troponin C induces a conformational change which results in the activation of myosin ATPase, ATP hydrolysis, and muscular contraction.

Termination of the IP_3–DAG–Ca^{2+} Signals

The increases in the cellular concentrations of IP_3, DAG, and Ca^{2+} which follow receptor activation are usually transient because of mechanisms which ensure the removal of the second messengers from their sites of action. IP_3 is subject to progressive dephosphorylation to yield inositol which is reincorporated into membrane-bound PIP_2. IP_3 is also converted by a specific kinase into inositol 1,3,4,5-tetrakisphosphate which, whilst subject to dephosphorylation, may have a second messenger function of its own, possibly by promoting the entry of extracellular Ca^{2+} into the ER.

As previously mentioned, DAG is converted to phosphatidic acid by DAG kinase. The product of the reaction, phosphatidic acid, has some attributes of a second messenger molecule, having been linked to the process of receptor-mediated exocytosis. For example, the degranulation of neutrophils, which is induced by bacterial chemotactic peptides, has been linked to the accumulation of phosphatidic acid in these cells. Phosphatidic acid is also formed by the actions of phospholipases C and D on membrane-bound phosphatidylcholine.

Following its influx into the cytoplasm from both extracellular and intracellular sources, the concentration of Ca^{2+} is eventually reduced by several mechanisms:

1. An ATP-dependent Ca^{2+} pump located in the membrane of the ER returns much of the Ca^{2+} to its storage sites within the vesicles of the ER.
2. The cytoplasmic membrane contains: (a) an ATP-dependent Ca^{2+} pump which extrudes Ca^{2+} into the extracellular space, (b) a Na^+–Ca^{2+} exchange system which also depletes cytoplasmic Ca^{2+}

The net result of these various activities is that the cytoplasmic concentration of Ca^{2+} falls to the resting level of <0.1 µM and the actions of the Ca^{2+}-dependent proteins are brought to a close.

3 SIGNALLING BY RECEPTOR TYROSINE KINASES

Amongst the most important regulators of cell growth, division and differentiation are the polypeptide growth factors. The activities of these factors are most clearly revealed when they are added, under appropriate conditions, to resting, non-dividing cells in tissue culture. A series of events is initiated which induce entry into the cycle of cell division. In this section we shall be concerned with the earliest biochemical events which follow the interaction of the growth factors with their surface receptors and which lead ultimately to alterations in transcriptional activity at the level of the genes or changes in cellular metabolism.

Many of the receptors for growth factors, including the insulin receptor, have intrinsic tyrosine kinase activity, *i.e.* the potential for phosphorylating the hydroxyl groups of sequence-specific tyrosine residues in target proteins. Ingenious protein engineering experiments involving the the receptor tyrosine kinases (RTKs) have shown unequivocally that this enzymic activity is essential for the signalling and biological activities induced by growth factors. RTKs are composed of three distinct domains: an extracellular, growth factor-binding region, a single membrane-spanning domain, and a cytoplasmic domain containing the kinase function as well as sequences essential for eventual interaction with proteins targeted for phosphorylation. There is a high level of sequence homology in the catalytic regions of the the known RTKs. Despite this similarity, inhibitors of kinase function, called tyrphostins, which are structurally related to tyrosine, have recently been described which are receptor-specific, indicating that the small differences in the catalytic regions are exploitable by medicinal chemistry. Despite their hydrophobicity and conserved length (22–26 residues), the membrane-spanning domains show no significant homology. As might be expected, the extracellular growth factor-binding domains exhibit major sequence and structural characteristics which are specific to their individual growth factors.

Following ligand binding, growth factor receptors cluster on the cell surface to form dimers, except in the case of the insulin receptor which is already dimeric (Figure 5). The formation of dimers, or a conformational change in an existing dimer, appears to be essential for the initiation of the next stage in the signalling sequence: the activation of the RTK which phosphorylates specific tyrosine residues in the cytoplasmic domain of the receptor itself. This autophosphorylation provides binding sites for target proteins in the cytoplasm which may then be subject to sequence-specific tyrosine phosphorylation.

SH2 and SH3 Domains

In recent years a diverse group of cytoplasmic enzymes and other proteins has been identified which share sequence-related regions known as SH2 [*src* (oncogene) homology] and SH3 domains. The SH2 domains, which consist of approximately 100 amino acids, mediate specific interactions between their host proteins and the autophosphorylated regions of the RTKs. The SH2 domains are recognised and bound by short sequences which flank the phospho-tyrosine residues. Conformational changes in the SH2-containing-proteins are induced by binding to the RTKs, which facilitate their phosphorylation and and activation or directly induce activation. The structures of some SH2 domains, alone and complexed with phosphopeptide sequences from the appropriate RTKs, have been examined by *X*-ray crystallography and by NMR spectroscopy to provide a

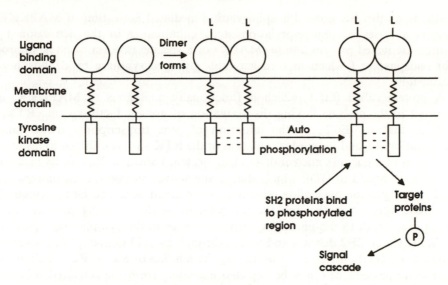

Figure 5: *A much simplified representation of the sequence of events following the binding of an agonist, or ligand (L), which is typically a cellular growth factor or mitogen, to the extracellular domain of a receptor–tyrosine kinase complex (RTK). Ligand binding promotes dimerisation of the RTK complex which leads to activation of the kinase function and autophosphorylation of the kinase itself. The resulting phosphotyrosine residues facilitate the binding to the kinase region of specific target proteins via their SH2 domains. Phosphorylation of the target proteins initiates a cascade of events culminating in the end biological response*

possible basis for the design of inhibitors of the binding process. SH3 domains, which contain about 50 residues, usually accompany SH2 domains and they also appear to be involved in mediating protein–protein interactions during signal transduction.

The identification of proteins containing SH2 domains, and which are presumably potential targets for RTK-mediated phosphorylation, continues apace, *e.g.* cytoplasmic kinases of both the tyrosine and serine/threonine classes, the Ras GTPase activator protein (GAP), phosphatidyl inositol-3-kinase (which generates phosphorylated lipid products which may themselves have second messenger activities), and phospholipase Cγ. Activation of the latter enzyme by phosphorylation leads to the hydrolysis of PIP_2 residues in the cell membrane and the release of the second messenger molecules IP_3 and DAG. The activation of PLCγ by RTKase explains the intracellular appearance of the IP_3 and DAG messengers following the stimulation of cells by growth factors such as epidermal growth factor (EGF) and platelet-derived growth factor (PDGF) in the absence of a G-protein mediated activation of PLC. Another important SH2 domain-containing protein which is a target for RTK-mediated phosphorylation is the extraordinarily named mitogen activated protein kinase kinase kinase (MAPKKK). The functional significance of this cumbersome name is that it is the first cytoplasmic enzyme in an extended signalling cascade leading from the RTK which is specific for insulin, to the characteristic activation of glycogen synthesis by this hormone. Phosphorylation-mediated activation of MAPKKK triggers a series of phosphorylation steps culminating in the activation by mitogen-activated protein kinase (MAPK) of a specific isoform of phosphoprotein phosphatase I which in turn activates glycogen synthase by dephosphorylating it !

A protein called Raf-1, which is functionally analogous to MAPKKK, is involved in the cascade linking the activation of growth factor-specific RTKs, such as that for EGF, to the initiation of gene transcription and cellular proliferation. Ligand-induced stimulation of the RTK has been shown to result in activation of a guanine nucleotide-binding protein known as Ras. In its inactive state Ras is bound to GDP which, during the activation event, is exchanged for GTP via a guanine nucleotide releasing factor called Sos. The latter protein is provoked into action through the intervention of the coupling protein Grb2 which binds both to the phosphotyrosine-rich sites in the cytoplasmic region of the RTK via an SH2 domain and to Sos through an SH3 domain. The exchange of GDP for GTP on Ras is facilitated by the binding of Sos to Ras. A chain of interacting proteins can now be depicted extending from the activated RTK to Ras:

Phosphotyrosine-rich region of RTK—Grb2—Sos—Ras

The Ras–GTP complex now activates the Raf-1 protein which initiates the subsequent down-stream events leading to mitosis by phosphorylating MAP kinase kinase in an analogous fashion to MAPKKK. There therefore appears to be an overlap between this cascade and that for insulin described earlier since both lead to the activation of forms of MAP kinase. Whilst the relationship between the two cascades is not clear at present, it should be remembered that insulin can also act as a mitogen in addition to its stimulation of glycogen breakdown.

4 FINAL COMMENTS

Five main systems of signal tranduction have been described, involving cAMP, cGMP, products of phospholipid hydrolysis, and Ca^{2+} ions as messengers, and the receptor tyrosine kinase initiated pathway. The extraordinary diversity of the proteins involved in what previously appeared to be convergent monolithic pathways may well present opportunities for therapeutically useful intervention. Although space has not permitted a serious analysis of the interactions, or 'cross-talk' between these systems, it must be remembered that they do not operate independently of each other. It is increasingly clear that normal cellular functioning relies upon a complex network of checks and balances amongst the myriad biochemical activities of cells. Many details of the workings of signal transduction mechanisms remain to be uncovered. Undoubtedly, nature has further surprises in store.

5 FURTHER READING

1. W.-J. Tang and A.G. Gilman, *Cell*, 1992, **70**, 869.
2. C.D. Nicholson, R.A.J. Challiss, and M. Shahid, *TiPS*, 1991, **12**, 19.
3. S.S. Taylor, J.A. Buechler, and W. Yonemoto, *Annu. Rev. Biochem.*, 1990, **59**, 971.
4. M. Chinkers and D.L. Garbers, *Annu. Rev. Biochem.*, 1991, **60**, 553.
5. T.M. Lincoln and T.L. Cornwell, *FASEB J.*, 1993, **7**, 328.
6. M.J. Berridge, *Nature*, 1993, **361**, 315.
7. K.Y. O'Neil and W.F. DeGrado, *TiBS*, 1990, **15**, 59.
8. J. Schlessinger and A. Ullrich, *Neuron*, 1992, **9**, 383.
9. M.D. Houslay, *Eur. J. Biochem.*, 1991, **195**, 9.
10. F. McCormick, *Nature*, 1993, **363**, 15.

CHAPTER 3

Enzyme Inhibitors

DAVID A. ROBERTS

1 INTRODUCTION

Enzyme inhibition represents a major strategy in drug design and almost one third of the current top fifty drugs by sales are enzyme inhibitors. The inhibition of an enzyme-catalysed reaction can enable the selective modulation of a variety of biochemical processes such as making cell growth, division, and viability untenable, or interrupting major metabolic pathways by blocking the formation of an essential or undesirable metabolite. Enzyme inhibition is complementary to receptor modulation *via* antagonists and in some cases can be used to potentiate the activity of a desirable species by inhibiting its degradation. Thus the biological activity of species 'B' can be attenuated *via* inhibition of the enzyme involved in its biosynthesis (Figure 1). The same overall effect can be achieved *via* antagonism of the receptor(s) for 'B'. A good example of this is the attenuation of the action of the vasoconstrictor peptide angiotensin II (AII) which can be achieved *via* inhibition of its biosynthesis by the angiotensin converting enzyme (ACE), or *via* AII receptor antagonism.

Given these choices for the attenuation of biochemical mechanisms, the medicinal chemist must firstly decide on whether enzyme inhibition is the most suitable strategy to achieve a particular goal. Various questions can be considered to guide the decision making process: what is known about the structure and mechanism of the enzyme? Is the primary amino acid sequence known? Has the structure been characterised by high-resolution X-ray crystal analysis or is there an opportunity to derive computationally a model structure based on homology with a related, characterised protein? Does the substrate of the enzyme possess biological activity and will its concentration increase and cause undesirable side-effects? Does the target enzyme have only one significant substrate or will other biological processes be affected if the enzyme is inhibited? Are there isoforms or mechanistically related enzymes present which might also be inhibited? If the enzyme is an essential component of an infecting organism, is it unique to that organism, or present in the host also?

Unfortunately, many of these questions will remain unanswered at the outset of a typical drug hunting programme. Nevertheless, if enzyme inhibition is judged to constitute an effective strategy the question arises as to how can the chosen enzyme be inhibited. An essential first step is to understand how enzymes in general, and the target enzyme in particular, work.

Enzymes are proteins which contain chiral recognition sites for specific substrates. They catalyse chemical reactions at these sites, often causing huge rate enhancements (10^{10}–10^{14} fold). In some cases their activity depends on the

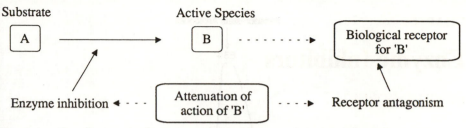

Figure 1: *Complementarity between enzyme inhibition and receptor antagonism*

presence of other organic molecules or ions called cofactors. There are some 10^6 functionally distinct enzymes, catalogued according to the Enzyme Commission Classification (see Appendix 3).

This vast array of enzymes share certain key properties which enable them to achieve catalysis and also provide the medicinal chemist with opportunities to derive general strategies for their inhibition. For example, enzymes contain catalytic functional groups, such as general acids and bases, nucleophiles, and metal ions (which can function as Lewis acids or redox systems). Proteases, for example, illustrate the range of functional groups employed by enzymes to facilitate the hydrolysis of peptide bonds, exploiting both general acid/base catalysis (aspartyl and metallo-proteases) and nucleophilic catalysis (serine and cysteine proteases). Enzymes also provide a relatively water-free, low dielectric constant environment, in which ionic forces are strengthened and transient intermediates which are unstable in aqueous environments have enhanced survival. In addition, enzymes stabilise the transition states of reactions, reducing the activation energy and hence increasing the rate of the reaction. In its simplest schematic form, the course of an enzyme-catalysed reaction can be considered to follow equation (1), in which E and S are free enzyme and free substrate respectively, ES the physically-bound complex of E and S (the Michaelis complex), P the product(s), and EP a physically-bound enzyme–product complex. All of these species lie in energy minima, while the transition state for chemical transformation ($ES^{\ddagger}$) of ES into EP lies at an energy maximum.

$$E + S \rightleftharpoons ES \rightarrow [ES^{\ddagger}] \rightarrow EP \rightleftharpoons E + P \qquad (1)$$

This equation can be expressed as a reaction profile (Figure 2) in which the free energy $\Delta G°$ is plotted versus the reaction co-ordinate showing (qualitatively) the progress of the reaction.

Until relatively recently enzyme inhibitors were designed predominantly on the basis of the substrate ground-state structure (so called substrate analogue inhibitors).

Similarly, the binding interactions available to the product structure can also be used in the design of putative inhibitors. There is little conceptual difficulty with these classes of agent since stable molecular structures (substrates or products) are used to design real (*i.e.* chemically stable) inhibitors. The strength of the enzyme–substrate interaction in the ground state is far outstripped by that

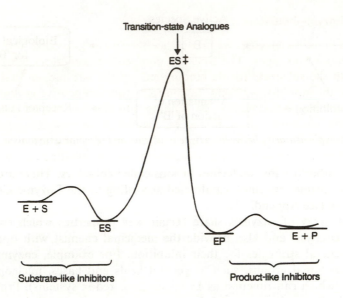

Figure 2: *Reaction profile of an enzyme-catalysed reaction*

in the fleeting transition state. Thus enzymes catalyse chemical reactions by virtue of their ability to sequester, specifically, the relevant transition state, thereby stabilising it and lowering the energy required by E and S to reach it. This suggests that inhibitors with very high enzyme affinity might be obtained if the geometric, steric, and electronic nature of the transition-state moiety is used as the basis for inhibitor design. A true transition-state analogue, with fleeting partial bonds, cannot be synthesised. However, derivatives which incorporate a number of the features likely to be required for transition-state binding can sometimes be prepared in stable form. The improvement in binding affinities of such 'transition-state analogues' is often striking, and will be illustrated by examples later in this chapter.

2 ENZYME INHIBITOR CATEGORIES

Enzyme inhibitors fall into two main types: reversible and irreversible. Reversible inhibitors usually bind *via* non-covalent or weakly covalent forces, and can be removed from the enzyme by dilution, gel filtration, or dialysis. They form a rapid equilibrium with the enzyme which results in a fixed degree of inhibition which depends on their concentration. Irreversible inhibitors generally bind covalently to the enzyme and are not removed by dilution/ dialysis and the degree of inhibition is time-dependent. The distinction between these two broad classes becomes blurred when considering exceedingly potent reversible inhibitors (*e.g.* non-covalent, very tightly bound, slowly dissociating), but this classification is still useful for describing many enzyme–inhibitor systems.

Reversible Enzyme Inhibitors

These agents bind to enzymes *via* non-covalent or weakly covalent forces, and fall into two major sub-types. The first are competitive inhibitors which compete directly with the substrate for its binding site on the enzyme, so that either the substrate or the inhibitor is bound. In contrast, non-competitive inhibitors do not compete with the substrate for its binding site on the enzyme and so both substrate and inhibitor can be bound independently. In practice, classical non-competitive inhibition is rare and more often mixed inhibition is encountered whereby inhibitor and substrate can be bound, but the binding of one affects the other. The nature of the inhibition taking place can be determined by enzyme kinetics. For example, consider the kinetics of the single substrate catalysed reaction in equation (2):

$$E + S \rightleftharpoons ES \xrightarrow{k_{cat}} EP \tag{2}$$

where k_{cat} is the first-order rate constant for the conversion of ES to EP. Assuming that the concentration of the enzyme is negligible compared with that of the substrate, then it is found experimentally that in most cases the initial rate (v) of formation of products or destruction of substrate by an enzyme is directly proportional to the concentration of the enzyme [E$_0$]. At sufficiently low substrate concentration [S], v increases linearly with [S] (Figure 3). But as [S] is increased, this relationship begins to break down and v increases less rapidly than [S] until at sufficiently high or saturating [S], v reaches a limiting value termed V_{max}.

This is expressed quantitatively in the Michaelis–Menten equation (3), the basic equation of enzyme kinetics, where $V_{max} = k_{cat}[E_0]$, and the concentration of substrate at which $v = \frac{1}{2} V_{max}$ is termed K_M, the Michaelis constant.

$$v = \frac{[E_0][S]k_{cat}}{K_M + [S]} \tag{3}$$

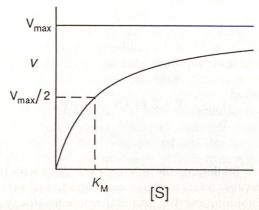

Figure 3: *Plot of v versus [S] for a reaction obeying Michaelis–Menten kinetics*

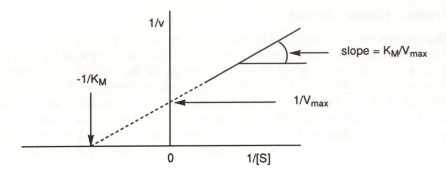

Figure 4:   *Lineweaver–Burk plot of $1/v$ versus $1/[S]$*

At low [S] the reaction rate depends upon substrate concentration and so is first order in substrate, whilst at high [S] the enzyme is saturated with substrate, and so the maximum velocity V_{max} is reached, and the reaction becomes zero order in substrate.

The Michaelis–Menten equation does not lend itself to the calculation of the constants V_{max} and K_M and so it is very useful to transform it into a linear form for analysing data graphically and detecting deviations from the ideal behaviour. One of the best known alternatives is the Lineweaver–Burk plot (equation 4), which is the inverse of the Michaelis–Menten equation.

$$1/v = 1/V_{max} + K_M/V_{max}[S] \qquad (4)$$

Plotting $1/v$ against $1/[S]$ (Figure 4) gives an intercept of $1/V_{max}$ on the y-axis as $1/[S]$ tends to zero, and $1/[S] = -1/K_M$ on the x-axis. The slope of the line is K_M/V_{max}. The effect of an inhibitor on these enzyme kinetic parameters allows the type of inhibition to be determined.

Reversible Competitive Inhibition

If an inhibitor I reversibly binds to the active site of the enzyme and prevents S binding and *vice versa*, I and S compete for the same site and I is said to be a competitive inhibitor (Figure 5). In the case of the simple Michaelis–Menten equation, an additional equilibrium must be considered (equation 5) described by the Lineweaver–Burk plot for this type of inhibition as shown in Figure 6.

$$E + S \rightleftharpoons ES \rightarrow E + P \qquad (5)$$
$$\updownarrow$$
$$EI$$

For competitive inhibition, the intercept on the y-axis (*i.e.* V_{max}) does not change. This is because a large enough concentration of substrate will overcome the reversible inhibition, and the maximal reaction velocity can be attained. A classical example of a competitive inhibitor which is a substrate analogue is

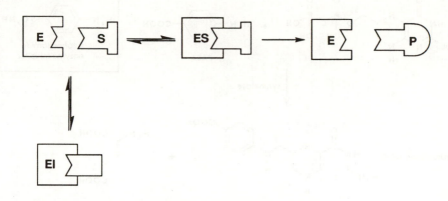

Figure 5: *Competitive inhibition; inhibitor and substrate compete for the same binding site*

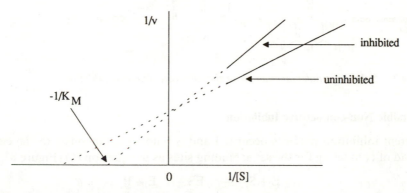

Figure 6: *Lineweaver–Burk plot showing competitive inhibition*

sulphanilamide which forms a tight complex with the enzyme 7,8-dihydropteroate synthetase with a dissociation constant of 10^{-9} M (Figure 7). One of the substrates for this folate synthesising enzyme is *p*-aminobenzoic acid (PABA) which has a structural resemblance to sulphanilamide and its analogues.

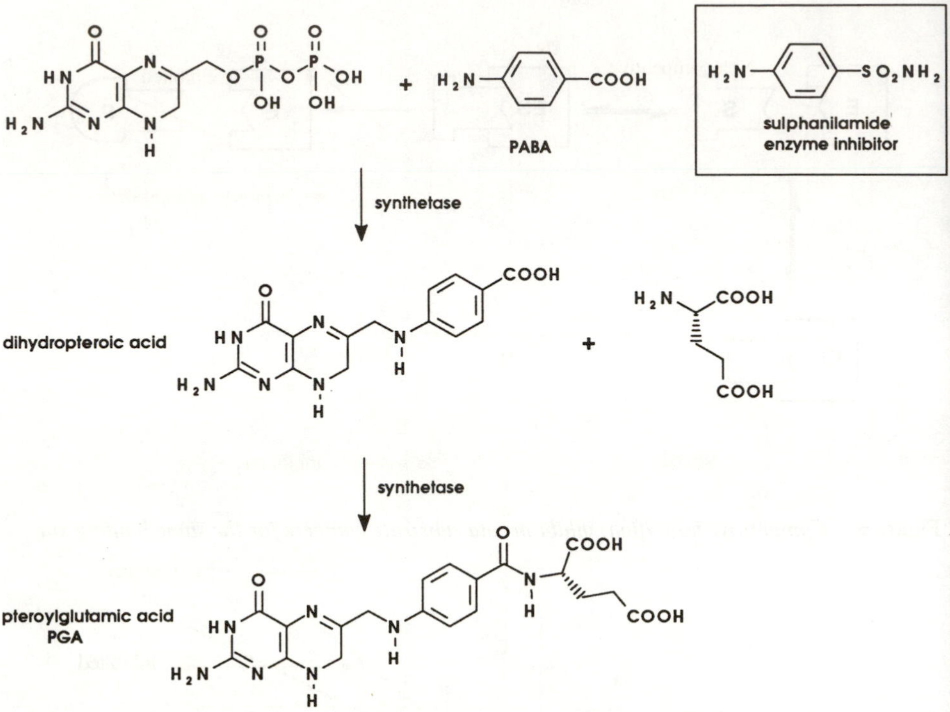

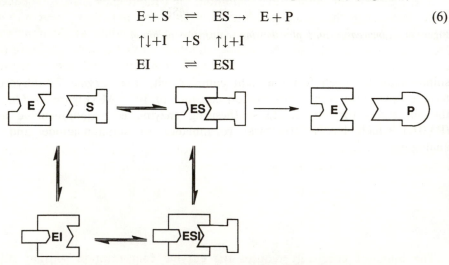

Figure 7: *Sulphanilamide; an example of the substrate analogue inhibitor*

Reversible Non-competitive Inhibition

Different inhibition patterns occur if I and S bind simultaneously to the enzyme instead of competing for the same binding sites as in equation (6) (Figure 8).

$$\text{E} + \text{S} \quad \rightleftharpoons \quad \text{ES} \rightarrow \quad \text{E} + \text{P} \tag{6}$$

$$\uparrow\downarrow +\text{I} \quad +\text{S} \quad \uparrow\downarrow +\text{I}$$

$$\text{EI} \quad \rightleftharpoons \quad \text{ESI}$$

Figure 8: *Non-competitive inhibition; inhibitor and substrate bind simultaneously*

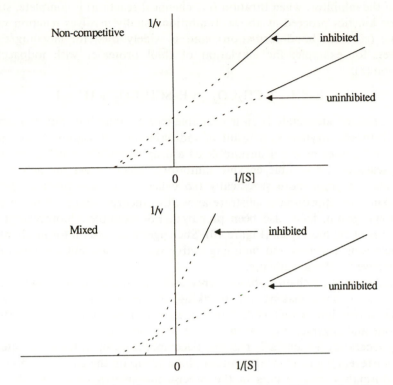

Figure 9 : *Lineweaver–Burk plots showing* (a) *non-competitive and* (b) *mixed inhibition*

The inhibition is only truly non-competitive when S and I bind completely independently. Lack of independence yields mixed inhibition (Figure 9).

In the case of non-competitive inhibition, the *y* intercept, *i.e.* V_{max} is reduced, since increasing the substrate concentration does not now overcome the inhibition because the substrate and inhibitor are binding at different sites. Hence K_M does not change. For mixed inhibition, both K_M and V_{max} have now changed and the plot clearly falls between the competitive and non-competitive situations.

Irreversible Enzyme Inhibitors

Irreversible enzyme inhibition is not reversible by dialysis, gel filtration or dilution and can be described in simple terms by equation (7).

$$E + S \; \rightleftharpoons \; ES \; \rightarrow \; E + P \qquad (7)$$
$$\uparrow\downarrow +I$$
$$EI$$

The inhibitor effectively reduces the enzyme concentration so that [E] is reduced to [EI]. Thus if the initial concentration of the enzyme was greater than that of the inhibitor, when titration (*i.e.* chemical reaction) is complete, standard enzyme kinetics proceed as above. Inhibition usually involves reaction with the enzyme (covalent bond formation), and is widely used for labelling catalytic residues, for example, the alkylation of thiol proteases with iodoacetate in equation (8).

$$E\text{-}SH + I\text{-}CH_2CO_2^- \rightarrow E\text{-}SCH_2CO_2^- + H^+ + I^- \tag{8}$$

In this case iodoacetate is an irreversible enzyme inhibitor, but its inability to select between enzymes as a result of indiscriminate alkylation of any reactive functional groups makes it unsuitable as a drug candidate. Later generations of more selective, irreversible enzyme inhibitors, which target the active sites of particular enzymes more specifically (so called active site-directed agents) by mimicking the appropriate substrate as well as incorporating a built-in reactive functional group, have also been prepared. For example, chloromethyl ketone inhibitors of chymotrypsin (Figure 10). Such agents are useful for mechanistically characterising enzymes and mapping active site residues, but are generally still too reactive for therapeutic use.

The design of mechanism-based, irreversible inhibitors uses knowledge of the chemical, *i.e.* bond making and breaking, mechanism used by the enzyme to catalyse a reaction as well as the binding energy of the non-reacting parts of the substrate and enzyme. These agents which are also known as 'suicide' inhibitors, act by generating a chemically reactive electrophilic group at the active site, which in turn irreversibly reacts with a nucleophilic group on the enzyme. This covalent bond formation thus occurs in the precise micro-environment of the enzyme active site. The advantage of this class of inhibitors is that they contain relatively unreactive groups until they undergo specific transformation by the enzyme, so enabling the design of agents that are more selective and non-toxic. There are many mechanism-based inhibitors of β-lactamase, the enzyme responsible for bacterial resistance to penicillins and other β-lactam antibiotics. An example of this class of drug is clavulanic acid which inhibits β-lactamase *via* formation of a stable acyl–enzyme–iminium complex (Figure 11) which can further react with a nucleophilic group on the enzyme.

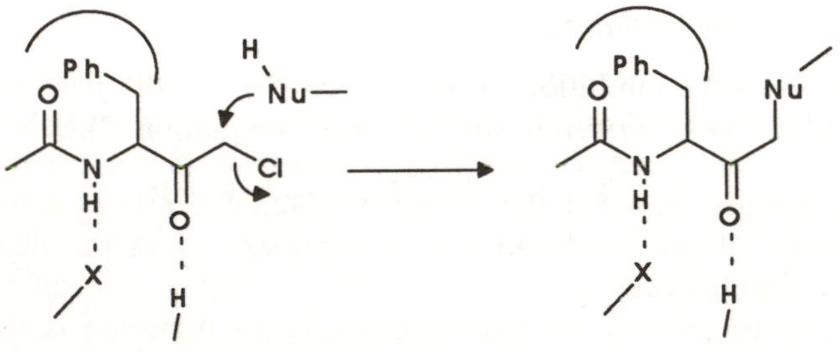

Figure 10: α-*Haloketone active site-directed, irreversible inhibitors*

penicillin substrate   acyl-enzyme complex   hydrolysis products

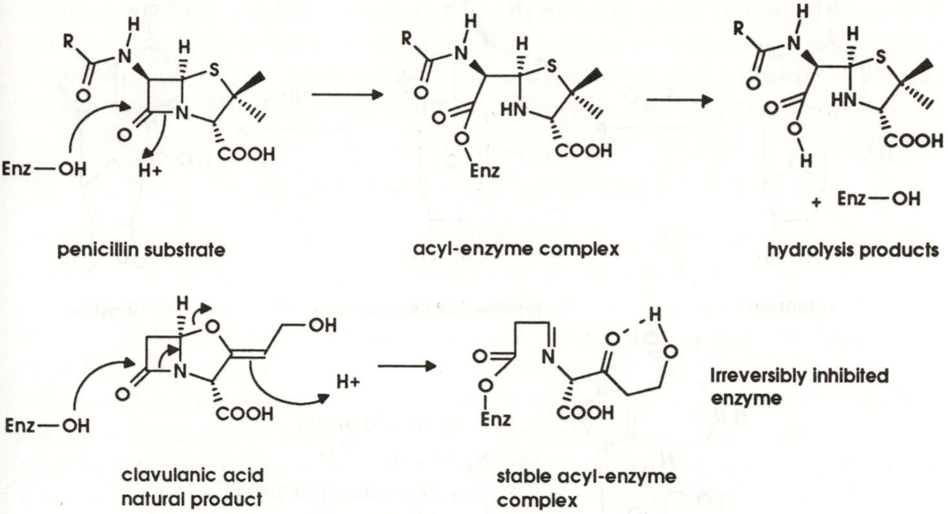

clavulanic acid   stable acyl-enzyme
natural product   complex

Figure 11: *Clavulanic acid; an example of a mechanism-based, irreversible inhibitor*

3 OPTIONS FOR DRUG DESIGN

The above discussion outlines various types of inhibitor and the question arises as to which is the most suitable for a particular drug target. Reversible, competitive inhibitors achieve high affinity for the target enzyme by fitting the active site well and so are more likely to be selective. Moreover, the design of such agents can be based rationally upon knowledge of the enzyme mechanism/ structure and the enzyme substrate. However, in many cases, detailed mechanistic/substrate information may not be available and the generation of active leads may be reliant upon random screening of compound collections or libraries. This approach is just as likely to identify compounds which inhibit by binding allosterically, away from the substrate binding site. Another potential problem with truly competitive inhibitors is that their activity can, in principle, be overcome by substrate accumulation. Reversible, non-competitive inhibitors do not suffer from the latter problem but there is no rational link with the enzyme mechanism and substrate (unless detailed information of the inhibitor binding site is available) and so inhibitor design tends to be more empirical (see above).

Irreversible inhibition can produce complete inactivation of the enzyme, which cannot be overcome. However, initial recognition by the enzyme involves only substrate-like affinity and so high drug concentrations must be achieved. Also, the enzyme usually processes the inhibitor quite efficiently as a substrate and in only a fraction of the enzyme–inhibitor complexes does the final nucleophilic attack and trapping occur.

Another, more recently recognised category of inhibitor is the slow, tight-binding type, which begin to mimic very effectively the transition state of the enzyme-catalysed reaction, referred to previously as transition-state analogue

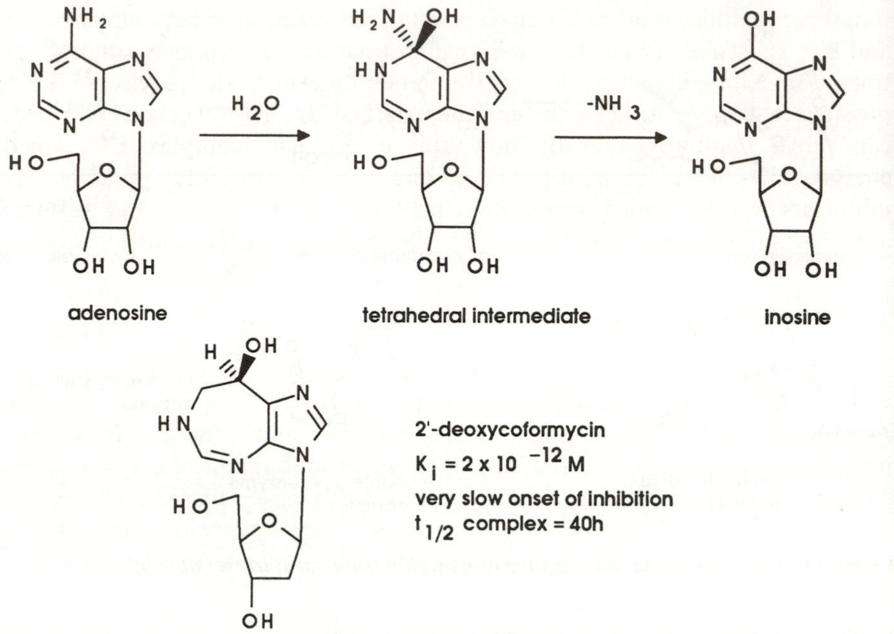

2'-deoxycoformycin

$K_i = 2 \times 10^{-12}$ M

very slow onset of inhibition

$t_{1/2}$ complex = 40h

Figure 12: *2'-Deoxycoformycin; a transition-state analogue inhibitor of adenosine deaminase*

inhibitors. A classical example is the adenosine deaminase inhibitor 2'-deoxyco-formycin, which inhibits the general base-catalysed addition of water to adenosine to give inosine (Figure 12). 2'-Deoxycoformycin exhibits some very unusual inhibitory properties, in addition to its extremely high affinity. Firstly, equilibrium with the enzyme is achieved very slowly, taking seconds or minutes rather than milliseconds as is normally the case. In addition, the enzyme–inhibitor complex is extremely long-lived. A modified kinetic analysis which can account for this behaviour, compared with classical competitive inhibition, is shown in equation (9).

$$
\begin{array}{ccccc}
E + S & \rightleftharpoons & ES & \rightarrow & E + P \\
\updownarrow & & & & \\
EI & \underset{k_b}{\overset{k_a}{\rightleftharpoons}} & EI^* & &
\end{array}
\tag{9}
$$

The EI* state of the enzyme–inhibitor complex is proposed to be attained *via* a conformational rearrangement of EI. The ratio of the rate constants k_a and k_b determines the extent to which EI* accumulates and its longevity. As k_b approaches zero, the inhibition becomes essentially irreversible. This is a very attractive phenomenon for a drug, since EI* is not in direct equilibrium with the substrate and so inhibition is not easily overcome. Furthermore, the binding in EI* can be extremely tight and so the duration of action can be very long. As indicated earlier, it seems likely that inhibitors which resemble the reaction transition state can bind extremely tightly to their target enzyme by exploiting the complementarity between the enzyme and the transition state. However, the initial recognition event in an enzyme-catalysed reaction is between the enzyme and the substrate, which it is designed by nature to recognise quickly. Since transition-state analogues do not resemble the substrate precisely, it seems possible that recognition by the enzyme may be slow. However, once formed, EI can move thermodynamically downhill to the new complex EI* which is energetically more favourable. Designing this feature into putative, stable inhibitors where detailed information on the enzyme structure and mechanism are known represents a real, but worthwhile challenge for the medicinal chemist.

4 EXAMPLES OF ENZYME INHIBITORS

There are many examples of successful drug hunting based on inhibition of a very wide range of enzyme classes including proteases, oxygenases, reductases, hydrolases, phosphodiesterases, topoisomerases, and kinases. It would be impossible to cover even a fraction of these various inhibitor types in a single chapter. Nevertheless it is instructive to consider at least a few recent examples of inhibitor design and discovery which have led either to successful marketed products or interesting and challenging medicinal chemistry.

Angiotensin Converting Enzyme and Renin Inhibitors

The renin–angiotensin–aldosterone system is a multi-regulated proteolytic cascade of enzyme-mediated events that converts angiotensinogen into angiotensin I (AI), angiotensin II (AII), and angiotensin III (AIII) and so provides a major regulatory mechanism for the control of blood pressure in mammals (Figure 13).

This cascade of events provides the medicinal chemist with the opportunity of blocking the formation of inappropriately high amounts of AII *via* inhibition of either the enzyme renin (aspartyl protease) or the angiotensin converting enzyme (zinc-dependent metallo-protease; ACE). Inhibition of ACE, which cleaves AI to AII, has demonstrated that obstruction of the system, prior to the formation of AII and AIII, can effectively lower blood pressure in a large majority of hypertensive patients. The key hypothesis in the development of ACE inhibitors, proposed by Ondetti and Cushman of the Squibb group, proposed that, since ACE is mechanistically related to the well-characterised metallopeptidase, carboxypeptidase A (CPA), CPA inhibitors could be modified to produce inhibitors of ACE. ACE is a membrane-bound metalloprotease which recognises and cleaves dipeptides from the *C*-terminus of AI and other related peptides. The enzyme contains a zinc ion at its catalytic site. Because there are no *X*-ray data available for the ACE active site, it was proposed that the zinc ion could co-ordinate the scissile bond of the substrate, activating it to nucleophilic attack by a conveniently placed water molecule, by analogy with the CPA mechanism (Figure 14).

This line of thought eventually led to the discovery and development of several commercially successful agents, the first three of which were captopril, enalapril, and lisinopril (Figure 15). These orally active, low molecular weight inhibitors

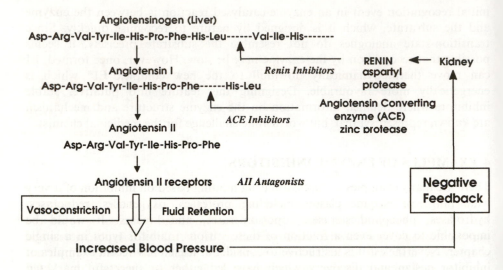

Angiotensinogen (Liver)

Asp-Arg-Val-Tyr-Ile-His-Pro-Phe-His-Leu------Val-Ile-His------

Angiotensin I   *Renin Inhibitors*   RENIN ← Kidney

Asp-Arg-Val-Tyr-Ile-His-Pro-Phe------His-Leu   aspartyl
                                                                 protease

                                                                 Angiotensin Converting
                                        ACE Inhibitors   enzyme (ACE)
Angiotensin II   zinc protease

Asp-Arg-Val-Tyr-Ile-His-Pro-Phe

Angiotensin II receptors   *AII Antagonists*   Negative
                                                                 Feedback
Vasoconstriction   Fluid Retention

Increased Blood Pressure

Figure 13: *Schematic representation of the renin–angiotensin–aldosterone system*

incorporate ligands (thiolate or carboxylate) to bind the zinc ion at the active site of the protease, thereby attaining high affinity.

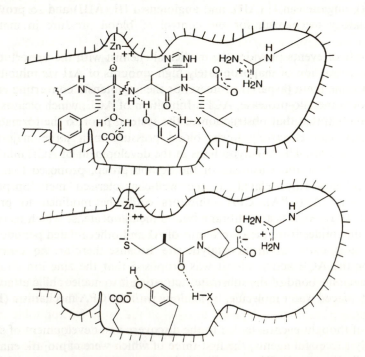

Figure 14: *Representations of the ACE active site showing substrate binding and inhibition*

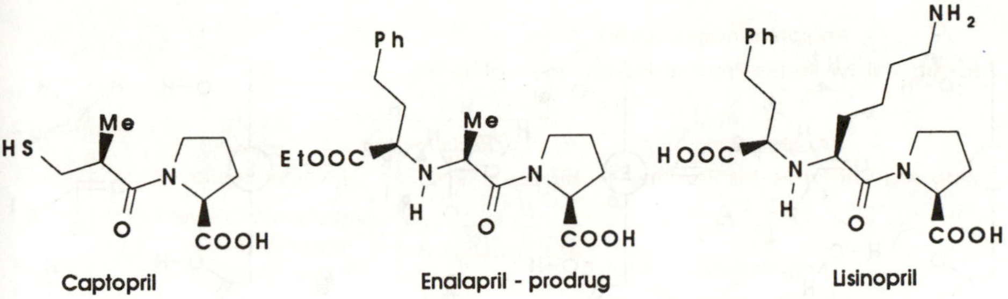

Captopril   Enalapril - prodrug   Lisinopril

Figure 15: *Commercially successful ACE inhibitors*

Despite their enormous clinical and commercial success, ACE inhibitors do suffer from a range of side-effects such as angio-oedema (mucosal lesions) and persistent cough. One possible explanation for this is that ACE is ubiquitous and unselective, and will also cleave a number of other biologically important peptides such as bradykinin and substance P. It follows therefore that ACE inhibition may potentiate the actions of these peptides and lead to undesirable side-effects.

The conversion of angiotensinogen to AI by the enzyme renin is the first, and rate-limiting step in the cascade. By contrast with ACE, renin has only one known substrate, being uniquely specific to angiotensinogen. Interruption of the cascade by renin inhibition could therefore be an extraordinarily specific pharmacological intervention, offering a valuable alternative to ACE inhibition, with the potential for fewer side-effects.

Renin belongs to the aspartyl protease mechanistic class of enzymes and is related in this respect to pepsin and cathepsin D (mammalian enzymes), and penicillopepsin and endothiapepsin (fungal enzymes). The primary amino acid sequence of human renin is known and early inhibitor design strategies focused on computer modelling work based on the substantial degree of homology displayed between renin and these two latter enzymes, for which high resolution X-ray crystal structures have been determined. More recently, a high-resolution X-ray analysis of the recombinant human protein has been obtained. These X-ray structures show that these enzymes have active sites containing two catalytic aspartates which can accommodate large peptidic substrates of eight amino acids or more. The postulated mechanism of action of this enzyme class (Figure 16) assumes that the ionised form of one of the aspartates acts as a general base to activate a water molecule to attack the scissile amide bond of the substrate, whilst the second protonated aspartate acts as a proton source for the developing tetrahedral transition state.

One major difference between the substrate recognition motifs of the renin and ACE active sites is that renin lacks the dominant zinc ion. This means that the overall binding of inhibitors depends heavily on the multi-hydrophobic interactions which the enzyme makes with the side-chain amino acid residues.

Although it is possible to prepare renin inhibitors based on the substrate structure, a much more attractive way to gain access to compounds with higher

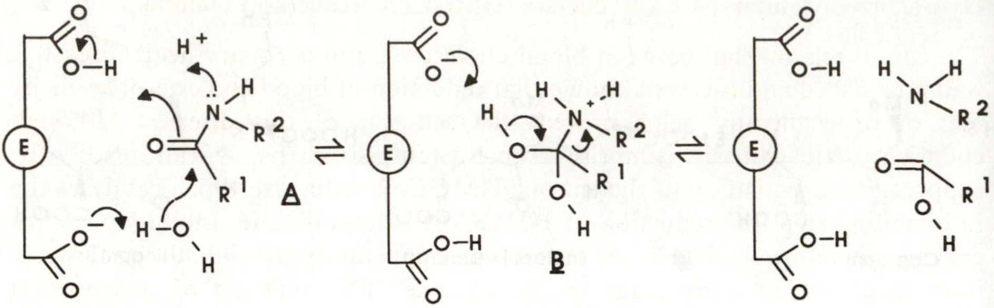

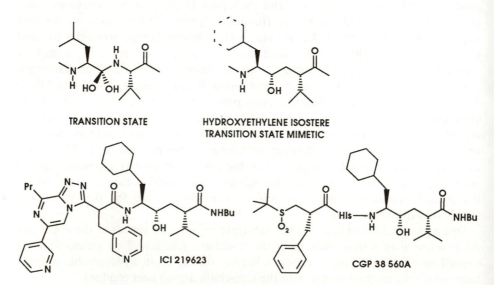

Figure 16: *Schematic representation of the mechanism of hydrolysis of substrate A by an aspartyl protease E via the transition state B*

affinity is to make chemically stable, non-hydrolysable analogues which resemble the transition state B in their geometry and electron distribution. This has been addressed by incorporation of the so called hydroxyethylene transition-state mimetic (Figure 17) into inhibitor structures such as the highly potent, non-peptidic renin inhibitor ICI 219623 (IC_{50} versus human renin 0.2 nM) and the pseudo-peptidic inhibitor CGP 38 560A (IC_{50} 0.7nM; Ciba-Geigy). Although these compounds display modest oral activity in primate models of hypertension, their poor bioavailability makes them unsuitable for further development and research efforts to find agents with markedly improved oral absorption and pharmacokinetics continue.

TRANSITION STATE

HYDROXYETHYLENE ISOSTERE
TRANSITION STATE MIMETIC

ICI 219623

CGP 38 560A

Figure 17: *Hydroxyethylene isostere transition-state mimetic and its incorporation into the potent renin inhibitors ICI 219623 and CGP 38 560A.*

Hydroxymethylglutaryl-CoA Reductase (HMGCoA Reductase) Inhibitors

The causal relationship between blood cholesterol and coronary heart disease is well established and it is well known that reduction of blood cholesterol levels by diet or drug therapy helps prevent the sequelae of this disease. Although cholesterol biosynthesis comprises some twenty-six steps, it can readily be suppressed by regulation of the enzyme HMGCoA reductase which catalyses the rate-limiting step, the reduction of HMGCoA to mevalonate. Inhibition of this enzyme therefore provides an attractive opportunity to inhibit cholesterol biosynthesis at an early stage in the cascade. The build-up of unprocessed substrate does not lead to toxicity problems, whereas earlier attempts to inhibit later stage enzymes in the cascade led to the accumulation of desmosterol in toxic levels. Very potent competitive inhibitors of HMGCoA reductase have become available from natural product isolation programmes. Thus, cultures of *Aspergillus terreus* yielded mevinolin (Figure 18) which is a very potent inhibitor (K_i 6.4×10^{-10}M), in which the secondary alcohol at the 5-position of the acidic side-chain is postulated to act as a putative mimetic of the tetrahedral transition state of the reduction reaction. As the pro-drug lactone, the compound is absorbed orally into the liver and efficiently inhibits cholesterol biosynthesis in man thereby lowering circulating low density lipoprotein (LDL) levels and elevating high density lipoprotein (HDL) receptor numbers. This profile has therefore led to the compound being widely used to control inappropriately high cholesterol levels in large numbers of patients, thereby reducing coronary risk factors such as atherosclerosis.

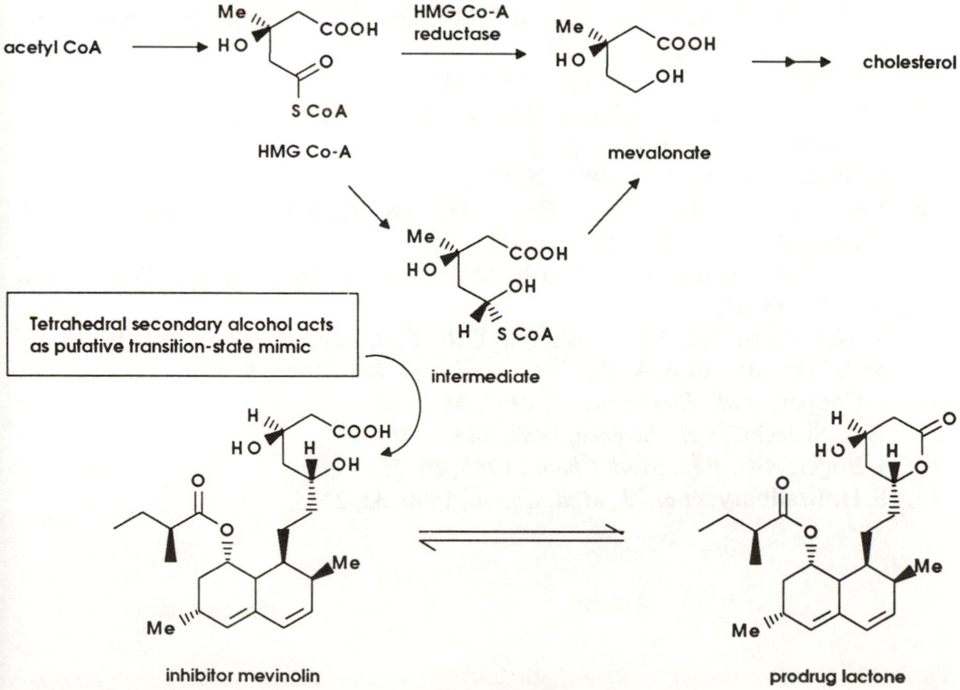

Figure 18: *Mevinolin; an inhibitor of HMGCoA reductase*

5 CONCLUDING REMARKS

Enzyme inhibition already constitutes a powerful strategy for the design of novel drugs by enabling the selective blockade of specific biochemical cascades. Historically, research on enzyme inhibition has been limited by the very poor availability of enzymes from various sources and by our inability to obtain them in sufficiently pure form. We are now entering an era where the importance of enzyme inhibition as a strategy for drug design is likely to grow as large numbers of pure enzymes become more readily available through molecular biology and their active sites are mapped using site-specific mutagenesis techniques. This growing target availability is being augmented by increasingly sophisticated protein NMR spectroscopic and *X*-ray crystallographic techniques, revealing more details of enzyme structure and mechanism and enabling the *de novo* design of enzyme inhibitors to become a reality.

6 ACKNOWLEDGEMENTS

The author is indebted to Dr Keith James, Pfizer Central Research, for providing some of the background material used in this chapter.

7 ADDITIONAL READING

1. 'Comprehensive Medicinal Chemistry', ed. P.G. Sammes, Pergamon Press, Oxford, 1st edition, 1990, Vol. 2.
2. A. Fersht, 'Enzyme Structure and Mechanism', Freeman, New York, 2nd edition, 1985, Chapter 3, p. 84.
3. K.T. Douglas, *Chem. and Ind.*, 1983, 311.
4. J.K. Seydel and K.J. Schaper, 'Enzyme Inhibitors as Drugs', ed. M. Sandler, Macmillan, London, 1980, p. 53.
5. C. Walsh, *Tetrahedron*, 1982, **38**, 871.
6 J.R. Knowles, *Acc. Chem. Res.*, 1985, **18**, 97; S.J. Cartwright and S.G. Waley, *Med. Res. Rev.,* 1983, **3**, 341.
7. J.F. Morrison and C.T. Walsh, 'Advances in Enzymology', Wiley, New York, 1988, **61**.
8. M.A. Ondetti and D.W. Cushman, *CRC Crit. Rev. Biochem*, 1984, **16**, 38.
9. M.J. Wyvratt and A.A. Patchett, *Med. Res. Rev.,* 1985, **5**, 483.
10. J. Cooper, *et al.*, *Biochemistry*, 1992, **31**, 8142
11. A.R. Sielecki, *et al.*, *Science,* 1989, **243**, 1346
12. J. Boger, *Ann. Rep. Med. Chem.*, 1985, **20**, 257.
13. R.H. Bradbury, *et al.*, *J. Med. Chem.*, 1990, **33**, 2335.

The Biological Evaluation of New Compounds

ROBERT A. COLEMAN

1 INTRODUCTION

In the pharmacological evaluation of new compounds, two questions must be addressed: 'Why do we want to evaluate these compounds?' and 'How do we go about it?'. The reasons why we should want to evaluate a new substance are various. Most importantly, we need to know whether the compound has any potentially therapeutic useful biological activity and, if it does, how potent it is. In addition, it is important to establish whether it has any other biological activity unrelated to that primary activity. And finally, we have to know whether it exhibits the desired biological activity *in vivo*, with the desired duration of action, when administered by the appropriate route.

In order to answer such questions, it is important to have a test strategy which will consist of a number of stages (Figure 1).

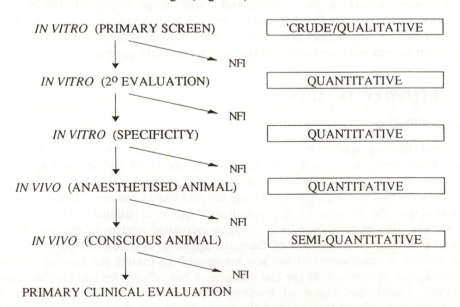

Figure 1: *A proposed test stategy. At each stage, a level of required activity is imposed. If the compound under test achieves or exceeds this predetermined level of activity, it will pass to the next stage. If however it fails to achieve the required activity level, it will be deemed to be of No Further Interest (NFI), and will not be tested further*

The first stage may be described as the primary screen, the object of which is to distinguish, from a large number of candidates, compounds worthy of further evaluation. This primary screen test is usually of a qualitative nature, being designed only to select compounds with activity at or below a certain concentration. In the secondary evaluation, the degree of that activity can be determined; this is a quantitative step. A compound with a desired degree of activity can next be tested for specificity of action; again this test may be conducted *in vitro*. Here, the compound is tested for activity other than that for which it is primarily required. Assuming that the compound has the desired level of primary activity, and it does not have any other potentially limiting effects, it may next be tested *in vivo*.

The use of *in vitro* techniques can provide a large amount of information about a new compound, but, however satisfactory its profile appears in such tests, it must still be tested in the complex, integrated system which is the whole animal. Quite often the first *in vivo* testing is conducted in anaesthetised animals, where effects on a number of different organs or systems can be studied in a quantitative fashion. After testing in anaesthetised animals, it may be appropriate to test the compound in a conscious animals where reflexes are intact, and behaviour may be studied. If the compound has a satisfactory profile in the *in vivo* tests, it may then go forward for clinical evaluation where it will first be tested in healthy volunteers, and then in patients.

I would now like to go over in some more detail how we would go about the biological evaluation of new compounds. Most primary evaluation of new compounds involves *in vitro* testing, and I will use predominantly the *in vitro* techniques to illustrate the biologist's approach to this task of drug evaluation. Commonly, *in vitro* studies may involve ligand binding studies, measurements of levels of second messengers, or evaluation of functional responses.

2 *IN VITRO* EVALUATION

Ligand Binding

Ligand binding studies may be carried out on whole tissue, on single or dispersed cells, or on cell membranes. The object of ligand binding is to determine the competition between the test molecule and a radiolabelled molecule which has high affinity for the binding site in question. Under control conditions, the binding of the radioligand alone is studied: increasing the concentrations of radioligand will result in increasing degrees of binding. From this, a suitable concentration of the radioligand is selected, and the ability of increasing concentrations of the test compound to inhibit the binding of this radioligand determined. If the test compound has affinity for the binding sites, it will inhibit the degree of binding obtained with the radioligand in a concentration-related fashion, and the concentration of the compound required to inhibit radioligand binding will give some idea its affinity for the ligand binding sites.

Each type of tissue preparation has it own advantages and disadvantages

Table 1 *The advantages and disadvantages of the use of various preparations for ligand binding*

	Advantage	Disadvantage
WHOLE TISSUE	simple	heterogeneous cell population limited availability?
SINGLE/DISPERSED CELLS	appropriate cell type	availability limited?
CULTURED CELLS	availability unlimited, minimal animal use	transformation of cells?
TRANSFECTED CELLS	relevant receptor	complicated, receptor not in native environment

(Table 1). Whole tissue has the advantage that it is simple to prepare, but it has the disadvantage that quite often whole tissues consist of a range of different cell types, and one can't be certain that the binding is taking place to the appropriate cell type. Dispersed cell preparations can be made from the appropriate cell type, but the availability of such cells may be limited, particularly if the cells are of human origin. Cultured cells have the advantage that they can be virtually unlimited in their availability, and of course the use of cultured cells reduces the necessity to use large numbers of experimental animals. However, the culture procedure itself is complicated, and may result in some transformation of the cells. Finally, one may use transfected cells, these being cells which are freely available and are easy to manipulate, and in which the appropriate receptor has been introduced. These have the advantage of course that the appropriate receptor is available for study, but have the disadvantage that it is a complicated process, and it is not certain at this time whether the receptor will behave exactly the same in a foreign membrane as it does in its native membrane.

A drawback with ligand binding studies themselves is that it is not always easy to distinguish whether a compound is an agonist or an antagonist, merely that it has an affinity for the receptor/binding site. This is an important point, so let us next consider *what is an agonist* and *what is an antagonist?*

An **agonist** is a molecule which not only has some affinity for a receptor, but also activates it thus causing a response, *i.e.* it has *efficacy.*

An **antagonist** is a molecule which has affinity for a receptor but fails to activate it, *i.e.* it has no *efficacy,* and thus causes no response. An antagonist will compete with an agonist for binding to the receptor, and thus prevents the agonist from interacting with the receptor and initiating agonist activity.

These definitions are rather simplistic, because in fact compounds do not necessarily exist as pure agonists and pure antagonists, but they may demonstrate a spectrum of activity from full agonists through partial agonists to antagonists, depending on their degree of *efficacy*. A full agonist will have high *efficacy*, a partial agonist will have moderate *efficacy*, and an antagonist will have no *efficacy*.

Measurement of Second Messengers

Now we consider briefly the use of the measurement of second messengers to quantify agonist activity. In the cell machinery, an agonist will interact with a receptor which will have some effect, often *via* a G-protein, on a second messenger system. There are a number of second messenger systems which are commonly found in life, but the most common are adenylyl cyclase and phosphatidyl inositol turnover, and one may measure the end product of these processes. In the case of adenylyl cyclase it is cyclic AMP, and in the case of phosphatidyl inositol turnover, it is inositol trisphosphate, IP3. Second messenger studies can be performed in whole tissues or in single or dispersed cells. The cells may be native cells, cultured cells, or transfected cells.

The measurement of these second messengers can be approached in a classical pharmacological fashion by which the relationship between increasing concentrations of agonist and production of increasing amounts of the second messenger may be studied. Further, the effects of increasing amounts of a potential antagonist on the ability of an agonist to produce elevated levels of second messenger can also be determined. Such studies are essentially no different from those in which we measure cell function, *e.g.* contraction, relaxation, or secretion. In functional studies on isolated tissues or isolated cells, it is possible to determine a number of parameters, for example, potency, specificity, and even in some cases duration of action.

Measurement of Functional Activity

Let us now consider functional testing on preparations of smooth muscle. I have chosen smooth muscle mainly because it is simple to use, experiments are simple to describe, and exemplify most aspects of primary drug evaluation, but the principles are similar to those in any functional assay, be that electrophysiological, chemokinetic or secretory. To maintain the smooth muscle in as healthy a state as possible, it must be immersed in an isotonic, physiological salt solution, its temperature must be maintained at the appropriate level, usually 37 °C, it must be oxygenated, usually achieved by bubbling the physiological solution with a mixture of 95% oxygen and 5% carbon dioxide, and its pH must be maintained at 7.4. In setting up the smooth muscle preparation, one must be aware of the orientation of the smooth muscle. Sometimes the smooth muscle cells lie in the longitudinal axis of the preparations, sometimes in the lateral axis. Thus sometimes it is appropriate to set-up a longitudinal preparation of a particular smooth muscle, and on other occasions a lateral or circular preparation. Some commonly used smooth muscle preparations are illustrated in Figure 2.

Quantification of Agonist Activity

The absolute potency of the drug is expressed in terms of the amount of drug required to produce a given effect. This is commonly the EC_{50} *i.e.* the concentration required to give a 50% maximum response. In order to determine

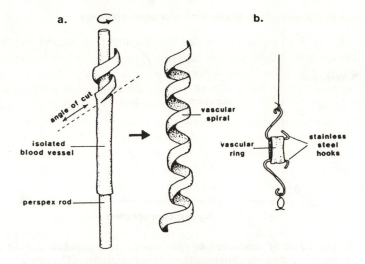

TRACHEAL RING PREPARATIONS

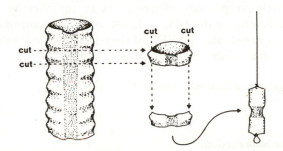

Figure 2: *Some commonly used smooth muscle preparations. Vascular smooth muscle cells are arranged in a circular fashion and thus isolated blood vessels may be prepared as spirals or rings. Spirals are mounted longitudinally by tying a thread to each end, one for fixing the preparation in the organ bath or other chamber and the other for attachment to a strain gauge. Tracheal smooth muscle serves to connect incomplete rings of cartilage and the smooth muscle cells are arranged in transverse fashion. Tracheas are therefore cut into rings consisting of one or more cartilaginous rings and the bulk of the cartilage cut away to leave the smooth muscle band with sufficient cartilage at each end to attach threads with which the preparation can be fixed and attached to a strain gauge*

the EC_{50}, it is necessary first to construct a concentration–effect curve, a plot of functional effect against concentration of agonist to produce that effect. From the concentration–effect curve, it is possible to determine the concentration which would produce the 50% maximum effect, *i.e.* the EC_{50} (Figure 3).

The problem with absolute potency is that it is influenced by tissue factors, and two different preparations containing the same type of receptor may show very different EC_{50}s for the same agonist depending on the efficiency of the coupling of the receptors to the second messenger system and/or the concentration or

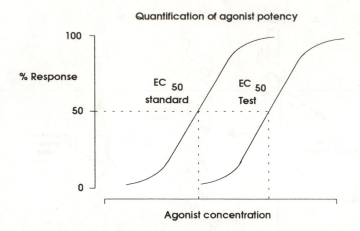

Figure 3: *A typical plot of concentration–effect curves to a standard agonist and a test agonist illustrating the determination of their respective EC$_{50}$ values*

density of the receptors available. Thus, a more useful means of quantifying agonist activity is relative potency, expressed as an equieffective concentration (EEC). In order to determine the EEC, it is necessary to incorporate a standard agonist in every experiment, and the EEC of the test agonist is a ratio of the EC$_{50}$ of the test agonist to that of the standard agonist.

$$Equieffective\ Concentration\ (EEC) = \frac{EC_{50}\ test\ compound}{EC_{50}\ standard}$$

Tissue Immersion or Superfusion?

The isolated smooth muscle can be mounted in an organ bath (immersion), or in a superfusion chamber (Figure. 4). Each of these two approaches has its own advantages and disadvantages. The main advantages with the immersion technique are the ease of setting up the preparation, and the ease of administering drug and maintaining a known concentration of drug in the bathing fluid. Disadvantages are removal of the drug from the bathing fluid, which involves emptying the bath and refilling it, a process which results in artefactual distortion of the record of tension changes of the tissue and a degree of stress to the tissues. Another disadvantage is the gradual build-up of toxic metabolites in the bathing fluid. The chief advantage of superfusion is that there is a constant removal of toxic metabolites from the tissue; thus the tissue remains healthier for longer. Also there is no necessity to wash the tissues, as they are being washed continuously. The chief disadvantage is in the difficulty of drug administration; they have to be added to the superfusion flow, and to maintain a particular drug concentration the drug must be infused for as long as administration is required, or added to the physiological fluid at source. The latter is clumsy, as modifications of drug concentrations in the fluid reservoir are complicated and slow.

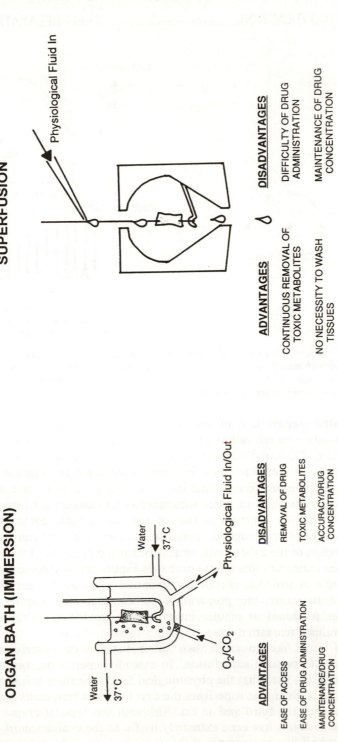

Figure 4: *Schematic illustration of an organ bath and a superfusion chamber, with an outline of the advantages and disadvantages of each technique*

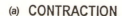

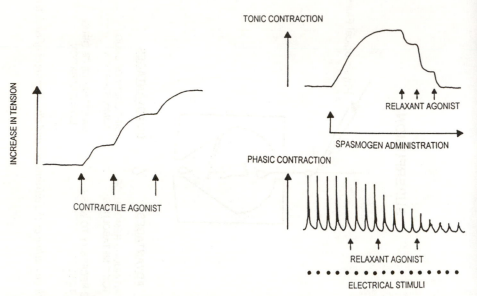

Figure 5: *Schematic illustration of contraction and relaxation of smooth muscle. As isolated smooth muscle is generally in a relaxed state, contraction is simple to achieve but to demonstrate a relaxation it is first necessary to precontract the preparation in either tonic or phasic fashion*

On isolated preparations of smooth muscle, measurements can be made of either contraction or relaxation. Of these two, contraction is usually the simpler, in the absence of external stimulation, as isolated smooth muscle is generally in a relaxed state, so it is easy to add a drug and measure a contraction as an increase in tension (see Figure 5a). Relaxation is less easy, as it is first necessary to contract the preparation in order subsequently to measure a relaxant response. Contraction may be achieved in one of two ways; tonic contraction, that is administration of a spasmogenic substance, *i.e.* one which will cause contraction, for the duration of the experiment, or at least for the duration of the construction of a relaxant concentration–effect curve (see Figure 5b), or **phasic** contraction, a good example of which is electrical stimulation to excite the nerves within the preparation to cause the preparation to contract (see Figure 5b). These contractions produced at regular intervals can provide a background against which to evaluate relaxant drugs.

I would now like to cover two distinct types of superfusion, cascade superfusion and parallel superfusion. In cascade superfusion, preparations are mounted in series, such that the physiological fluid superfuses this series from the top and that the fluid that superfuses the first tissues subsequently superfuses the second and then the third and so on. Although this type of preparation is not widely used today, it has been extremely useful in the evaluation of compounds with a short half-life; an example of this is thromboxane A_2, a prostanoid with a

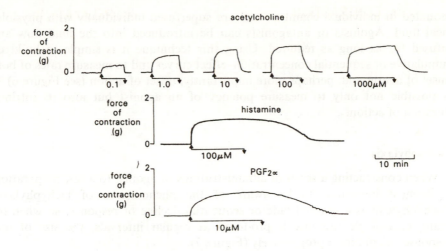

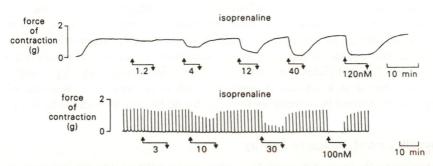

Figure 6: *Typical sequential concentration–effect curves to agonists on superfused preparations of guinea-pig trachea illustrating its use in determining not only potency, but also time course of both onset and offset of action. In descending order: a full contractile concentration–effect curve to acetylcholine (0.1–1000 μM) and single contractile responses to histamine and prostaglandin $F_{2}\alpha$ illustrating different time courses of contraction and relaxation: a full relaxant concentration–effect curve to isoprenaline on a tonically-contracted preparation: a full relaxant concentration–effect curve to isoprenaline on a phasically-contracted preparation*

half-life of 30 seconds. Such compounds can be generated enzymatically at the head of the cascade, and can be evaluated virtually simultaneously on a number of preparations. The cascade may consist of a range of different preparations, or of similar preparations in the presence of different concentrations of antagonists or other modifying drugs. The original application of this technique was to attempt to identify substances in tissue extracts; by including the appropriate preparations in the cascade, one can evaluate a whole range of biological activities simultaneously. However, as today there are far more efficient means of achieving such evaluation, the use of cascade superfusion has declined.

In contrast, the technique of parallel supervision which is more akin to the use of the organ bath is more widely used. In this technique, preparations are mounted in individual chambers and are superfused individually with physiological fluid. Agonists or antagonists can be introduced into the fluid flow and infused for as long as required. Using this technique it is simple to build up cumulative or sequential concentration–effect curves and to measure rates of both onset of action and, perhaps more importantly, offset of action (see Figure 6). It is possible not only to measure potency of an agonist but also its intrinsic duration of action.

Tachyphylaxis

When constructing a series of administrations of agonist to a test preparation, it is most important to be aware of the phenomenon of tachyphylaxis. Tachyphylaxis is a gradual fade or sequential decline of response, so when for example, a single response is produced at regular intervals, the size of that response will diminish progressively (Figure 7).

Similarly, if one repeats full agonist concentration–effect curves, these curves will progressively decline or be depressed. Steps must be taken to prevent this phenomenon of tachyphylaxis influencing the determination of potency of an agonist; this may necessitate increasing the interval between successive concentration–effect curves, or constructing only a single concentration–effect curve on each preparation, and comparing concentration–effect curves obtained on tissues in parallel. Tachyphylaxis is not a phenomenon which occurs on all preparations, but on some it is a particular problem, and only experience will tell which preparations should be avoided and which should be treated with particular care.

Quantification of Antagonist Activity

Antagonist activity is determined as a function of the ability of a compound to prevent the actions of an agonist. In order to determine this, the effect of the agonist has to be determined, first in the absence, and then in the presence of the

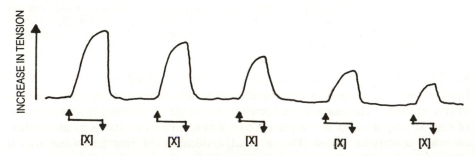

Figure 7: *The development of tachyphylaxis where the response to the repeated administration of a particular agonist declines progressively with successive administrations. Some preparations are particularly prone to tachyphylaxis while others appear resistant. There are a number of reasons for the development of tachyphylaxis including uncoupling of receptors from the intracellular second messenger and simple decline in receptor number*

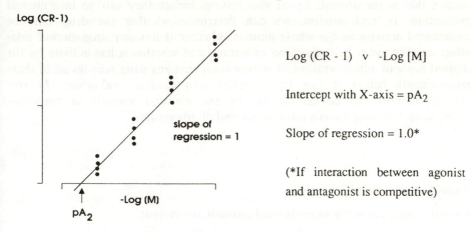

Schild Plot for pA$_2$

Log (CR-1)

slope of regression = 1

-Log (M)

pA$_2$

Log (CR - 1) v -Log [M]

Intercept with X-axis = pA$_2$

Slope of regression = 1.0*

(*If interaction between agonist and antagonist is competitive)

Figure 8: *The calculation of pA$_2$, a measure of the affinity of an antagonist for a particular receptor by the method of Arunlakshana and Schild (1959). Concentration-effect curves to an agonist are repeated first in the absence, then in the presence of increasing concentrations of antagonist and a plot of log (concentration-ratio – 1) against log [molar concentration of antagonist] constructed.*

antagonist. A commonly used measure of antagonist potency is the pA$_2$ which is a measurement of the compound's affinity for the receptor. The pA$_2$ is the log molar concentration of antagonist required to cause a two-fold rightward shift of an agonist concentration–effect curve. The pA$_2$ is normally derived from an Arunlakshana and Schild plot, that is a plot of log (concentration ratio − 1) against log (molar concentration of antagonist). If this plot has a slope of unity, it is evidence of a competitive interaction, and the point at which the plot crosses the concentration axis, the abscissa, determines the pA$_2$ (Figure 8).

Alternatively, if only a single antagonist concentration is used, antagonist potency (affinity) may be expressed as an apparent pK$_B$ (pK$_B$ app.) which is determined from the equation:

pK$_B$ app = log (concentration-ratio − 1) − log (molar concentration of antagonist)

The pA$_2$ and the pK$_B$ should have the same value, both being a measure of affinity of the antagonist for the receptor. However, in the above equation for pK$_B$ app., the assumption is made that the interaction between antagonist, agonist and receptor is competitive (*i.e.* the slope of the Schild plot is 1.0), an assumption not made in the determination of pA$_2$.

3 IN VIVO TESTING

Drugs are developed for use in animals and humans, and, while *in vitro* tests can provide an immense amount of information about their pharmacological profile, ultimately the compounds will have to be evaluated in the whole, integrated system that is the animal, *i.e. in vivo* testing, before they can go into clinical evaluation. In such studies, we can determine whether the drug has the anticipated activity in the whole animal, whether it has any unsuspected side-effect liability, what is its duration of action, and whether it has activity by the desired route of administration. It is important that any drug satisfies all of these requirements before it can be accepted into clinical evaluation. *In vivo* experimentation can be carried out in anaesthetised animals or conscious animals, each having its own advantages and disadvantages.

Anaesthetised Animals

The advantages of using anaesthetised animals are various:

1. The animal is easy to manipulate,
2. It is possible to measure a wide range of parameters,
3. There is ease of access to a variety of routes of drug administration, because one can cannulate any vessel which is appropriate.

The chief disadvantages relate to the fact that anaesthesia compromises the physiological relevance, many reflex processes are inhibited, and obviously one cannot measure any behavioural effects. Finally, in an anaesthetised animal, there will usually be a need to administer further anaesthetic to maintain a sufficient depth and duration of anaesthesia, and this administration can interfere with the progress of the experiments.

In experiments on anaesthetised animals, many of the principles outlined for *in vitro* experimentation can be employed. Thus, agonist dose–response curves can be constructed on a range of parameters simultaneously, these curves can be repeated until reproducible responses are obtained, and then a further curve to a test agonist may be constructed. From such an experiment, both the absolute and relative potencies of the agonists can be determined on a range of parameters. Alternatively, after completion of the curves to the standard agonist, antagonist may be administered by an appropriate route, and curves to the standard agonist repeated in its presence, thus enabling the determination of antagonist potency *in vivo*.

In essence, the use of an anaesthetised animal preparation may be regarded as a more complex version of an *in vitro* experiment. Thus responses can be measured directly from strain gauges or pressure transducers, and drugs may be administered either directly to a particular organ of interest, or systemically, that is into the whole system *via* the blood stream, such that the whole body receives the same dose of drug virtually simultaneously. Phenomena such as tachyphylaxis, which can complicate the interpretation of experiments *in vitro*, can also occur *in vivo*, and the experimenter must be aware of this and take the necessary steps in experimental design to eliminate or at least to minimise this complicating factor.

Conscious Animals

The testing of drugs in conscious animals is usually the last stage in drug evaluation prior to testing them in humans, whether healthy volunteers or sick patients. It is of crucial importance to ascertain that activities that are demonstrated in isolated tissues and/or anaesthetised animals are similarly expressed in a whole animal in as relevant a physiological state as possible to the patient who will be expected to receive the compound in the form of a new medicine.

In addition to the fact that conscious animal testing has the advantages that it is less invasive and more relevant to the clinical state, it also has other advantages: there is the possibility of almost unlimited duration (depending on the nature of the experiment, an experiment may last for just a few minutes or over the life span of the animal), and of course, if appropriate, one can study behaviour. The disadvantages are that only a limited number of parameters can be measured, and the difficulty of drug administration. Certain routes are relatively easy, for example, intramuscular, intradermal, subcutaneous, but routes such as intravenous and intra-arterial can prove substantially more difficult, particularly in animals that are by their nature uncooperative.

There are means by which drug administration and many physiological measurements can be made much more simple in a conscious animal, for example by implanting catheters into blood vessels, and mounting strain gauges on particular organs, and exteriorizing the appropriate connections at a point where the animal will not interfere with them, *e.g.* at the back of the neck. However, this is beyond the scope of the present chapter.

4 CONCLUSIONS

I have attempted to describe some of the approaches used by the pharmacologist to identify the biological activity of new compounds, including the use of a test strategy which will maximise the chances of identifying important activities and minimise the time wasted taking forward compounds with inadequate or inappropriate profiles of action. I have also described, largely using smooth muscle as an example, how the pharmacologist uses the tools available to him to make measurements and thus judgements on the compounds that he has to work with. It is of crucial importance to realise, however, that success results from teamwork, and that the pharmacologist cannot work alone. Thus any research programme will only succeed if the pharmacologist makes the most of the drugs that he is provided with, from whatever original source, and the medicinal chemist works with him to optimise desirable activities and if possible to eliminate the undesirable ones. I hope therefore that this chapter will give the medicinal chemist a little insight into the way in which the pharmacologist works and some of the problems that he will encounter, as it is only with understanding that such an important relationship can prosper.

5 BIBLIOGRAPHY

1. O. Arunlakshana and H.O. Schild, *Br. J. Pharmacol.*, 1959, **14**, 48.
2. W.C. Bowman and M.J. Rand, 'Textbook of Pharmacology', Blackwell, Oxford, 1980, Ch. 39.
3. R.A. Coleman in 'Prostaglandins and related substances – A Practical Approach', ed. C. Benedetto, R.G. McDonald-Gibson, S. Nigam, and T.F. Slater, IRL Press, Oxford. 1987, pp. 267–303.
4. E.E. Daniel and D.M. Paton, 'Methods in Pharmacology, Vol. 3. Smooth Muscle', Plenum Press, London, 1975.
5. R.F. Furchgott, *Adv. Drug Res.*, 1966, **3**, 21.
6. E.C. Hulme and N.J.M. Birdsall, in 'Receptor–Ligand Interactions – A Practical Approach', ed. D. Rickwood and B.D. Hanes, IRL Press, Oxford. 1992, pp. 63–176.
7. H.P. Rang and M.M. Dale, 'Pharmacology', Churchill Livingstone, Edinburgh, 1991, Ch. 1.
8. C.M. Smith and A.M. Reynard, 'Textbook of Pharmacology', Saunders, Philadelphia, 1991, Pt. 1.

CHAPTER 5

Pharmacokinetics

ROBERT M.J. INGS

1 INTRODUCTION

Definitions

Many definitions have been proposed for 'pharmacokinetics' but the simplest is probably the best:

Pharmacokinetics – the study of the movement of drugs within the body and encompassing absorption, distribution, and elimination, *i.e.* WHAT THE BODY DOES WITH THE DRUG.

Another closely allied subject is pharmacodynamics.

Pharmacodynamics - the study of the pharmacological response to a drug, *i.e.* WHAT A DRUG DOES WITH THE BODY.

Pharmacokinetics is of most value when it is used predictively and in order to perform this effectively, pharmacokinetics and pharmacodynamics should be used together. Normally, pharmacokinetics is only meaningful if one chemical species is being examined so that our analytical methods must be SPECIFIC. Unfortunately, total radioactivity measurements are invariably non-specific and are **NOT** normally suitable for pharmacokinetic analysis.

ALL THE FOLLOWING ASSUME SPECIFIC ANALYSES UNLESS OTHERWISE STATED:

Absorption   the process by which a drug moves into the body from its site of administration to its site of measurement.

Distribution   the reversible transfer of a drug from the site of measurement (usually blood or plasma).

Elimination   the irreversible transfer of a drug from the site of measurement, including:
      metabolism
      renal excretion
      biliary excretion
      lungs
      sweat
      milk, *etc.*

The Pharmacokineticist in Industry

How can pharmacokinetics help us in drug development? Its objectives can be summarised as follows:

1. To provide *in vivo* evidence for the optimisation of dosage form, *i.e.* bioavailability.
2. To design rational dosage regimens which maximise efficacy and minimise side-effects.
3. To recommend adjustment of dosage regimen in disease states and with age.
4. To make recommendations to minimise possible effects of drug–drug interactions.
5. To assist in the design of new drugs by optimising their pharmacokinetics, *e.g.* avoiding compounds with large first pass effects.

Physical Chemical Properties of Drugs and Their Pharmacokinetics

All drugs have to cross cell membranes to be absorbed, distributed or eliminated. There are three main mechanisms by which a drug can cross a cell membrane:

1. Passive diffusion
2. Facilitated diffusion (carrier mediated)
3. Active transport (carrier mediated)

The carrier mediated transport mechanisms tend to be for those compounds which closely resemble natural substances. The most general method for the transport of drugs is, therefore, passive diffusion. The cell membrane is a bimolecular lipid layer associated with protein (Figure 1) with the hydrophobic ends of the lipid pointing inwards. Thus, any substance wanting to cross the membrane must first dissolve in the lipid layer, *i.e.* it must show lipid solubility. There are also small pores within the membrane (aqueous pores) through which some low molecular weight water-soluble compounds can diffuse. The number of these pores will depend on the type of tissue.

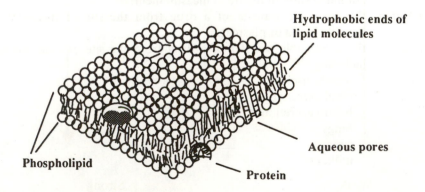

Hydrophobic ends of lipid molecules

Aqueous pores

Phospholipid

Protein

Figure 1:   *A diagram of a cell membrane*

A good indicator of how a drug will transport *in vivo* is to look at its partition between an organic solvent (*e.g.* octanol) and an aqueous medium (usually buffer at a physiological pH). Most drugs are organic molecules with one or more substituents which confer on them acid, basic or amphoteric properties. Drugs with acidic or basic properties can exist in ionised or un-ionised forms:

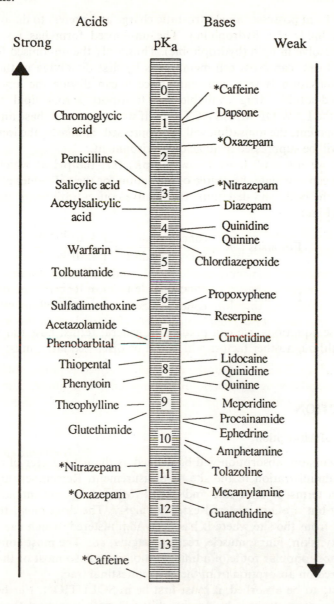

Figure 2: *pKa of different drugs*

Acidic drugs :
$$[HA + H_2O] \quad \rightleftharpoons \quad [H_3O^+] + [A^-]$$
un-ionised   ionised

Basic drugs :
$$[B + H_2O] \quad \rightleftharpoons \quad [BH^+] + [OH^-]$$
un-ionised   ionised

The ionised form possesses an electrostatic charge and prefers to dissolve in water rather than lipids (*i.e.* hydrophilic). The un-ionised form has no charge and prefers to dissolve in lipid (hydrophobic). Thus, only the un-ionised form, unlike the ionised form, can cross cell membranes by first dissolving in the lipid. The degree of ionisation is very important since it can dictate the amount of un-ionised, lipid-soluble drug available for transport across lipid membranes. Remember the LAW OF MASS ACTION. If we have a weak base and put it in a basic environment, the ionisation will be suppressed. Similarly, the ionisation of a weak acid will be suppressed in an acidic environment.

How can we use this? If we know the pK_a (*i.e.* the pH at which it is 50% ionised), we can calculate the degree of ionisation for the pH values at the various sites within the body and determine the relative concentrations on each side of a membrane (Figure 2).

$$\text{For acids : } R = \frac{\text{conc. on side 1}}{\text{conc. on side 2}} = \frac{1 + 10^{pH_1 - pK_a}}{1 + 10^{pH_2 - pK_a}}$$

$$\text{For bases : } R = \frac{\text{conc. on side 1}}{\text{conc. on side 2}} = \frac{1 + 10^{pK_a - pH_1}}{1 + 10^{pK_a - pH_2}}$$

With these equations, we can predict, in general terms, how our drug might transport, although other factors which will be discussed later, must be borne in mind.

2 ABSORPTION

Mechanism of Absorption

For this discussion, absorption will be defined as the net transfer of a drug from its site of administration to the site of measurement. Remember, absorption is measured in terms of both rate and extent. Most drugs are intended to work systemically but are administered extravascularly. The drug must, therefore, be transported from the site where it has been administered, which can include the buccal cavity, skin, lungs, muscle, rectum, vagina, *etc.* The most convenient and hence the most popular route of administration is oral, so most of the discussion will be centred on absorption from the gastrointestinal tract.

For a drug to be absorbed, it must first be in SOLUTION. Furthermore, the absorption of most drugs is by passive diffusion with transport through a lipid cell membrane from an area of high concentration to an area of low concentration. This requires no energy and shows no saturation, no competition

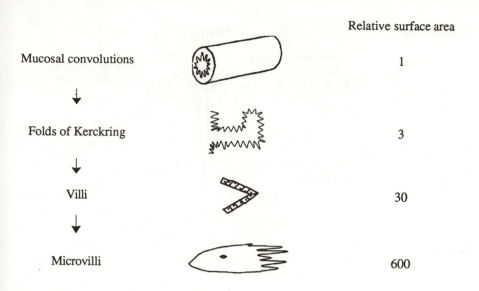

	Relative surface area
Mucosal convolutions	1
Folds of Kerckring	3
Villi	30
Microvilli	600

Figure 3: *The influence of villi on the area of the absorptive surface*

or specificity. The drug must dissolve in the lipid membrane first, which usually means it has to be in its un-ionised lipid soluble form. The pH of the different regions of the gastrointestinal tract is, therefore, an important determinant in the absorption of the drugs. For instance, it would be expected that acidic drugs would be better absorbed from an acidic environment. This is known as the pH-PARTITION HYPOTHESIS.

Does this mean that acidic compounds, such as aspirin, are best absorbed from the stomach where the pH is 1? In theory yes, since the acidic conditions of the stomach should suppress any ionisation. In practice, no, since the area of the absorptive surface is of far more importance. Although the stomach has folds within it, there are not the folds of Kerckring, the villi, and the microvilli found in the intestine which increase the relative surface area up to 600 times (Figure 3).

Absorption of acidic compounds, such as aspirin, tends to be relatively low from the stomach with the majority from the duodenum where the pH is still low enough. THE pH-PARTITION HYPOTHESIS IS THEREFORE ONLY A 'RULE OF THUMB'.

Since absorption from the stomach tends to be low, the rate of gastric emptying can have a profound effect on the absorption process. It would be expected that drugs which delay gastric emptying (propantheline) would slow absorption whilst those which promote gastric emptying (metoclopramide) would increase absorption (Figure 4).

Food, also, can delay gastric emptying and so might slow absorption of some drugs, although if dissolution is rate-limiting the opposite may be true. Blood flow and factors which influence blood flow also affect the absorption of some drugs (perfusion rate-limited). For those drugs which are diffusion rate-limited (*i.e.* diffusion across the membrane in the slowest step), blood flow has little effect.

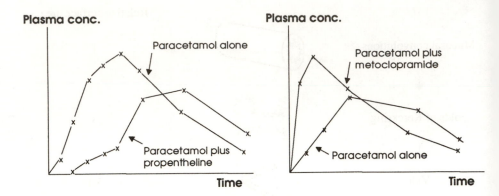

Figure 4

Incomplete Absorption

The discussion so far has been limited to the absorption of compounds which are already in solution. Most drugs, however, are given in a solid dosage form (a tablet or capsule) and can be subject to even more limiting factors. Investigations into the efficiency of absorption from various dosage forms are generally classed as BIOAVAILABILITY STUDIES.

Bioavailability. The rate and extent to which the intact drug or the active constituent reaches the systemic circulation.

Absolute Bioavailability. This is when the total quantity of drug reaching the systemic circulation is measured and is usually performed by comparing the bioavailability of the test formulation with that of an intravenous dose where complete bioavailability can be assumed. This is because all the dose is administered into the systemic circulation. COMPLETE BIOAVAILABILITY CAN NOT BE ASSUMED FROM ORAL SOLUTIONS.

Relative Bioavailability. This is when the total quantity of drug reaching systemic circulation is not measured but the bioavailability of test formulation is compared with that of another formulation which is NOT administered directly into the systemic circulation and where complete bioavailability cannot be assumed (*e.g.* a comparison of two oral formulations).

The measure of availability must reflect both the rate and extent to which the drug appears in the systemic circulation. Normally this includes maximum plasma/blood levels, time to maximum and area under the curve (AUC) to INFINITE TIME if a single dose. If sufficient of the drug is excreted unchanged in urine, this can be used as a measure of extent of bioavailability. For blood/plasma levels, however, the following equations are used:

$$\text{Absolute bioavailability (F)} = \frac{\text{AUC}_{po}}{\text{AUC}_{iv}} \times \frac{\text{Dose}_{iv}}{\text{Dose}_{po}} \times 100\%$$

$$\text{Relative bioavailability} = \frac{\text{AUC}_{po}\text{ (test)}}{\text{AUC}_{po}\text{ (standard)}} \times \frac{\text{Dose}_{po}\text{ (standard)}}{\text{Dose}_{po}\text{ (test)}} \times 100\%$$

The pharmacokinetics of one drug must be linear for this relationship to hold (see later). Several mathematical methods are available to calculate AUC but the most commonly used are direct integration and the trapezoidal rule.

Why should there be incomplete bioavailability?

instability	} *e.g.* benzylpenicillin in the acid conditions of the stomach
gastrointestinal transit time	} insufficient time at the absorptive surface
microfloral metabolism gut wall metabolism first pass hepatic metabolism	} presystemic metabolism
biopharmaceutical factors	

The fraction of the dose finally escaping metabolism (*F*) and which appears in systemic plasma (Figure 5) is:

$$F = F_{\text{Intestine}} \times F_{\text{Gut}} \times F_{\text{Liver}}$$

Hepatic first pass metabolism is perhaps the best known and will be discussed later. Because of this BEWARE: DON'T USE TOTAL RADIOACTIVITY TO DETERMINE BIOAVAILABILITY – USE SPECIFIC ASSAYS. Remember, a drug can be 100% absorbed but show 0% bioavailability.

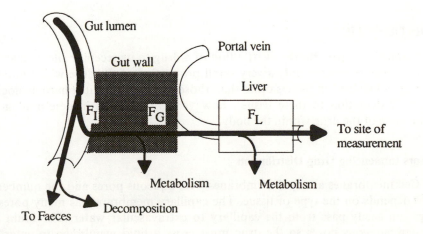

Figure 5: *Presystemic metabolism*

Biopharmaceutical Factors

Solid formulations can be modified by various excipients to either speed up or slow down dissolution. However, as a drug has to be in solution before it can be absorbed, it is often assumed that a solution of the drug is the most bioavailable form. Usually this is true, but if a compound is highly insoluble in the acid conditions of the stomach it may precipitate, giving a suspension of variable particle size with poor dissolution. In such a case a well defined micronised solid formulation may well show a better dissolution.

Animal Models to Determine Absorption

There are a variety of *in vitro/in situ* animal models for following the absorption of drugs from the gastrointestinal tract. However, these should not be confused with bioavailability methods which specifically measure intact drug in the intact animal. Animal models can, however, be useful early in a drug discovery/ development programme for selecting the best from a series of candidate drugs. In summary, these include:

Type	Method	
In vitro	Everted gut sac	
In situ	Closed loop, *e.g.* Doluisio technique	
In situ	Perfused loop	increasing
In situ	Isolated intestinal loop with complete mesenteric blood collection	complexity
In situ/In vivo	Thiry–Vella loop (dog)	

For routine work it is best to start with the simplest (*e.g.* everted gut sac or closed loop) and move to a more complicated technique if the simple ones fail.

3 DISTRIBUTION

Most concern is spent on the distribution of a drug to its receptor site. Generally, however, this represents only a very small proportion of the dose whilst more of the drug is localised in tissues other than those involved with its pharmacological action. Distribution to these tissues, however, is important in determining the time-course of the drug within the body.

Factors Influencing Drug Distribution

pH. Cell membranes are lipid membranes with aqueous pores and the number of pores depends on the type of tissue. The capillary membrane has many pores so drugs can easily pass from the capillary to extravascular water. The brain has very few aqueous pores so the drug must cross a lipid membrane to enter the brain and to do so must first dissolve in the lipid. Moreover, since drugs tend to be acids or bases which can exist in ionised or un-ionised forms, the extent of ionisation and the proportion of the un-ionised, lipid soluble form will dictate how the drug will distribute.

Does the pH in the body vary enough at different sites to influence distribution? YES – plasma is slightly more basic than tissues so that for basic drugs ionisation is suppressed more. Thus, more un-ionised drug is available to move from plasma to tissues where it then becomes ionised and can't get back. The opposite is true for acids – 'RULE OF THUMB' – basic compounds tend to distribute out of plasma into tissue more than acidic drugs.

Binding to Macromolecules. Most emphasis is put on plasma protein binding because it is easy to measure, but tissue binding is just as important. A major factor in drug distribution is the ratio of plasma to tissue binding. Acidic drugs bind to albumin which is found both in plasma and tissues. Basic drugs bind to α_1-acid glycoprotein (a stress protein) and lipoprotein. Some endogenous compounds also bind mainly to globulins. The rates of association and disassociation for reversible protein binding are very rapid so that the bound and unbound form of the drug can be considered to be in equilibrium at all times. Only unbound drug diffuses into and out of tissues; hence the importance of the ratio of tissue to plasma binding.

Volume of Distribution. Measurements must be SPECIFIC for the drug when considering this term. The volume of distribution is simply a term that relates the amount of drug within the body at any one time to its concentration. Often we wish to relate the concentration of a drug in the plasma, which is usually measured, to the total amount in the body. Normally, intravenous data have to be used for the calculations.

As an example, consider a drug which has been administered intravenously as a bolus. The amount in the body at zero time must be the amount dosed, since none of the drug will have been eliminated. If the concentration of drug is estimated at zero time (C_{po}) by extrapolating the plasma level curve back, the volume can be easily calculated by:

$$V_i \text{ (litre)} = \frac{\text{Dose} \quad (\text{mg})}{C_{po} \ (\text{mg/litre})} \qquad \text{Note how units are derived, } i.e. \text{ litre}$$

initial distribution volume

There are other volumes of distribution terms ($V_{(area)}$ and V_{SS}) which are perhaps more useful:

$$V_{(area)} = \frac{\text{Dose}}{\text{AUC} \times \lambda_z}$$

where λ_z is the slope (exponential constant) of the terminal phase.

This volume term is calculated once distribution is complete and approximates to V_{SS}. However, it is also dependent on the elimination kinetics.

$$\text{For a bolus injection } V = \text{Dose} \ \frac{\sum\limits_{i=1}^{n} C_i / \lambda^2_i}{\text{AUC}^2}$$

where C_i is the exponential coefficient and λ_i is the exponential constant. As the name suggests, it is the volume of distribution at steady-state and, ideally, is the parameter which should be measured since it is independent of elimination kinetics.

It is often asked 'Does the volume of distribution relate to physiological volumes?' Usually NO – it is a mathematical balancing term which sometimes might approximate to plasma volume (3 litres for man). This low value would tell you that the drug does not distribute very well. For other drugs it might approach the volume of extracellular water (18–22% of body weight) or total body water (60% of body weight). However, beware of concluding too much on how the drug distributes if it happens to approach these values, especially without considering plasma protein binding, since it is only the unbound drug which distributes. Often for basic drugs the volume of distribution exceeds body weight because of avid uptake by the tissues. Examples of volumes of distribution for different drugs are given in Figure 6.

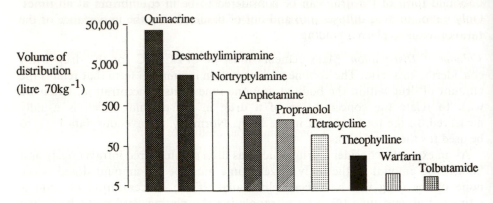

Figure 6:   *The variation of volume of distribution, plotted on a logarithmic scale, between different drugs in man*

4 ELIMINATION

Route of Elimination

Elimination is defined as the irreversible transfer of a drug from the site of measurement and includes:

    metabolism
    renal excretion
    biliary excretion
    lungs
    sweat, milk, *etc.*

Thus if elimination includes metabolism, what happens when we administer radioactive drug?

When a drug is changed chemically by metabolism, the original drug substance is no longer present and has, therefore, been eliminated. If we want to examine the pharmacokinetics of the metabolite, we have to look at it separately, *i.e.* specific measurements.

Renal Excretion. All low molecular weights compounds WHICH ARE NOT BOUND TO HIGH MOLECULAR WEIGHT PROTEINS are glomerular filtrated. The rate at which this occurs in man is approximately 125 ml min^{-1} and is termed the glomerular filtration rate (GFR), often measured by creatinine or inulin clearance. Glomerular filtration always occurs in the healthy kidney but some compounds are also actively secreted from plasma into the tubular lumen, mainly along the proximal tubule.

Tubular secretion is an active process with a separate mechanism for acids and bases. However, within each group it is relatively non-specific with competition between compounds. The most common example is the competition between the tubular secretion of β-lactam antibiotics (*e.g.* cephalosporins) and probenecid. In fact, probenecid, as well as being used experimentally to demonstrate renal tubular secretion of drugs (Figure 7), is used to inhibit the tubular secretion of some antibiotics in order to reduce their elimination and to increase their duration of action.

Active tubular secretion, unlike glomerular filtration, is not dependent on plasma protein binding since the drug tends to be stripped from the protein molecule with the former process.

A final but very important factor when considering overall renal excretion is reabsorption, which takes place for most drugs by passive diffusion throughout the length of the nephron of the kidney. The ability for a drug to be reabsorbed will depend on its ability to cross lipid membranes and hence its polarity and degree of ionisation at the pH of tubular contents. Polar compounds, such as the

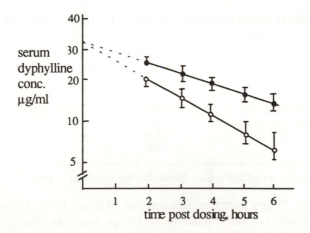

Figure 7: *Kinetic consequences of concomitant dyphylline-probenecid use. Semilog plot of serum dyphylline concentration/time relationship. Closed circles represent dyphylline elimination in the presence of probenecid. Bars represent ± SD*

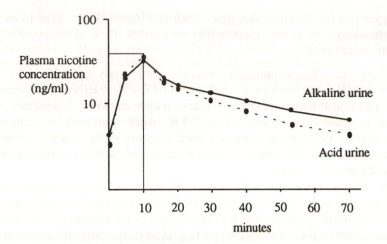

Figure 8: *Mean plasma nicotine concentrations with alkaline and acid urine*

β-lactams, have difficulty in crossing back and therefore tend to be extensively renally excreted. If the 'urine' is acid, basic compounds become ionised and can't cross back so their net renal excretion increases. Conversely, more reabsorption occurs with bases when the urine is made basic, resulting in decreased renal excretion such as with nicotine (Figure 8). Urinary pH is therefore very important.

In summary:

net rate of renal excretion = rate of filtration + rate of secretion − rate of reabsorption

Think of each process in relation to the drug.

Table 1: *Molecular weight threshold for biliary excretion*

Species	Molecular weight
Rat	325
Dog	325
Guinea Pig	400
Rabbit	475
Monkey	500
Man	500

Note that for rat and dog the threshold is low compared to man.

Biliary Excretion. Biliary excretion (elimination of drugs in the bile) is a complex process which is still not fully understood. Drugs which are biliary excreted are secreted into bile against a concentration gradient requiring an active process for which there is competition.

Factors affecting the degree of biliary excretion include polarity (a strongly polar group aids biliary excretion) and structural considerations. One of the most important factors, however, is molecular size, since for all compounds with a molecular weight <300 or with very high molecular weights (proteins) there is little biliary excretion. Between a molecular weight of 300 and 500 there appears to be a species difference (Table 1).

Other Routes These are usually of minor importance and include sweat, mammary secretions, and expired air. Mammary secretions are important because, even if the total amount involved is small, there is the possibility of ingestion by the neonate. Therefore, its determination forms an integral part of drug development.

Clearance

Clearance (*Cl*) is one of the most important and useful parameters in pharmacokinetics and can only be calculated when SPECIFIC measurements have been made. It is defined as the volume of blood/plasma/serum completely cleared of total drug/unbound drug per unit time (*e.g.* ml min^{-1}) and relates the rate of elimination to the concentration of total drug/unbound drug in blood/plasma/serum. It is calculated by:

$$Cl = \frac{F.\text{Dose}}{AUC_\infty}$$

F = Fraction of dose absorbed
AUC_∞ = area under blood/plasma/serum curve to infinite time for total drug or free drug

ALWAYS SPECIFY WHICH CLEARANCE IS BEING MEASURED AND CORRECT IF MOVING FROM ONE TO ANOTHER, *E.G.* FOR PLASMA TO BLOOD CORRECT WITH BLOOD TO PLASMA RATIO.

Normally clearance is calculated from intravenous data when $F = 1$, since with oral data, F is not often known.

Clearance is additive, *i.e:*

$$Cl = Cl_R + Cl_{Bil} + Cl_M$$

Cl_R = renal clearance; Cl_{Bil} = biliary clearance; Cl_M = metabolic clearance

Renal clearance is calculated by:

$$Cl_R = \frac{U_t}{\text{AUC}_t}$$

U_t = amount of drug excreted unchanged in urine in time t, and AUC_t = area under the blood/plasma/serum curve for the same time.

Using renal and total clearance the total amount of drug to be excreted in urine unchanged (f_e) can be calculated:

$$f_e(\%) = \frac{Cl_R}{Cl} \times 100$$

Clearance is also related to the blood flow of the eliminating organ (Q) and the extraction ratio for the drug (ER).

$$Cl = Q.ER$$

Extraction ratio is a measure of how efficient an organ is at eliminating the drug (Figure 9).

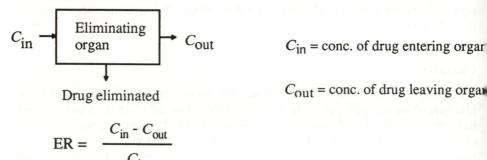

$$ER = \frac{C_{in} - C_{out}}{C_{in}}$$

Figure 9

If the organ is not very efficient $C_{out} \approx C_{in}$. Therefore:

$$ER = \frac{C_{in} - (\sim C_{in})}{C_{in}} = \frac{0}{C_{in}} = 0$$

If the organ is very efficient $C_{out} = 0$. Therefore:

$$ER = \frac{C_{in} - 0}{C_{in}} = \frac{C_{in}}{C_{in}} = 1$$

The extraction ratio may, therefore, range between 0 (no elimination) and 1 (total elimination). Let us consider the situation of the eliminating organ being the liver, which is extremely efficient at removing a drug. Thus when administered orally, very little drug will escape the liver since all of it must go through the liver *via* the portal blood system on its first pass, *i.e.* first-pass metabolism. Thus for drugs that undergo high hepatic first-pass metabolism the ER of the liver approaches 1 so the blood clearance (measured from i.v. data) must approach hepatic blood flow:

$$Cl = Q.ER$$
when $ER \rightarrow 1$ and $Cl \approx Q$

To determine whether a drug will be subject to high first pass metabolism, administer it intravenously and determine if blood clearance approaches hepatic blood flow, assuming all elimination is hepatic.

Let us now consider a drug in routine clinical use where it is normally administered repetitively. Generally, in pharmacokinetics it is believed that the

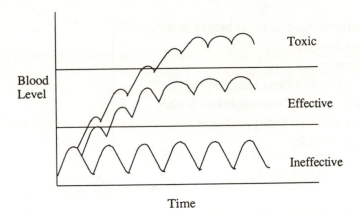

Figure 10: *Relationship between plasma level and effect with repeated dosing*

pharmacological response, either desired (therapeutic) or undesired (toxic) is related to plasma levels (Figure 10).

At steady-state on repeated dosing

$$\text{rate in} = \text{rate out}$$
$$= Cl \times C_{\text{pss}}$$

If you know clearance from intravenous studies and you know the steady-state plasma level you require (*i.e.* within the effective therapeutic window), you can very simply calculate the rate to be administered (mg day^{-1} *etc*). A similar procedure can be used for constant rate infusions. Note that only clearance is used for this, NOT volume of distribution.

If clearance, volume of distribution, or absorption changes, the kinetics are termed as non-linear. Obviously, if clearance is being used to calculate dosage regimen, studies must be performed to ensure that it does not change with dose (dose-dependent kinetics) or time (time-dependent kinetics). Checks for dose-dependent kinetics are usually performed by increasing the dose and determining whether the AUC increases in direct proportion (Figure 11).

Alternatively, each plasma level can be normalised to one dose to see whether they become superimposable. Time-dependent kinetics are determined by monitoring for steady-state plasma levels and checking whether they increase (inhibition) or decrease (induction) with time. Diurnal variations can also occur within a 24 hour period (*e.g.* diazepam and clobazam).

Half-life is defined as the time taken for the concentration of a drug to decrease by one half, and if the process is a single exponential, it is constant at any concentration (Figure 12). To calculate it, plot the data on semi-logarithmic paper (plasma level on the log *y* axis and time on the linear *x* axis) and measure

A.   an elimination process has become saturated
      (eg. phenytoin)
B.   linear kinetics
C.   if orally administered, absorption may be
      saturated, but if administered intravenously,
      plasma protein binding is saturated
      (eg. naproxan)

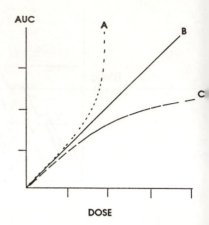

Figure 11

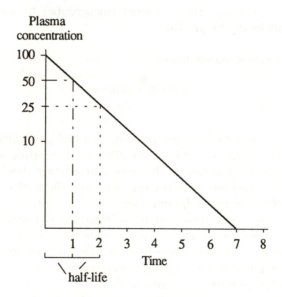

Figure 12: *A semilogarithmic plot of plasma levels of drug versus time showing determination of half-life*

the time that the concentration takes to decrease by half (*e.g.* between 90 and 45, 50 and 25, 20 and 10, 5 and 2.5, *etc*).

More often than not, however, when data are plotted on semi-logarithmic paper, the plot is still curved. This is because the decline of the drug is composed of several exponential processes, each with its own straight line but which, when added together, form a curve. You can separate out each line by 'feathering' or 'peeling', more formally called the method of residuals. To attempt this, it must

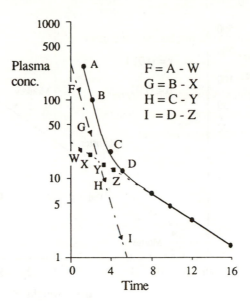

Figure 13: *Calculations for the method of residuals*

be established that the terminal portion is really log-linear as it is assumed that this is the true slope of the terminal exponential phase (Figure 13). Sampling should continue for at least 3 half-lives for the assumption to be valid.

Extrapolate the log-linear portion back to zero time and measure the extrapolated concentration (W to Z) at the same times as the respective observed values A to D. To remove the influence of the terminal exponential from the first exponential, simply subtract the value from the extrapolated line from the observed value. Plot values F to I and this will give you another line which, if straight, is the second exponential line. If it is still curved you continue the process. The slope of the lines gives you the half-life of each phase.

It is often asked 'Is half-life the most important measure of elimination or clearance?' Half-life is probably the most well known pharmacokinetic parameter but is not necessarily the best measure of elimination. Half-life is not a primary pharmacokinetic parameter but is a hybrid parameter and a function of volume of distribution and clearance.

$$t = \frac{0.693 \times V_D}{Cl}$$

If half-life changes it could be a change in volume of distribution, clearance or is it both? You can't tell from half-life alone and you must dose the drug intravenously to determine which of the parameters is changing (*e.g.* diazepam in the elderly). If clearance changes, steady-state plasma levels on repetitive dosing also change, but if volume of distribution changes, they don't. Adjustment would be needed for the former but not the latter. Half-life does, however, determine the time to reach steady-state (approximately 4 to 5 half-lives).

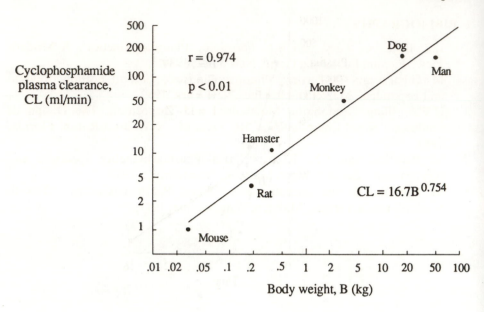

Figure 14: *Allomeric relationship between cyclophosphamide plasma clearance and body weight*

5 CONCLUSIONS

Now we have most of the basic pharmacokinetic parameters, is there any way we can use them predictively, especially for drug design? More and more it is becoming necessary to select out not only those compounds with undesirable toxicological or pharmacological profiles but also those with poor pharmacokinetic profiles, *e.g.* low absorption, high first-pass metabolism, or wrong half-life (too long or too short). To undertake this, a method is needed to extrapolate pharmacokinetic parameters from animal experiments to those for man. This can be done by scaling since the pharmacokinetics of a drug (*e.g.* Cl, V_D or $t_{1/2}$) can be related by a power function to the body weight.

$$\text{Pharmacokinetic parameter} = \text{coefficient} \times \text{body weight}^{\text{power}}$$

The power function and coefficient are specific for each pharmacokinetic parameter and each compound. In practice, simply plot the log of the pharmacokinetic parameter against the log of the body weight. The value of the parameter for man can then be extrapolated (Figure 14). The power function for volume of distribution tends to 1, that for clearance to 0.75 and that for half-life to 0.25.

6 BIBLIOGRAPHY

1. L.Z. Benet, G. Levy, and B.L. Ferraiolo, 'Pharmacokinetics - A Modern View', Plenum Publishing Corp., New York, 1984.
2. M. Gibaldi and D. Perrier, 'Pharmacokinetics – Second Edition, Revised and Expanded', Marcel Dekker Inc., New York, 1982.
3. H.P.A. Illing, 'Xenobiotic Metabolism and Disposition, The Design of Studies on Novel Compounds', CRC Press Inc., NW Boca Raton, Florida, 1989.
4. M. Rowland and T.N. Tozer, 'Clinical Pharmacokinetics. Concepts and Applications', Lea & Febiger, Malvern, Pennsylvania, 1989.
5. M. Gibaldi, 'Biopharmaceutics and Clinical Pharmacokinetics – Fourth Edition', Lea & Febiger, Malvern, Pennsylvania, 1991.

CHAPTER 6

Drug Metabolism

COLIN VOSE

1 INTRODUCTION

This chapter is intended as a general overview of drug metabolism for the medicinal chemist. References and bibliography have been included at the end to provide sources of further more detailed information.

Drug metabolism is an important elimination pathway. It may be defined as 'The chemical alteration of a drug by a biological system with the principal purpose of eliminating it from the system'. Mammals use exogenous compounds for the synthesis of their essential components and the maintenance of life. When a foreign compound cannot be assimilated into these pathways it will be eliminated. Drug elimination may occur directly by excretion in urine or bile for intrinsically water soluble drugs, indirectly by metabolism followed by the excretion of the metabolites in urine and bile or by a combination of these processes. Metabolism generally produces products which are more water soluble and more easily excreted. The metabolic fate of a drug can influence its pharmacodynamics and toxicology.

2 DRUG METABOLISM PATHWAYS

The metabolism of drugs may be classified into two types: Phase I and Phase II reactions.

Phase I reactions are those which produce or introduce a new chemical group on a molecule (Table 1). There is a wide range of Phase I reactions which generally yield a product (metabolite) more water soluble and thus more easily excreted than the drug and may also produce metabolites which are substrates for the

Table 1: *Phase I metabolic pathways*

Reaction type	Pathway
Oxidation	Aliphatic or aromatic hydroxylation
	N- or S-oxidation
	N-, O-, or S-dealkylation
Reduction	Nitro reduction to hydroxylamine, amine
	Carbonyl reduction to alcohol
Hydrolysis	Ester to acid and alcohol
	Amide to acid and amine
	Hydrazides to acid and substituted hydrazine

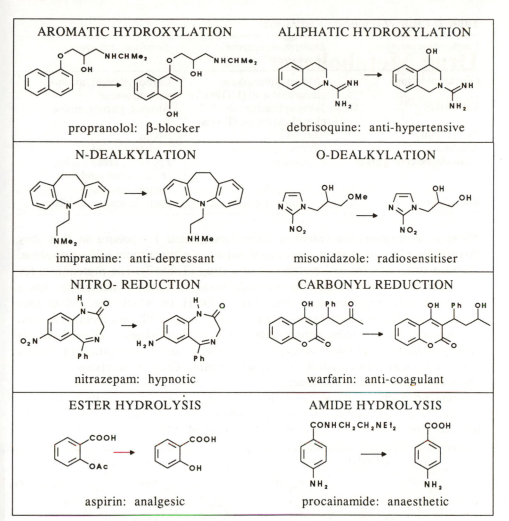

Figure 1: *Examples of Phase 1 metabolism*

Phase II reactions. However, with some drugs these pathways may also produce reactive, potentially toxic metabolites.

Oxidations, which are the commonest Phase I reactions, include hydroxylation, *e.g.* propranolol, debrisoquine, oxidation at nitrogen or sulphur atoms, *e.g.* nicotine, sulindac, and *N*- or *O*-dealkylation, *e.g.* imipramine, misonidazole (Figure 1). The dealkylation pathway is oxidative, as the initial step is hydroxylation in the alkyl group adjacent to the heteroatom with subsequent cleavage of the C–heteroatom bond.

Reduction of nitro or carbonyl groups leads to amines and alcohols respectively (Figure 1) with a consequent increase in water solubility. Similarly hydrolysis of esters or amides yields the more water soluble acids, alcohols and amines.

Table 2: *Phase II conjugation pathways*

Conjugation reaction	Endogenous reagent or substrate	Xenobiotic substrate
Glucuronidation	Uridine diphosphate glucuronic acid (UDPGA)	Carboxylic acid, alcohol, phenol, amine
Sulphation	3'-Phosphoadenosine5'-phosphosulphate (PAPS)	Alcohol, phenol, amine
Acetylation	Acetyl-CoA	Amine
Amino acid	Glycine, glutamine	Carboxylic acid
Glutathione conjugation	Glutathione	Epoxides, arene oxides, chloro compounds, quinone-imines
Methylation	S-adenosyl methionine	Phenols, amines, thiols

Phase II or conjugation reactions differ from Phase I reactions in that they involve the addition of an endogenous molecule, *e.g.* glucuronic acid or sulphate, onto the drug or a Phase I metabolite of a drug (Table 2). The prerequisite for conjugation reactions is that the molecule (drug or Phase I metabolite) has a suitable chemical group, *e.g.* OH, NH_2, COOH to which the endogenous substrate can be attached. The conjugation of a drug or Phase I metabolite with glucuronic acid, sulphate, amino-acids or glutathione (Figure 2) increases its water solubility. Additional conjugation pathways are *N*-acetylation of amines and *O*-, *N*-, and *S*-methylation. These, unlike other Phase II reactions, generally result in a more lipophilic product.

Some products of Phase II conjugation reactions may contribute to drug toxicity, *e.g.* glucuronide or sulphate conjugates of certain substituted *N*-hydroxyamides are implicated in the induction of bladder cancer.

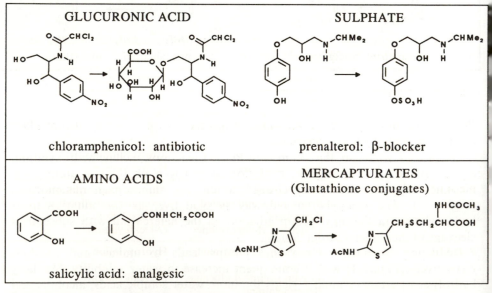

Figure 2 examples:

GLUCURONIC ACID — chloramphenicol: antibiotic

SULPHATE — prenalterol: β-blocker

AMINO ACIDS — salicylic acid: analgesic

MERCAPTURATES (Glutathione conjugates)

Figure 2: *Examples of Phase II metabolism (conjugation)*

3 SITES OF DRUG METABOLISM

Drug metabolism can occur in most tissues and organs of the body, *e.g.* liver, kidneys, gut, blood, plasma. The liver is probably the most efficient metabolising organ, having a high capacity for most metabolic reactions. The kidneys and gut wall are important sites for Phase II or conjugation reactions. Hydrolysis of esters and amides may occur in most tissues as well as blood and plasma.

Within the cell the complex metabolic pathways may occur in the endoplasmic reticulum (microsomes), mitochondria, and the cell cytosol. Many oxidative reactions are carried out by the membrane-bound mixed-function oxidases or cytochrome P-450 enzymes in the microsomes. The cytochrome P-450 enzymes are dominant in the Phase I metabolic pathways and within each animal species including man a number of different isozymes are expressed, each showing some substrate specificity. Thus inter-species differences in metabolism reflect in part the properties of the P-450 isozymes expressed. Three isozyme families appear to be most important in the metabolism of drugs in man, P-450 IIIA, P-450 IID, and P-450 IIC (Table 3), and are also expressed in other mammalian species, *e.g.* rat and dog.[1,2] The data in Table 3 show that there is overlap in substrate specificity even between these major isozyme families.

Some metabolic pathways, *e.g.* N-acetylation, occur in the mitochondria, and conjugation (Phase II) reactions may occur in the cytosol or on membrane-bound enzymes. The enzymes involved in most other drug metabolism pathways also exist in multiple forms (isoenzymes) which may show differing substrate specificities.

Table 3: *Substrates for and some metabolic pathways catalysed by the more important P-450 isozyme families*

Isozyme	Substrate	Metabolic pathway
P-450 IIIA	Dihydropyridines	Aromatization
	Cyclosporine, Erythromycin, Ethylmorphine, Lidocaine	Dealkylation
	Steroids	Aliphatic and aromatic hydroxylation
	Benzodiazepines	Hydroxylation
P-450 IID	Debrisoquine	Alicyclic hydroxylation
	Propranolol and related β-blockers	Aromatic and aliphatic hydroxylation
	Codeine, Ethylmorphine	O-Dealkylation
P-450 IIC	Phenytoin, Tolbutamide, Retinol	Hydroxylation
	Ethylmorphine, Lidocaine, Benzphetamine	N-Dealkylation

4 RELATIONSHIP BETWEEN STRUCTURE AND EXTENT OF METABOLISM

The extent of drug metabolism is dependent on two factors:

- Water solubility of the drug
- Availability of sites for metabolism

These are reflected in the lipophilicity (log $D_{7.4}$) and the chemical structure of a drug. Thus, the antidepressant drug chlorpromazine (Figure 3) is very lipophilic with poor water solubility and has many potential sites of metabolism. It undergoes N-dealkylation, aromatic hydroxylation, sulphoxidation, N-oxidation and a combination of these processes. Some of the resulting Phase I metabolites are also substrates for Phase II conjugation reactions, *e.g.* glucuronidation, sulphation. This produces many metabolites which are excreted in urine and bile with little or no excretion of unchanged drug. In contrast, the more water soluble atenolol is excreted predominantly unchanged in urine. Only a small amount ($\leqslant 5\%$ dose) is excreted as its hydroxy metabolite.

The extent of metabolism of many drugs lies between these two extremes, with a mixture of parent drug and metabolites being excreted. Within a series of compounds, *e.g.* β-blockers, the importance of metabolism as an elimination route generally increases with increasing lipophilicity.[3]

chlorpromazine	atenolol
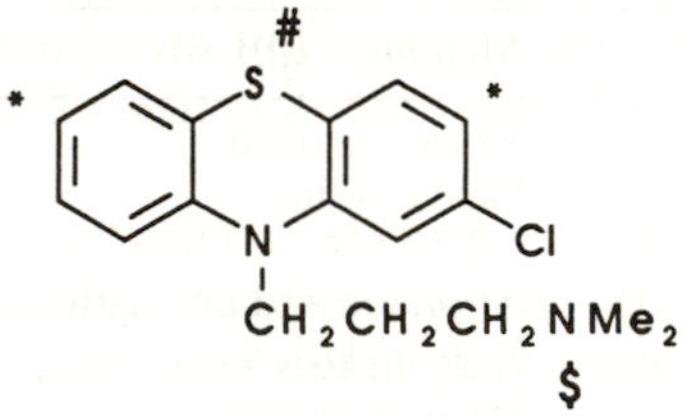	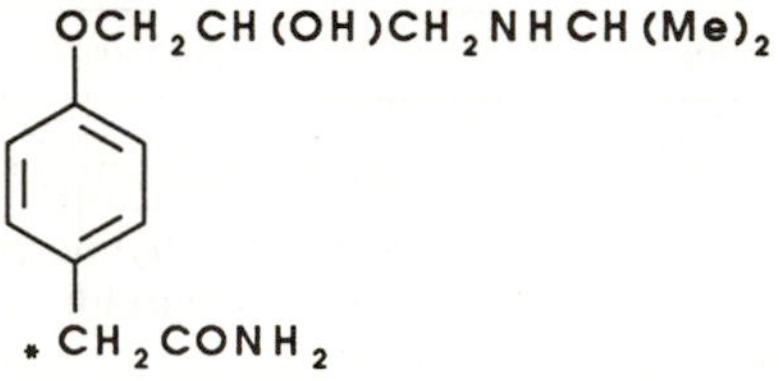
$ ⇒N-O # ⇒S-O ⇒NH-Me ⇒NH$_2$ * ⇒-OH plus combinations and conjugation	* ⇒-OH

Figure 3: *Examples of metabolism of lipophilic (chlorpromazine) and hydrophilic (atenolol) drugs*

5 HOW IS DRUG METABOLISM STUDIED?

The metabolic fate of a drug can be studied by a combination of techniques including:

- Radiolabelled drug (^{14}C, ^{3}H, ^{35}S) and measurement of total radioactivity
- Extraction and chromatographic techniques, *e.g.* HPLC, TLC, GC
- Specific analytical methods for drug and/or metabolites
- NMR and mass spectrometry

The use of radiolabelled drugs provides a technique to detect and quantify all drug-related material in the complex mixture of endogenous compounds in biological samples. Measurement of total radioactivity in plasma, urine and faeces gives information on the absorption and routes and rates of excretion of drug related material. A combination of extraction and chromatographic procedures can be used to provide information on the extent of metabolism in the biological samples. These methods also allow isolation and purification of metabolites for identification by suitable spectroscopic techniques, *e.g.* NMR and mass spectrometry.

It may also be possible to carry out direct NMR analysis of biological samples (*e.g.* urine) with minimal sample preparation. This can provide very rapid metabolic information when relatively high doses have been administered and urinary excretion of drug and metabolites is rapid and extensive. Thus it may be possible to identify metabolites and estimate their concentrations in small urine volumes following freeze-drying and dissolution in D_2O using proton NMR spectroscopy. Alternatively solid-phase extraction and elution with appropriate solvents may provide concentration and partial purification of metabolites from biological samples prior to NMR analysis.

Drug metabolism may be studied *in vivo* or *in vitro*. Thus it is possible to use liver preparations, *e.g.* microsomes, hepatocytes, liver slices, to assess the potential metabolic fate of compounds in a series early in drug candidate selection to compare species differences in drug metabolism, and predict possible fate in man.

Specific analytical methods for drug and metabolite(s) then allow measurement of their concentrations in biological fluids and thus the kinetics of drug absorption, distribution, and elimination.

Radioisotope techniques can also be used to provide qualitative and quantitative distribution of drug derived material by whole body autoradiography. It does *not* define the distribution of parent drug unless combined with methods to estimate drug and metabolite concentrations, *e.g.* extraction and chromatographic analysis.

6 WHY DO WE STUDY DRUG METABOLISM?

Drug metabolism information provides a link between the animals used in pharmacology and toxicology studies and man. A comparison of the drug's fate in all species studied allows the interpretation of the relevance to man (Figure 4).

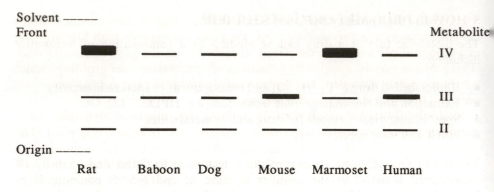

Figure 4: *Comparative metabolism in different species*

Metabolites may be:
> Inert
> Toxic
> Pharmacologically active

Figure 5

Thus, the species which most resemble man in their metabolism of a compound provide the most relevant data.

Pharmacologic activity may result from the production of an active metabolite, as may unwanted side effects (Figure 5). By understanding the metabolism of a drug, it may be possible to correlate pharmacologic (pharmacodynamic) and toxicologic effects with the pharmacokinetics of the drug and of its metabolite(s). However, a measurement of the total radioactivity alone in plasma or other samples does not give an accurate assessment of drug concentration or pharmacokinetics. Total radioactivity is the sum of the concentrations of the drug (if present) and any radiolabelled metabolites, as shown for plasma in Figure 6. Thus analytical methods to determine the proportion of drug and metabolites are essential to interpret total radioactivity data.

Drug metabolism information can assist drug discovery programmes. Thus poor bioavailability due to poor absorption or extensive 'first-pass' metabolism may

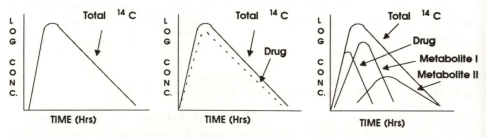

Figure 6: *Relationship between total ^{14}C measured and metabolic fate of drug*

yield low *in vivo* potency for compounds showing high *in vitro* potency. Many potent antibiotics, *e.g.* cephalosporins, are polar compounds with low log D at physiological pH and thus are poorly absorbed from the gastrointestinal tract. This problem may be avoided by formation of appropriate ester pro-drugs which are much better absorbed, and hydrolysed during first-pass metabolism in gut wall and liver to release the active species.

Similarly if rapid metabolism is limiting the pharmacodynamics of a compound, modification of the structure may be used to reduce this effect. This can produce a more effective drug candidate for development. This approach was used to design the β_1-adrenoceptor antagonist betaxolol, which had a bioavailability of 80% and a half-life in man of 14–22 h, by modifying the *p*-substituent in metoprolol (bioavailability $\sim 50\%$; $t_{1/2}$ 3.5 h). This work used *in vitro* metabolism studies in liver preparations (*e.g.* microsomes, homogenates) to select the most metabolically stable compounds.[4]

Application of drug metabolism techniques to a series of imidazolyl and aryl substituted propan-1-one drugs, designed to inhibit anti-anaerobic bacteria showed that *in vitro* activity correlated with the extent to which they were converted to the corresponding propenone analogues.[5] However, their activity *in vivo* did not correlate with that found *in vitro*. It was shown that this was due to the reactive propenone products being removed by reaction with tissue nucleophiles, and thus unable to inhibit bacterial replication.

7 WHAT FACTORS CAN MODIFY DRUG METABOLISM?

Dose Level

As the dose of drug increases, the capacity of the metabolic enzyme systems may be saturated. This can lead to alternative pathways coming into operation and/or to a disproportionately higher concentration of drug or of a toxic or active metabolite being present. This can result in toxicity. Thus paracetamol (Figure 7) is eliminated by conjugation with glucuronic acid and sulphate at normal

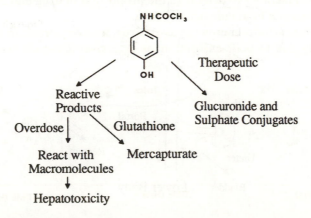

Figure 7: *Dose dependent effects: paracetamol*

therapeutic doses. At higher doses, sulphate and glucuronide conjugation become saturated and formation of a mercapturic acid by conjugation of reactive Phase I metabolites with glutathione is also observed. Intentional overdose saturates glucuronidation and sulphation and depletes the glutathione. The reactive intermediates accumulate and cause damage to cell macromolecules with resultant liver and kidney toxicity. These types of effect can be important in interpreting pharmacology and toxicology data, and assessing its relevance to man.

Route of Administration

Drugs given orally have to pass the gut microflora and digestive enzymes in the gut lumen, and drug metabolising enzymes in intestinal wall and liver before reaching the systemic circulation (Figure 8).

Metabolism may occur at any or all of these sites and can reduce the drug concentration (amount) in the systemic circulation. If the drug itself is the active compound, this will affect the intensity of its pharmacodynamic effects. When this pre-systemic metabolism occurs in gut wall or liver, it is called the 'first-pass' effect.

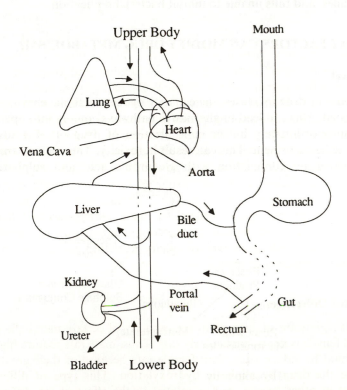

Figure 8

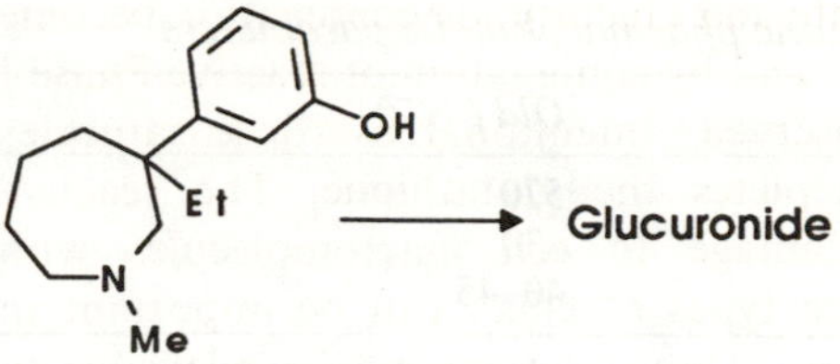

meptazinol: analgesic

Peak Plasma Level after 50mg dose

Orally   <0.01 µg/ml
Rectally 0.05-0.2 µg/ml

Figure 9

Meptazinol (Figure 9) is an analgesic drug subject to a very high first-pass effect *via* glucuronide conjugation. This is by-passed if the drug is administered rectally since blood drainage from the rectum avoids the hepatic portal vein. Thus, less drug is eliminated before reaching the systemic circulation and higher concentrations are obtained for a given dose.

The 'first-pass' effect may for extensively metabolised drugs contribute to between- and within-subject variability.

Species

There are frequently quantitative differences in the Phase I pathways between species. These are at present difficult to predict and interpret. The general conclusion is that in man the rate of the P-450 pathways is about 20 times slower than in rat and about 6 times slower than in dog, although this may vary for particular compounds owing to species differences in isoenzymes.

A number of qualitative differences are seen for Phase II pathways. Dogs are unable to acetylate aromatic amines and are more sensitive to the pharmacologic and toxic effects of such compounds. Cats lack the ability to form glucuronide conjugates and only primates form amino-acid conjugates with glutamine. These differences can have implications for the screening of compounds in animal species other than man. Differences in biliary excretion also occur. As a broad generalisation, compounds (drugs or metabolites) with MW $\geqslant 325$ will undergo extensive biliary excretion in rat and dog, whereas MW $\geqslant 500$ is required in man.

Sex-related Differences

There are significant differences in the capacity of certain metabolic pathways in male and female rodents, particularly rats. Thus, male rats require higher doses of hexobarbital to induce sleep than female rats because of their greater ability to inactivate the drug by aliphatic hydroxylation. This type of difference is less important in other species, and is related to the effect of sex differences in the expression of cytochrome P-450 isozymes in the rat.

Table 4: *Age-dependent effects on imipramine pharmacokinetic parameters*

	Young	*Old (> 70)*
Clearance (ml/min)	950	570
Half-life (h)	17	30
C_{max} (ng/ml)	10–20	40–45

Volume of distribution and protein binding were unchanged; the decreased clearance is due to the reduced ability of the old liver to N-dealkylate

Age

This is an important determinant of drug metabolism and is best studied in man. At either end of the age range, the liver (and other tissues) is (are) generally less capable of metabolic reactions, than in the subjects aged 18–45 used in early clinical studies. For example, neonates are essentially unable to conjugate chloramphenicol with glucuronic acid (see Figure 2).

This results in an accumulation of drug leading to toxic cardiovascular effects (grey baby syndrome). Similar problems can occur in the aged liver (Table 4) with the reduced clearance of imipramine in the liver requiring changes in the administered dose, to avoid excessive drug accumulation and hence increased side-effects.

Disease

Drugs which are mainly eliminated by metabolism can show changes in their kinetics in patients with liver disease. Propranolol is more bioavailable in cirrhotic patients because of a much reduced first-pass effect. Similarly, conversion of a pro-drug to active compound may be decreased in liver disease. However, it is difficult to predict the effect of a particular liver disease on the fate of a specific drug.

Drug Interactions

Other drugs administered concomitantly can alter the metabolism of a drug because they affect drug metabolising enzymes, *e.g.* cytochrome P-450, glucuronyl transferase. This can result in increased (induction) or decreased (inhibition) metabolism of the co-administered drug. Phenytoin and cimetidine, respectively, are examples of drugs which cause these effects. Such compounds may also modify their own extent of metabolism and hence kinetics on repeated administration.

Genetics

This results in individual difference in expression of different isoenzymes involved in drug metabolism and may lead to wide population differences in the metabolic fate of a compound. Some 10% of the population are unable to hydroxylate debrisoquine (Figure 1) and other drugs metabolised by the same P-450 enzyme (P450 IID6) with potential effects on their activity and side effects. Similarly, there are genetic differences in the ability to *N*-acetylate certain classes of drug, *e.g.* dapsone, isoniazid. Some people have a much lower capacity to carry out this reaction which in turn influences the activity and side-effects of such compounds.

8 CONCLUSIONS

Drug metabolism is an important elimination route for many compounds. An understanding of drug metabolism pathways and the factors which influence them provides information about mechanisms underlying changes in the kinetics, toxicity, and pharmacodynamics of drugs in animals and man. Information on the log $D_{7.4}$, pK_a and structural complexity of a drug allows some prediction of metabolic fate. Extrapolation across species is not precise for metabolic pathways. However, in general, the small (shorter life span) species are more adept at Phase I oxidative pathways, producing a wider range of metabolites. Thus in man metabolite profiles are often less complex than in animals. These differences tend to reflect the decrease in basal metabolic rate with increasing body weight. An understanding of the relationship between drug metabolism, pharmacology, and toxicology can be applied to aid the design of drug candidates.

Preliminary information on metabolism can be of value in selecting drug development candidates and in designing compounds with improved kinetic and thus pharmacodynamic profiles.

9 REFERENCES

1. D. Smith, *Drug Metab. Rev.*, 1991, **23**, 355.
2. M. Murray, *Clin. Pharm.*, 1992, **23**, 132.
3. G.R. Bourne, in 'Progress in Drug Metabolism', ed. J.W. Bridges and L.F. Chasseaud, Wiley, London, 1981, Vol. 6, pp. 77–110.
4. P.M. Manoury, *et al.*, *J. Med. Chem.*, 1981, **30**, 1003.
5. G. Dean and C.W. Vose, in 'Methodological Surveys in Biochemistry and Analysis', Vol. 20, ed. E. Reid and I.D. Wilson, Royal Society of Chemistry, Cambridge, 1990, pp. 207–210.

10 BIBLIOGRAPHY

'Drug Disposition and Pharmacokinetics', S.H. Curry, Blackwells, Oxford, 1980.
'Drug Metabolism from Microbes to Man', ed. D.V. Parke and R.L. Smith, Taylor and Francis, London, 1977.
'Drug Metabolism from Molecules to Man', ed. D.J. Benford, J.W. Bridges, and G.G. Gibson, Taylor and Francis, London, 1987.

CHAPTER 7

Physicochemical Properties and Drug Design

NIGEL P. GENSMANTEL

1 INTRODUCTION

One of the many difficulties encountered by medicinal chemists is to understand how the many different physical, molecular and atomic properties of a compound can influence how it interacts with its target receptor. In so far that the biological properties of a compound are directly related to its chemical and physical properties then it is theoretically possible to select compounds for synthesis that vary those properties efficiently. When a compound is presented directly to its receptor then several interactions contribute to the enthalpy of binding. The affinity of a compound for its receptor is characterised by the binding constant of that compound. Reversible binding can be divided into a number of interaction types:

i.   Electrostatic interactions; coulombic interactions which are favourable.
     ion–ion $^+NH_3$ .... ^-O_2C
     ion–dipole $^+NH_3$ .... $^{\delta-}O=C$
ii. Hydrophobic interactions; binding results from non-polar lipophilic regions coming together. The stability of the interaction is associated with the degree of order of surrounding water molecules.
iii. Hydrogen bonding; short-range directional interactions which contribute to the specific interactions that a drug molecule makes with its receptor.
     dipole–dipole $N–H^{\delta+}$ .... $^{\delta-}O=C$

It is beyond the scope of this chapter to review all aspects of these interactions. Emphasis will be placed on the ability to measure, modify, and predict the above 'classical' molecular properties, electronic, lipophilic, steric, and hydrogen bonding. There are a large number of excellent reviews that will stimulate the interested reader.[1-5]

2 ELECTRONIC PROPERTIES AND IONISATION CONSTANTS

The acidity and basicity of a compound have a major role to play in controlling the transport of a compound to its site of action and the binding at this target site. The un-ionised form is involved in hydrogen bonding while the ionised form also influences the strength of salt bridges and ion–dipole interactions.

Many drugs have acidic and basic centres and for weak acids and bases the equilibria between the protonated forms are defined by K_a, the equilibrium constant.

For a weak acid:

$$CH_3COOH \overset{K_a}{\rightleftharpoons} CH_3COO^- + H^+ \qquad K_a = \frac{[CH_3COO^-][H^+]}{[CH_3COOH]}$$

For a weak base:

$$CH_3NH_3^+ \overset{K_a}{\rightleftharpoons} CH_3NH_2 + H^+ \qquad K_a = \frac{[CH_3NH_2][H^+]}{[CH_3NH_3^+]}$$

Defining pH $= -\log_{10}[H^+]$ then:

For an acid: $pK_a = pH + \log[CH_3COOH] - \log[CH_3COO^-]$
For a base: $pK_a = pH + \log[CH_3NH_3^+] - \log[CH_3NH_2]$

Many methods can be used to determine ionisation constants experimentally. Potentiometric titration is the most commonly used method, although other methods such as spectrophotometry, conductometry, pH-partition, and NMR have also been used. The methods available have been reviewed by Albert and Serjeant,[6] and this book provides a useful experimental text.

Table 1: *Ionisation constants for some typical acids and bases*

	pK_a		pK_a
CH_4	40	benzoic acid	4.2
ROH	16–20	RCOOH	4.0–5.0
$RCONH_2$	16–18	aniline.H^+	4.6
RNH_3^+	10–11	$CH_2(NO_2)_2$	3.6
CH_3NO_2	10.2	2,4-dinitrobenzoic acid	1.4
phenol	10.0	$Cl_2CHCOOH$	1.3
p-nitrophenol	7.2	p-nitroaniline.H^+	1.02
pyridine.H^+	5.2	CF_3COOH	0

3 HAMMETT RELATIONSHIP

The work of Albert[7] in the mid 20th century was the first real attempt to correlate the degree of ionisation of a compound with its biological activity. Physical chemists first became involved in the 1930s, when Hammett[8] undertook the systematic study of a series of benzene derivatives to establish a set of quantitative parameters that were transferable and could be used for the prediction of other systems. This was largely an empirical approach and was initially concerned with aromatic systems. In 1937 Hammett published σ_{meta} and

σ_{para} substituent constants for benzoic acids having defined a susceptibility constant ρ (slope of the line) to be one. Hydrogen was used as the standard substituent ($\sigma_H = 0$). It was found that σ values for a given substituent in the *meta*- and *para*-positions need to be different since the observed electronic influence of a substituent at the *meta*- and *para*-positions are different. Hammett observed that *meta*-substituents produced large inductive effects while *para* substituents showed enhanced resonance effects. Electron-releasing substituents have negative σ values and electron-withdrawing substituents have positive σ values. For *meta*- and *para*-substituted benzoic acids:

$$pK_a = 4.20 + \rho\Sigma\sigma$$

where 4.20 is the pK_a of benzoic acid at 25 °C, and σ is the substituent constant.

Hammett type relationships have been successfully applied in a wide variety of physiochemical studies. Substituent effects have been correlated with chemical reactivity, NMR shift data, and UV and IR spectra; the list is almost endless. Unfortunately the original parameter set is limited and problems can arise when there is a resonance interaction between the substituent and reaction centre, or the contributions of inductive and mesomeric effects are not constant within a series, or when there are steric interactions between the substituent and the reaction centre, as with *ortho*-substituted benzoic acids.

The original pioneering work of Hammett was taken further by Taft[9] in the early 1950s. He derived a set of parameters that specifically addressed deficiencies in the original data set of Hammett, *i.e.* no *ortho*-substituents in aromatic systems and poor explanation of aliphatic systems. Taft derived a set of σ^* values that were designed to separate out the polar, steric, and resonance effects for a give substituent. The values were derived from an analysis of the acid- and base-catalysed hydrolysis of aliphatic esters.

$$\sigma^* = 0.403 \, [\log(k/k_0)_{base} - \log(k/k_0)_{acid}]$$

where k_0 represents the methyl derivative, k the substituted compound, and 0.403 is a scale factor to put σ^* constants on the same scale as aromatic polar effects.

Taft substituent values assume that only base hydrolysis is sensitive to inductive effects and that both acid and base hydrolysis are equally affected by steric and resonance effects. Equally Taft σ^* values have been shown to be additive and correlate with measured ionisation constants of aliphatic acids and bases:

$$pK_a(R_1R_2R_3CCOOH) = 5.10 - 0.81\Sigma(\sigma^*)$$
$$pK_a(R_1R_2R_3NH^+) = 9.61 - 3.30\Sigma(\sigma^*)$$

Purely inductive effects, σ_I, are difficult to establish. However, measurement of the ionisation constants (pK_a values) of bicyclo[2.2.2]octane-1-carboxylic acid[10] and quinuclidine,[11] where steric effects are minimal and no resonance effects can occur, have allowed scales of σ_I to be developed and subsequently used in quantitative structure–activity relationship (QSAR) analysis of aliphatic systems.

Hammett aromatic σ constants are a combination of inductive and resonance effects and different values are required for a substituent depending on its position of substitution. Swain and Lupton[12] defined new electronic constants, a field constant F, a measure of the inductive effect, and a resonance constant R, to try to explain all σ scales. Swain and Lupton derived F and R values for each substituent and a linear combination was assumed.

$$\sigma = aF + bR$$

where a and b are weighting factors.

Other Hammett-like parameter scales[13] have also been developed over the years:

i. σ_p^+ from solvolysis studies
ii σ_p^- from ionisation constants of phenols and anilines
iii σ_p from alkaline hydrolysis of non-conjugate systems
iv   modified F and R values[14]
v   parameters relevant to free radicals
vi   charge transfer constants

4 HYDROPHOBIC INTERACTIONS AND LIPOPHILICITY

The hydrophobic effect[15] has been a source of debate for many years and the hydrophobic interaction has become synonymous with lipophilicity.[16] Why are we interested in lipophilicity? Lipophilicity is an important factor affecting the distribution and fate of drug molecules. Increased lipophilicity has been shown to correlate with increased biological activity, poorer aqueous solubility, increased detergency/cell lysis, increased storage in tissues, more rapid metabolism and elimination, increased rate of skin penetration, increased plasma protein binding, faster rate of onset of action and in some cases shorter duration of action.

The thermodynamics of these non-polar interactions are complicated and many. Initially when a solute molecule is placed in water a cavity has to be created for the solute and stronger water–water interactions are formed around the cavity whilst weaker interactions occur between water and solute molecules. The solvent water molecules become more ordered, and hence there is an unfavourable entropy of dissolution. The association of non-polar solute molecules reduces the non-polar surface area in contact with water, reduces the amount of water around the solute, and results in a favourable entropy of association. Hydrophobic interactions are considered to be entropy driven and the effect is related to the non-polar surface area of the solute molecules. Experimental data suggest that the free energy for methylene groups to associate in water is 0.7 kcal mol^{-1}, whilst for benzene the value is 2.0 kcal mol^{-1}.

5 PARTITION COEFFICIENT AS AN INDEX OF LIPOPHILICITY

The partition coefficient, P, is simply a measure of the affinity of a molecule for a lipid phase versus that for water, *i.e.* the concentration in the octanol phase divided by the concentration in the aqueous phase.

$$[DRUG]_{aqueous} \overset{P}{\rightleftharpoons} [DRUG]_{octanol} \qquad P = \frac{[DRUG]_{octanol}}{[DRUG]_{aqueous}}$$

1-Octanol has become the standard solvent for the determination of partition coefficients although solvents such as hexane, chloroform, and butanol have been used. Hansch[17] chose octanol as the reference solvent for $\log P$ measurements because of its superficial similarity with lipids: a long alkyl chain plus a functional group having both hydrogen bond accepting and donating characteristics. Hydrocarbon solvents such as hexane are of limited use in that most drug molecules have a low solubility in these solvents and self association can be a problem.

The shake flask method is the conventional experimental approach used for the determination of partition coefficients. To obtain accurate values by this method it is necessary to:

i.   mutually saturate the octanol – water solvents; saturated octanol contains 27% water on a mole fraction basis
ii. correct for molecular association of the solute molecules
iii. avoid the use of high volume ratios of solvent to water, and *vice versa*
iv. avoid temperature changes to minimise changes in solvent miscibilities

Although the classical method of Hansch and Fujita[18] still features prominently in the measurement of lipophilicity a number of other experimental techniques have been developed. Automated and semi-automated methods have been developed based on the filter probe method as well as flow injection extraction methods. Lipophilicity scales have also been developed based on reversed phase thin layer and HPLC measurements.[19]

6 IONISATION AND ITS EFFECT ON THE PARTITION COEFFICIENT

If a solute can ionise then the simple distribution of the un-ionised form into the octanol phase is dependent on the pH of the experiment. The distribution coefficient, $\log D$, is defined as the effective or nett lipophilicity of a compound at a given pH, and is a function of both its lipophilicity when un-ionised and the degree of ionisation.

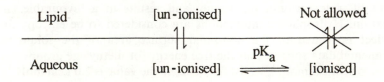

For an acidic compound $\qquad$ $HA \rightleftharpoons H^+ + A^-$ $\qquad$ $D = \dfrac{[HA]_{org}}{[HA]_{aq} + [A^-]_{aq}}$

For organic bases $\qquad\qquad$ $BH^+ \rightleftharpoons H^+ + B$ $\qquad$ $D = \dfrac{[B]_{org}}{[B]_{aq} + [BH^+]_{aq}}$

For a weak acid, the pH-partition curve follows a simple relationship:

$$\log(P/D - 1) = pH - pK_a$$

According to the simple pH-partition hypothesis, only the un-ionised form of the compound is able to partition into the non-aqueous phase. If correct then the compound should show maximum lipophilicity below the pK_a of an acid and above the pK_a of a basic compound and the distribution coefficient should be pH dependent. See Figure 1.

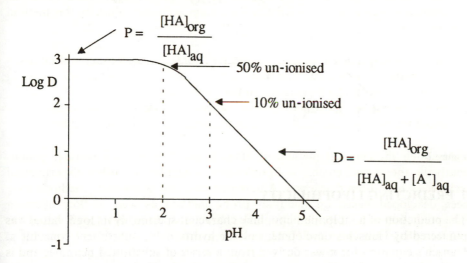

Figure 1: *Relationship between logD, pH and the % un-ionised for an acidic compound of logP = 3 and pK$_a$ = 2*

The partitioning of zwitterions, compounds containing both an acidic and basic centre, is more complex still.

A mono acid or base still ionises as a function of pH

Lipid	[un-ionised]	Not allowed
Aqueous	[un-ionised] $\overset{pK_a}{\rightleftharpoons}$ [ionised]	

but for an amphoteric compound it is the electrically neutral species that partitions

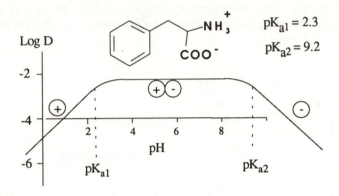

Any amphoteric compound will exhibit maximum lipophilicity when overall neutrally charged. Below pK_{a1} or above pK_{a2} of the compound the mono ionised species dominates and the distribution coefficient decreases with unit slope. (Figure 2)

Figure 2

7 PREDICTING LIPOPHILICITY

The prediction of a molecule's lipophilic character, specifically its $\log P$ value, was pioneered by Hansch's development of the hydrophobic substituent constant π. Hansch's equation for π was derived from a series of substituted benzenes and is similar to that used by Hammett to explain electronic effects:

$$\pi_X = \log P_{RX} - \log P_{RH}$$

where P_{RH} and P_{RX} are the partition coefficient of the parent and substituted compound respectively and π_X is the change in the log of the partition coefficient when the hydrogen atom of the parent is replaced by substituent X. The original Hansch and Leo approach fails because the electronic, steric, and hydrogen bonding environment affects the contribution that a substituent makes.

Fujita and Hansch[18] suggested that the hydrophobic constant π and $\log P$ were linear free energy related variables by analogy with the Hammett electronic substituent constant. Analysis of large sets of biological data by Hansch and co-workers gave some support to this LFER view. Following on from the work of

Hansch and Fujita, Nys and Rekker[20] used regression analysis of experimental log P data to derive a new lipophilicity parameter f:

$$\log P = \Sigma f$$

The new fragmental constants included environment effects and they gave a more general method to estimate the log P value. As with electronic effects, substitution in a given system was found to be additive and for any compound log P can easily be calculated:

$$\log P_{(x,y,z)} = f_x + f_y + f_z + f_{\text{environment}}$$

The Rekker fragmental system and the Hansch and Leo π values are linked:

$$f_x = \pi_x + f_{\text{hydrogen}}$$

In the late 1970s Hansch and Leo[21] adopted the fragmental approach of predicting log$P$ values and developed the program CLOGP, designed to calculate the lipophilicity of any molecule using the method of additivity. Hansch and Leo have compiled tables for aromatic and aliphatic substituents based on many series of compounds. Extensive tables of fragmental constants are available and are exemplified in Table 2.

The lipophilicity of a compound can be adjusted in several ways, for example:

- introduction of a suitable ionising group
- if the compound is already an acid or base then modification of the pK_a will affect the distribution coefficient at a given pH
- introduction of a suitable functional group with the appropriate fragmental value

There are many occasions when the simple additivity rule fails. If a compound contains a fragment not yet parameterised this method will fail. When a

Table 2

	Polar - HYDROPHILIC	
	Aliphatic	*Aromatic*
$CONH_2$	−2.11	−1.26
OH	−1.64	−0.44
NH_2	−1.54	−1.00
NO_2	−1.16	−0.03
COOH	−1.11	−0.03
H	**0.23**	**0.23**
Cl	0.06	0.94
CH_3	0.88	0.88
C_6H_5	1.92	1.92
	Non-polar - LIPOPHILIC	

compound contains groups that interact due to electronic, steric, and/or hydrogen bonding interactions between substituents then large errors can occur. In the case of amino acids where charge separation can influence all of the intramolecular effects listed, large errors can arise between the measured and predicted $\log P$ values.[22]

For example a simple amino acid (^+H_2N—$(CH_2)_n$—COO^-)

Number of carbon atoms	Correction Δ_{zw}
1-4	−2.3
5	−2.9
6	−3.4
7	−3.8

Likewise alkylation of the amino group does not lead to the expected increase in lipophilicity.

The octanol – water partition system is by no means the only system of interest and Leahy *et al.* have investigated the partition of solutes in four systems:[23]

i.   octanol – water, H-bond donor and acceptor
ii.   chloroform – water, H-bond donor
iii. propylene glycol dipelargonate – water, H-bond acceptor
iv.   alkane – water, inert

The difference between partitioning of solutes into two different partition systems was found to correlate with a number of biological processes; *e.g.* $\Delta \log P$ correlates with brain and skin penetration.

8 STERIC PARAMETERS

The steric features of a molecule are closely related to a compound's ability to bind to its receptor and thus elicit its biological activity. The intermolecular interactions between a ligand and its receptor can lead to favourable binding if atoms in the molecule occupy a cavity in the receptor. If part of the ligand needs to occupy volume required by the receptor then binding becomes less favourable.

Several steric parameters have been developed to reflect the steric influence of a substituent on molecular properties. Taft's steric parameters E_s were derived from the study of the acid-catalysed hydrolysis of aliphatic esters[9]

$$E_s = \log k_x / k_0$$

where k_x is the rate constant for the substituted compound and k_0 is the rate constant for the methyl analogue. At the same time Taft also developed E_s^0 substituents for *ortho*-substituted benzoic acid esters.[9] The work of Hancock (1961) suggested that modified E_s values were required to take into account hyperconjugation effects. E_s^c values were derived by studying the reactions of systems such as aliphatic amines.[24] Taft and Hancock substituent constants are experimentally derived and there is a limited data set available for use in QSAR studies.

On the other hand parameters that can be computed easily allow any substituent to be considered. The van der Waals radius of a substituent is a useful measure of the steric bulk of a group, but assumes that substituents are spherical. An extension of this approach was adopted by Verloop who devised a parameter set that would also account for the shape of the substituent.[25] These STERIMOL parameters are a set of distances, L, the length that a substituent extends from the parent using the connecting bond between the parent and the substituent as the direction, and a set of width values, $B_1 - B_4$, perpendicular to each other and with B_1 set to the smallest width. STERIMOL parameters have been tabulated for a large number of simple substituents and have proven to be extremely useful in QSAR studies and substituents whose values are not available can be calculated easily.

Molar refractivity (MR), though not really a size parameter, has also been used extensively in QSAR studies. The molar refractivity is related to the molar volume, V, through:

$$MR = \frac{(n^2 - 1)V}{(n^2 + 2)}$$

where n is the refractive index. MR values are readily calculated using the CMR program from Daylight. The list of steric parameters is not endless but parameters such as minimal steric difference, MSD,[26] minimal topological difference, MRD,[27] and shape descriptors[28] V_0, S_0, and L_0 have all had some success in QSAR studies.

9 HYDROGEN BONDING

Hydrogen bonds are the most important short-range interaction in biological systems and are responsible for maintaining the tertiary structure of proteins. Unlike electrostatic interactions, hydrogen bonds have a directional component and the hydrogen bond strength decreases as the geometry becomes less optimal. Hydrogen bond donors are in general OH, SH (aromatic), NH, and activated CH groups while hydrogen bond acceptors are electronegative atoms such as N, O, S, and F. The separation distance between the heavy atoms forming the hydrogen bond is 2.5–2.7 Å and the strength of a hydrogen bond in aprotic solvents has been estimated at between 2 and 5 kcal mol^{-1}.

In proteins the major interactions are between carboxyl, hydroxyl, carbonyl, amino, imino, and amido groups. As proton acceptors carboxylates are better than carbonyls in amides, ketones, or un-ionised acids while as proton donors ammonium ions are better donors than hydroxyl groups which are in turn better than amide groups. Other atoms or functional groups can participate in hydrogen bonds but are generally much weaker, *e.g.* an alkyl thiol group is a negligible proton donor.

Del Bene's[29] theoretical studies suggested that for a series of hydrogen bond donors (X–A–H) and acceptors (B–Y)

$$X-A-H + B-Y \overset{K_{hb}}{\rightleftharpoons} X-A\cdots H\cdots B-Y$$

where X and Y vary from H, CH_3, NH_2, OH through to F then:

i.   as X goes from H to F then X–A–H becomes a better proton donor
ii. as Y goes from F to H then B–Y becomes a better acceptor

This trend can be rationalised on the basis of electrostatic effects, *e.g.*:

i.   as X becomes more electronegative, the more δ^+ on the proton, the better the proton donor
ii. as Y becomes more electronegative, the less the electron density on B and hence B forms a weaker H—B bond

Rubin and Panson[30] studied hydrogen bonding between substituted phenols and pyridines in carbon tetrachloride and found a good correlation between the pK_a of the donor (phenol) and the acceptor (pyridine) as substitutions were made in the donor–acceptor series. Over a wide range of acidity and basicity it does appear that the strength of a hydrogen bond is related to the pK_a of the donor or acceptor. A more detailed analysis of the data reveals that within this general-isation a number of families exist which show a significant variance from the line of best fit for all the data. Recently, detailed studies have been performed to establish a more general scale capable of predicting hydrogen bond strengths for all donors and acceptors. The initial step requires the selection of a common acceptor or donor and an experimental method. Experimentally, hydrogen bond strength has been shown to be related to 1H NMR and IR shifts.

Taft and Schleyer[31] derived acceptor–donor strengths based on the equilibrium constant between 4-fluorophenol in CCl_4 and the acceptor of interest.

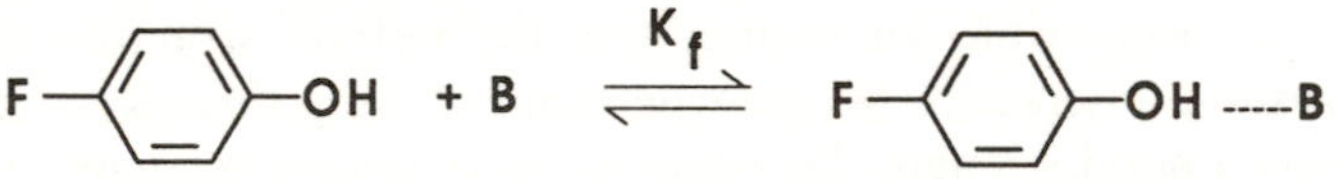

The more recent comprehensive study of Abraham *et al.*[32] used *N*-methylpyrro-lidone (1) as a common acceptor in $MeCCl_3$ to determine the pK_{HB} for proton donors and 4-nitrophenol (2) to determine pK_{HB} of proton acceptors.

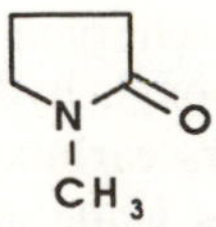

(1) 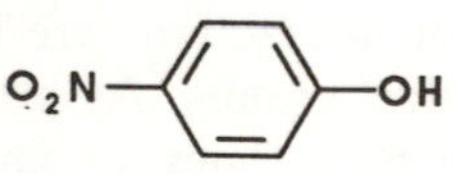   (2)

Experimentally it was found that pK_{HB} values do not correlate with pK_a values of the donor or acceptor. As a result of their work they defined pK_α scales for proton donors and pK_β scales for proton acceptors.

10 PREDICTION OF DRUG–RECEPTOR INTERACTIONS

The experimentally observed ΔG of binding can be considered as a summation of a series of intermolecular forces as discussed earlier.

Favourable interactions:

i. Electrostatic
ii. Hydrophobic
iii. Hydrogen bonding

Unfavourable contribution:

i. Loss of rotational and translational entropy upon binding.

It has been argued by Page that the strength of a specific bond can be obtained by comparing the binding energies of pairs of compounds containing a single different functional group. The 'Anchor Principle'[33] assumes that the loss of rotational and translation entropy is invariant to the substituent.

Mutagenesis Studies

The strength of interaction made by a specific functional group can be probed by protein engineering in a number of ways. Estimation of the strength of hydrogen bonds has been studied by:

Modification of the Enzyme. Fersht[34] has used mutagenesis studies of tyrosyl-tRNA synthetase enzyme to calculate hydrogen bond energies and in general found:

i. Hydrogen bond strengths between enzyme and uncharged group are in the range of 0.5–1.5 kcal mol^{-1}
ii. Hydrogen bond strength to charged groups are of the order of 3.5–4.5 kcal mol^{-1}

Modification of the Ligand. Binding studies of deoxy sugars at glycogen phosphorylase[35] supported the view that hydrogen bond strengths for interactions with neutral species and with charged species were similar to those above.

Mutation studies on subtilisin[36] estimated the average free energies for ion pair interactions of 1.8–2.5 kcal mol^{-1} and showed that the electrostatic effects were additive. The interaction energies appear low when compared with theoretical studies, but reflect the negative effect of desolvating a charged species before it can bind.

Ligand Binding Studies

Ligand binding studies of small peptides, *N*-Ac-D-Ala-D-Ala, binding to the antibiotic ristocetin A have allowed Williams[37] to define a series of favourable as well as unfavourable binding energies.

Favourable binding interactions:

i.   Hydrogen bonds
             amide–amide   4.8 kcal. mol^{-1}
             amide–hydroxyl   2.9 kcal mol^{-1}
             amide–carboxylate   6.7 kcal mol^{-1}
ii.   Solvent contact surface
             removal of a methyl group   1.18 kcal mol^{-1}

Unfavourable binding interactions:

i.   Translation and rotation (size dependent)   11.9–14.8 kcal mol^{-1}
ii.   Number of internal rotations   1.2–1.9 kcal mol^{-1}

The results are broadly in agreement with mutagenesis studies.

Statistically Derived Group Contributions

Andrews *et al.*[38] analysed statistically data from 200 non-covalent drug–receptor interactions and expressed the experimental free energy of binding, ΔG, using the simple formula:

$$\Delta G = T\Delta S_{r,t} + n_{DOF}E_{DOF} + n_x E_x$$

where:

$T\Delta S_{r,t}$ represents the unfavourable entropy term for a ligand binding to its receptor, assumed to be constant, and estimated to be 14 kcal mol^{-1}
n_{DOF} represents the internal degrees of conformational freedom, rotatable bonds in the ligand
E_{DOF} represents the average entropy loss on binding per rotatable bond
n_x represents the number of times that the functional group x appears in the ligand
E_x represents the derived average intrinsic binding energy for group x.

Analysis allowed the evaluation of the average intrinsic binding energy for 10 common functional groups (Table 3).

By summing the intrinsic binding energies for a given compound and deducting the negative entropy terms, *e.g.* unfavourable entropy of binding and loss of degrees of rotational freedom, then an estimate can be made of the expected binding energy. Compounds that have a high affinity for their receptor will show binding energies in excess of the predicted values based on the average intrinsic binding energies derived by Andrews. When a compound is not the best fit for its receptor then the predicted binding energy will be significantly higher than the experimental value.

Table 3: *Intrinsic binding energies (kcal mol^{-1}) (from Andrews[38])*

Group	Energy	Range	Group	Energy	Range
Charged			Neutral		
N^+	11.5	10.4–15.0	$C = O$	3.4	3.2–4.0
$PO_4{}^{2-}$	10.0	7.7–10.6	OH	2.5	2.5–4.0
$CO_2{}^-$	8.2	7.3–10.3	Halogen	1.3	0.2–2.0
			N	1.2	0.8–1.8
			O,S	1.1	0.7–7.0
			C (sp^3)	0.8	0.1–1.0
DOF	−0.7	−0.7 to −1.0	C (sp^2)	0.7	0.6–0.8

11 CONCLUSIONS

The rational design of novel bioactive compounds relies on the understanding of molecular properties. QSAR studies involve the use of substituent parameters to model changes in molecular properties as substituents are changed at defined positions within the compound of interest. Properties such as lipophilicity have been shown to correlate with many biological processes, for example the transport of organic molecules across cell membranes and absorption into cells. Introduction of an acidic or basic site into the compound changes the physical properties of that compound. Absorption in particular is dependent on the amount of un-ionised compound and for acidic or basic compounds the pH of the surrounding environment will influence the availability of the compound. Acidic compounds with a low pK_a will prefer to be ionised unless at very low pH; therefore, absorption will only occur in the stomach. In the gastrointestinal tract, where the pH is much higher, the amount of un-ionised material is much lower and absorption will be reduced. It is clear that subtle changes in lipophilicity and ionisation can result in significant changes in biological activity. The binding of small molecules to their receptor depends on the compound having optimal electrostatic, hydrogen bonding and hydrophobic interactions. All these interactions can be manipulated by appropriate synthesis and it is the role of the medicinal chemists to understand and exploit the underlying molecular properties that control biological activity.

12 ACKNOWLEDGEMENTS

I should like to thank Dr. A. Davis and Mrs C. N. Manners for their contributions, helpful comments, and suggestions on the content of this lecture and manuscript.

13 REFERENCES

1. M.A. Tute, 'History and Objectives of Quantitative Drug Design', in 'Comprehensive Medicinal Chemistry', ed. C. Hansch, P.G. Sammes, and J.B. Taylor, Pergamon Press, Oxford, 1990.

2. Y.C. Martin, 'Quantitative Drug Design', Marcel Dekker, New York, 1978.
3. 'Correlation Analysis in Chemistry, Recent Advances', ed. N.B. Chapman and J. Shorter, Plenum Press, New York, 1978.
4. 'Medicinal Chemistry', a series of monographs: 'Drug Design', ed. E.J. Ariens, Academic Press, 1971.
5. 'Physical Chemical Properties of Drugs', ed. S.H. Yalkowsky, A.A. Sinkula, and S.C. Valvani, Marcel Dekker, New York, 1980.
6. A. Albert and E.P. Serjeant, 'The Determination of Ionisation Constants', Chapman and Hall Ltd, 1972.
7. A. Albert *et al.*, *Br. J. Exp. Pathol.*, 1945, **26**, 160.
8. L.P. Hammett, 'Physical Organic Chemistry', McGraw-Hill, New York, 1940.
9. R.W. Taft, 'Steric Effects in Organic Chemistry', Wiley, New York, 1956.
10. J.D. Roberts and W.T. Moreland, *J. Am. Chem. Soc.*, 1953, **75**, 2167.
11. C.A. Grob and M.G. Schlageter, *Helv. Chim. Acta*, 1976, **59**, 264.
12. C.G. Swain and E.C. Lupton, *J. Am. Chem. Soc.*, 1968, **90**, 4328.
13. O. Exner, in 'Correlation Analysis in Chemistry, Recent Advances', ed. N.B. Chapman and J. Shorter, Plenum Press, New York, 1978, Chapter 10.
14. F.E. Norrington *et al.*, *J. Med. Chem.*, 1975, **18**, 604.
15. F. Franks, 'Water', Royal Society of Chemistry, London, 1983.
16. H. Kubinyi, *Progr. Drug. Res.*, 1979, **23**, 97.
17. A. Leo, C. Hansch, and D. Elkins, *Chem. Rev.*, 1971, **71**, 525.
18. T. Fujita, J. Iwasa, and C. Hansch, *J. Am. Chem. Soc.*, 1964, **86**, 5175.
19. N. El Tayar *et al.*, *J. Chromatogr.*, 1989, **556**, 181.
20. R.F. Rekker, 'The Hydrophobic Fragmental Constant', Elsevier, Amsterdam, 1977.
21. C. Hansch and A.J. Leo, 'Substituent Constants for Correlation Analysis', Wiley, New York, 1979.
22. D.W. Payling and C.N. Manners, unpublished data.
23. D.E. Leahy, P.J. Taylor, and A.R. Wait, *Quant. Struct. Act. Relat.*, 1989, **8**, 17.
24. C.K. Hancock, E.A. Meyers, and B.J. Yager, *J. Am. Chem. Soc.*, 1961, **83**, 4211; C.K. Hancock, *J. Org. Chem.*, 1973, **38**, 4239.
25. A. Verloop, W. Hoogenstraaten, and J. Tipker, 'Drug Design', Vol. VII, ed. E.J. Ariens, Academic Press, New York, 1976, p. 156.
26. A.T. Balaban, et al. 'Steric Fit in Quantitative Structure Activity Relationships', Lecture Notes in Chemistry, Vol. 15, Springer-Verlag, Berlin, 1980.
27. Z. Simon *et al.*, *Eur. J. Med. Chem.*, 1980, **15**, 521.
28. A. J. Hopfinger, *J. Am. Chem. Soc.*, 1980, **102**, 7196.
29. J. Del Bene, *J. Am. Chem. Soc.*, 1973, **95**, 5460.
30. J. Rubin and G.S. Panson, *J. Phys. Chem.*, 1965, **69**, 3089; 1964, **68**, 1601.
31. R.W. Taft *et al., J. Am. Chem. Soc.*, 1969, **91**, 4801.
32. M.H. Abraham *et al.*, *J. Chem. Soc., Perkin Trans. II*, 1989, 1355.
33. M.I. Page, *Angew. Chem. Int. Ed. Engl.*, 1972, **16**, 449.
34. A.R. Fersht, R.J. Leatherbarrow, and T.N.C. Wells, *TiBS*, 1986, **11**, 321.
35. A.R. Fersht *et al.*, *Nature (London)*, 1985, **314**, 235.

36. J.A. Wells *et al.*, *Proc. Nat. Acad. Sci.*, *USA*, 1987, **84**, 1219.
37. D. H. Williams *et al.*, *J. Am. Chem. Soc.*, 1991, **113**, 7020. A.J. Doig and D.H. Williams, J. *Am. Chem. Soc.*, 1992, **114**, 338.
38. P.R. Andrews, D.J. Craik, and J.L. Martin, J. *Med. Chem.*, 1984, **27**, 1648.

CHAPTER 8

Quantitative Structure–Activity Relationships

ANDREW M. DAVIS

1 INTRODUCTION

The discovery of a novel drug molecule is a long, expensive, and tortuous process with no guarantee of success. Clearly, out of the almost infinite number of possible compounds, only a finite number can ever be synthesised for testing within a given time and the skill of the medicinal chemist is in deciding which of those compounds to make first. Of course, there is then the small problem of how to make them! In order to make that decision, the mass of biological data produced for compounds already tested needs to be analysed in such a way that features which are important for the biological activity/activities can be identified and then built into future molecules. The aim of QSAR is to find predictive relationships between quantitative descriptions of physical properties of compounds and the response of the biological system under consideration. The response could be the K_i measurement of an inhibitor in an enzyme assay, the pED_{50} of a receptor agonist, or even just whether the compounds are active/inactive in the biological screen. Hopefully the resulting QSAR will lead to an understanding of the molecular features/properties most important in determining activity, and guide the optimisation of biological activity within the compound series.

The birth of QSAR as we know it came with the work of Hansch and co-workers in the early 1960s,[1] but this was more of a coming of age, and Hansch's ideas were based on work stretching back to the middle of the last century. It was in 1868 when Crum-Brown and Fraser noted that the Curare-like paralysing properties of a series of quaternised strychnines depended upon the quaternising group, and proposed that physiological activity was some function of the constitution of the molecules.[2]

$$\text{Physiological activity} = f(\text{constitution})$$

In 1869 Richardson showed that toxicities of simple ethers and alcohols were inversely related to their water solubility,[3] and in 1893 Richet[4] noted that the narcotic effect of alcohols varied in proportion to their molecular weight. But probably the most influential of these early investigators were Overton[5,6] and Meyer.[7] They independently concluded that the narcotic action (on tadpoles) of many compounds depended solely upon the oil–water partition coefficient. This indicated that narcosis was being induced by the partitioning of the compound into the lipid constituent of cells, and the effect the compounds had upon the

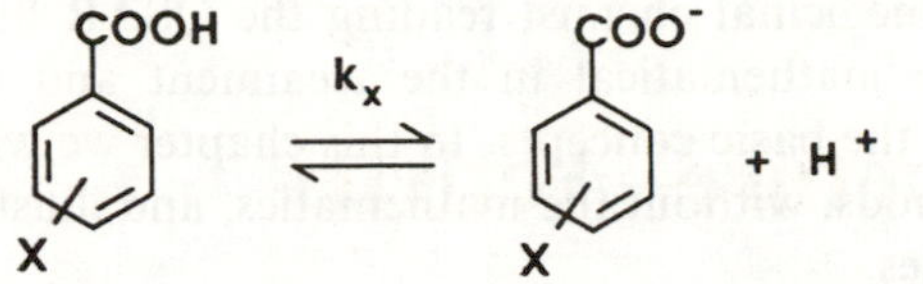

$$\log k_X/k_H = \sigma \cdot \rho$$

Figure 1: *Hammett used the ionisation constant of benzoic acids as the standard reaction for defining the σ scale, i.e. ρ = 1 by definition*

physical state of those lipids. This was the first indication that lipophilicity was important in controlling biological effect.

The potential importance of ionisation was demonstrated by Albert in 1939.[8] He showed that, for a series of acridines, their antiseptic action depended upon the proportion of cationic form in solution and, once allowance had been made for the differing pK_as of the series, all compounds studied showed similar activities.

Physical organic chemistry provided the descriptors for electronic effects and steric effects in the 1940s and 1950s with the work of Hammett[9] and Taft.[10,11] Hammett demonstrated that the electronic effect of a substituent, σ, on an aromatic system was a function of the substituent, and the sensitivity of the particular organic reaction, ρ, to the electronic effect, (Figure 1).

Taft was able to parameterise substituent effects of aliphatic systems by studying the effect of substituents upon the acid- and base-catalysed hydrolysis of esters. Because the acid-catalysed hydrolysis of esters is virtually independent of the electronic effect of the substituent, and only depends upon its steric influence, he was able to extract a similar substituent constant σ* and also the steric effect of the substituent, which he termed E_s.

Hansch's contribution was to realise that it was unlikely that one property alone would be enough to describe biological activity, but that a multi-parameter approach was needed. He utilised the σ and E_s parameters of Hammett and Taft to describe electronic and steric effects and created a new substituent constant π, defined in a similar way to Hammett and Taft's σs, for the difference between the n-octanol–water partition coefficient for the substituted and unsubstituted benzene. Later the use of π was discontinued because it did not take into account the effects that close proximity of substituents could have upon their lipophilicity contribution. He applied the statistical procedure multiple linear regression to identify relationships between biological activity and the lipophilic, electronic and steric properties of molecules. Many data sets were identified where biological activity could be described by linear relationships with these physical properties[12] and many data sets where a non-linear dependence upon π was observed.[13] In order to describe this, $(\pi)^2$ terms were also included in the regression analysis. Hansch hypothesised that in order for a drug to reach its receptor it must pass many lipophilic membrane barriers and on its way may be bound specifically or non-specifically to blood or membrane proteins, or partition into fat stores. This transport rate would then be limiting upon the activity observed for the drug. Hansch termed this the 'random walk' of the drug to the receptor.

Since Hansch's pioneering work QSAR has come a long way, and many new statistical descriptors and techniques have been introduced, so that now it can be confusing or off-putting to the medicinal chemist reading the QSAR literature. Many statistical texts are quite mathematical in the treatment and make it incredibly difficult to understand the basic concepts. In this chapter we will try to describe the concepts of the methods, without the mathematics, and illustrate the techniques with literature examples.

2 SAR *vs* QSAR ?

What are the advantages to the medicinal chemist of QSAR? The SAR approach is intuitively appealing and often successful, but in general relies on pair-wise comparisons of the activity of compounds of interest. This approach makes no allowance for errors in the measure of biological activity and for outliers, *i.e.* compounds that show unusually high or low activity and which are difficult to identify. Changes in structure cause changes in a number of physical properties at once and pairwise comparisons make it difficult to identify which of these properties is most likely to be controlling activity.

In contrast QSAR generally considers the data-set as a whole. The method assumes that biological error exists, but as long as the error is small compared with the range of biological activities the QSAR approach can be successful. Outliers can generally be easily identified and dealt with appropriately. Often the outlier, if it is a true outlier and not some spurious result from the screening, can be very informative. It is likely that this compound contains uniqueness that is important for the receptor in a positive or negative sense. QSAR can ensure that the compounds synthesised cover as wide a diversity of structure as possible (*i.e.* that the property space has been well spanned.) Finally if the correlation with activity can be made then this can often be used to give a mechanistic interpretation of the biological activity and can always be used predictively to guide the optimisation of activity.

The commonest statistical tools are indicated in Table 1. They can be divided into two classes, *pattern recognition techniques*, which can be used to identify how compounds group in property space, or how the descriptors group if intercorrelation exists in the x-descriptor set, and *correlation methods*, which identify quantitative relationships between these x-descriptors and biological activity and are the workhorses of QSAR methods.

Table 1: *Commonly used statistical methods*

Pattern recognition	Correlation analysis
Cluster Analysis	Multiple Linear Regression
Principal Component Analysis	Principal Components Regression
Non-linear Mapping	Partial Least Squares Regression
Neural Networks	Neural Networks

Hansch first used multiple linear regression (MLR) and it is still the most widely used statistical tool in QSAR today. But MLR is limited to using less than

20 parameters (although this does depend on the numbers of compounds in the set) because of the risk of finding chance correlations. It assumes that the descriptors are all independent of each other (*i.e.* they are not correlated) and that they are all important to activity. In many cases all these rules are broken.[14] Often the descriptors are intercorrelated, sometimes because the descriptors are chemically related but often by chance. This can lead to multiple statistically similar MLR models which can be chemically misleading. Often too many descriptors are used which increases the risk of finding a chance correlation. In the 1980s the growing use of computers to calculate properties of molecules led to a plethora of descriptors that could be used in QSAR analysis including MO energies, partial atomic charges, dipole moments, molar volumes, surface areas, *etc*. With more than a few descriptors, intercorrelation can cause problems for MLR, as indicated above. Techniques such as principal components analysis, principal components regression (use of extracted components in an MLR), and factor analysis (similar to PCA/PCR) were beginning to be utilised. More recently the method of partial least squares analysis has been introduced specifically for QSAR problems and is finding widespread applicability.

The role of the statistical method is to identify correlations between physical properties (descriptors) and activity. It has to give confidence that the correlation identified could not have arisen by chance, *i.e.* to show that there is a real relationship between physical properties and activity.

3 LINEAR REGRESSION AND MULTIPLE LINEAR REGRESSION

It is relatively easy to draw a straight line through a set of points. Linear regression routines will calculate the 'line of best fit' through the data. This line

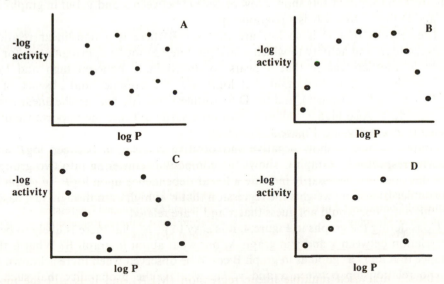

Figure 2: *Graphs A-D datasets show low or zero r^2 values between x and y*

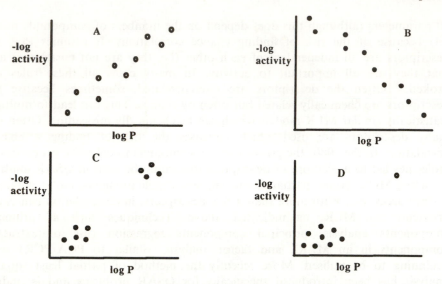

Figure 3: *Graphs A–D datasets show high or unit r^2 values between x and y*

ensures that there is equal residual variation above and below the line. How well the line summarises the data is described by the coefficient of variation, the r^2 value. This varies from 0 for no correlation between x and y to 1.0 for perfect fit of the line to the data. (In some published regressions the correlation coefficient, r, is quoted instead of r^2. This is probably because r, being the square root of r^2, is always bigger and so makes the correlation appear better!) Inspection of r^2 alone can be misleading. The observation that the r^2 value is low or zero does not necessarily indicate that there is no relation between x and y. For example, in Figure 2 all four data-sets show a low or zero r^2 between x and y, but in graphs B, C, and D there obviously is a relationship.

The reasons that r^2 is so low are that for B there is a non-linear relation between $\log P$ and activity to which a straight line cannot be approximated, for C there is another feature that appears to discriminate between high and low activity that is more important that $\log P$ (*e.g.* the presence and absence of a methyl group for instance), and for D an outlier is heavily biasing the linear best-fit procedure. Also high r^2 values do not necessarily indicate the importance of a variable to activity, *e.g.* Figure 3.

Graphs A and B show negative and positive correlation between $\log P$ and activity respectively. Graph C shows the compounds clustering into two groups, but this does not necessarily indicate a linear dependence upon $\log P$. In graph D the outlier so heavily weights the regression that r^2 is high even though, just based on this data, one would not guess that x and y are related.

Considering the graphs in Figure 4, it is easy to guess that there is likely to be a correlation between x and y in graph A, but what about in graph B? What is the chance that an r^2 as good as in graph B could be observed when there is known to be no relationship between x and y, *i.e.* what is the probability that such a relationship could have arisen by chance?

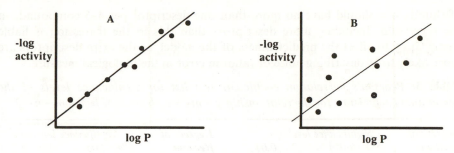

Figure 4: *In graph A there is a strong relationship between x and y, but what about graph B?*

A simulation with a large enough set of random variables can give an indication of such levels of chance. Table 2 shows the results from correlating 999 columns of random numbers for 10 compounds with the 1000th column of random numbers which we shall call the biological activity.

It can be seen that most of the columns show very low r^2 values, but from this sample of 1000 columns, four columns show an r^2 of 0.7–0.8 and two 0.8–0.9! From this example we may guess that two times out of every 999 one could obtain a correlation with an r^2 value of 0.8–0.9 when no causal relationship exists between x and y, *i.e.* the correlation is just a chance correlation. Statisticians know about these levels of chance or significance, and much of statistics is based on such knowledge of the distribution of errors.

Table 2: *Distribution table showing the results from taking 999 sets of 10 random numbers and correlating with the 1000th set of random numbers to simulate the likelihood of chance correlation in linear regression.*

r^2 range	0–0.1	0.1–0.2	0.2–0.3	0.3–0.4	0.4–0.5	0.5–0.6	0.6–0.7	0.7–0.8	0.8–0.9	0.9–1.0
No. of columns in range	616	187	90	47	37	12	3	5	2	0

Most statisticians are willing to accept a correlation that is good enough to ensure that, on average, it could only have arisen by chance one time in 20 or better (5% significance level). For example tabulations of critical levels of r^2 suggest that for 10 compounds one would need $r^2 > 0.4$ to assure a significant correlation at 5% level, and $r^2 > 0.59$ at 1% level (the Pearson's correlation test lists significance levels of the correlation coefficient r, Table 3). The simulation just described gave 59 out of 999 columns with $r^2 > 0.4$ (5.9%) and 10 out of 999 (1.001%) with $r^2 > 0.6$, in good agreement with statistical theory.

In multiple linear regression, another variable is included that can hopefully describe a significant amount of the residual variation about the correlation of the previous variable/s with y. Obviously the more variables included in a regression the better the model describes the data. For 10 compounds, 10 descriptors could describe the data perfectly (one for each compound). As a rule of thumb, one should have no more than one descriptor per 4–5 compounds in the regression. Including more descriptors than this in the regression is liable significantly to affect the predictiveness of the model, as the extra descriptors are more likely to be describing noise or random error in the biological measure.

Table 3: *Pearson's correlation coefficient test list for significance levels of the correlation coefficient r for the relationship y = mx + c, degrees of freedom = n − 2*

Degrees of freedom	Significance level of r		Degrees of freedom	Significance level of r	
	5% (0.05)	1% (0.01)		5% (0.05)	1% (0.01)
2	0.950	0.990	11	0.553	0.684
3	0.878	0.959	12	0.532	0.661
4	0.811	0.917	13	0.514	0.641
5	0.754	0.875	14	0.497	0.623
6	0.707	0.834	15	0.482	0.606
7	0.666	0.798	20	0.423	0.537
8	0.632	0.765	30	0.349	0.449
9	0.602	0.735	40	0.304	0.393
10	0.576	0.708	60	0.250	0.325

Multiple linear regression was used to guide the optimisation of the structure activity relationships of a series of calcium channel agonists[15] (Figure 5).

These compounds are of considerable interest for the treatment of heart failure, since calcium plays a central role in excitation–contraction coupling. Increase in intracellular calcium concentration leads to a corresponding increase in the force of contraction. One method of achieving this is to open the cardiac calcium channel. Compounds were tested for their ability to increase the force of contraction of a 1 Hz paced guinea pig atrial strip, and recorded as a concentration of drug to produce 50% of the developed tension of an isoprenaline standard. It was found that substituent changes on the 2-position of the phenyl ring gave the most promising compounds. From an initial test set of 8 compounds the following MLR relationship was identified.

$$\log (\text{force}) = 0.42(\text{fragmental lipophilicity}) + 0.33(B_x) - 1.97$$
$$n = 8; \; r^2 = 0.79; \; F = 9.3 \; p = 0.02; \; sd = 0.24$$

The equation shows that this two variable model described 79% of the overall variation in log (force) from eight points. Beneath the equation are the statistical

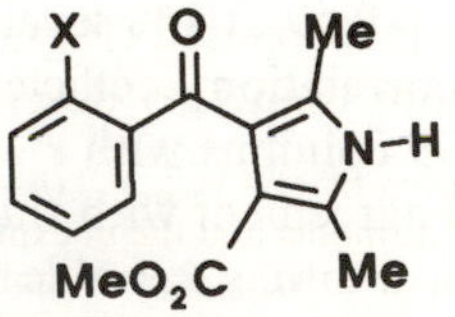

$$X = F, H, Me, Br, I, CF_3, NO_2, OMe, COOMe, -O_2C-(2-HO-C_6H_4)$$

Figure 5: *Use of MLR on a set of calcium channel agonists*

parameters of the model most often quoted in published regression equations; the number of points n, the overall model r^2, the F value, the model significance p and the final residual standard deviation, *i.e.* the average deviation of y values from the final correlation. The 'F' value is used to test the significance of the resulting multiple regression model. In linear regression, significant levels of the correlation coefficient are tabulated, as discussed earlier, but for a multiple regression model r^2 alone does not take into consideration the number of terms in the regression equation. The F test represents a generalised test of model significance for multiple regression models containing any number of cases and variables. By definition it is the ratio of the variation in y explained by the model to the unexplained residual variation in y.* In the crudest sense, the larger F, the more likely the model is significant. From tabulations of significant levels of F, the model above was found to be significant at the 2% level, *i.e.* only two times in 100 would one expect to find an eight-point, two variable multiple regression model as good as this to arise by chance. Most multiple regression packages list the model significance directly.

The equation showed that most of the observed activity changes could be explained by considering the steric bulk of the substituent and its lipophilicity. This correlation led to the suggestion to synthesise the benzyl substituent, which was discovered to be a very potent calcium channel agonist.

4 DESIGNING THE INITIAL SYNTHETIC TARGETS – CLUSTER ANALYSIS

The calcium channel agonist dataset was an example where MLR proved successful, but MLR under certain circumstances can give confusing results. Intercorrelation of the original descriptor set is often the reason for this. In the calcium channel receptor example, the initial synthetic targets were carefully chosen so that the descriptors were not correlated. Hence each was describing a 'unique' physicochemical feature of the compound set, and amongst the eight compounds they spread across the property space as widely as possible. In this case a unique MLR solution will be identified if one or any of the descriptors prove relevant. But how can one ensure that when picking the initial synthetic targets, the physical properties being varied are uncorrelated and spread across property space as widely as possible with the least number of compounds? If one is trying to consider only two descriptors, for instance $\log P$ and σ, then a plot of $\log P$ *vs* σ can be used to pick substituents that effectively cover this 2-D property space causing $\log P$ and σ to be uncorrelated (Figure 6.)

When one is considering more than two descriptors this graphical approach

---

* The total variation/variance in y is given by $(y - y_{mean})^2 / (n-1)$. In regression the total y variance is partitioned between that explained by the model and the unexplained residual variation.
Explained variation in $y = (y_{predicted} - \text{mean of } y_{predicted})^2 / \text{number of variables in regression model}$
Unexplained variation in $y = (y_{predicted} - y_{observed})^2 / (n - \text{number of variables in regression model} - 1)$
$F = $ explained variation in y / unexplained residual variation in y
In this case, $F = 9.3$, the critical level of F at the 5% level with two and five degrees of freedom is 5.79 and at the 1% level 13.27. The computer program generating the model computed the significance to be 2%.

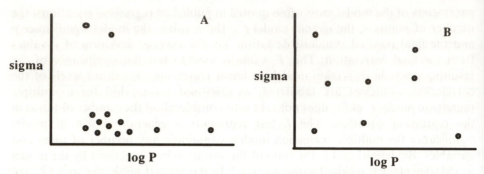

Figure 6: *Graph A exemplifies a bad experimental design where 2-D property space is not well covered with too many compounds with too similar properties. Graph B shows a good example: properties are well spread with low correlation between the two descriptors*

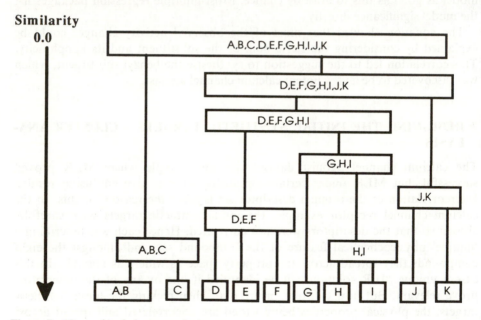

Figure 7: *Hierarchical cluster analysis*

becomes quite cumbersome. A number of pattern recognition techniques have been used to aid target selection, and one of the most useful is cluster analysis.[16,17] This technique aims to group compounds together that appear similar based on the physical property descriptors being considered. Cluster analysis is the generic title for a wide number of different but related techniques. Hierarchical cluster analysis starts off with the assumption that all compounds are in the same group, *i.e.* all are similar, as measured by some similarity criterion. In a stepwise fashion it then makes its similarity cut-off more and more stringent and so splits the set up into smaller and smaller groups (Figure 7). At the extreme, each compound is in its own group. In between these two extremes one can choose a number of different splitting levels giving a number of different groups. The usual approach is to take a substituent database which may contain 100s of substituents and cluster to get the same number of groups as the number of compounds you initially want to synthesise. In the calcium channel data set described above this was eight. One can then simply pick a substituent from each group. This should ensure that the eight compounds spread the property space as widely as possible. One should also check that the descriptor sets for these eight compounds are still not correlated and they can then be synthesized.

5 PROGRESSIVE METHODS – PRINCIPAL COMPONENTS ANALYSIS (PCA)/ PRINCIPAL COMPONENTS REGRESSION (PCR)

As mentioned previously, when more than a few descriptors are used in MLR one can run into problems because of chance correlations between the descriptors leading to more than one MLR model being extracted. A number of approaches can be taken to identify the intercorrelations in the descriptor set and to use these to identify new variables that can summarise the information content of the descriptor set in a far smaller number of descriptors. One such technique is PCA. In Table 4, the price, top speed, acceleration (0–60), and brake horse power is given on four cars, a Maclaren F1 racing car (estimated), a Ford RS Cosworth, a Ford Escort XR3i, and a Lada Riva.

Table 4: *Data on four cars*

Model	Price/£	Top speed/mph	0–60 mph/s	bhp
MacLaren F1	2 000 000*	180 + *	3.0*	470*
Ford RS Cosworth	24 000	140	5.7	227
Ford escort XR3i	12 500	115	10.6	105
Lada riva	4 000	95	14	66

* estimated

As can easily be seen just by inspection, all these four descriptors are strongly correlated. We could replace all four by a new descriptor, engine performance, which in one way or another all the original descriptors were measuring. This is basically what PCA does. It identifies 'underlying' descriptors which best summarise the information content of the original descriptor block. To a greater or lesser extent all descriptors make some contribution to the component extraction. Figure 8 shows this in graphical terms.

The three descriptors, in this case $\log P$, molar volume, and MR, are strongly related. The principal component would be a vector on this graph that passes through as much of the data as possible and is shown as PC1. In the graphical sense it corresponds to a rotation and translation of the axes that are our frame of reference for looking at the data. Subsequent components are identified as orthogonal directions to PC1 so they investigate directions that are independent of, *i.e.* non-correlated to, PC1 *etc.* This one vector can be used to replace the

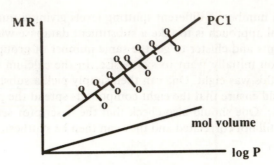

Figure 8: *3-D Graph showing how compounds spread over logP, molar volume, and MR and their projection onto a new summary variable, Principle Component 1 (PC1)*

Table 5: *Training set for pyrethroid insecticides*

R^1	R^2	R^3	R^4	R^5	R^6
Me	F	F	F	F	F
Cl	F	F	F	F	F
Me	Me	Me	Me	Me	Me
Cl	Me	Me	Me	Me	Me
Me	H	I	H	H	H
Cl	H	I	H	H	H
Me	H	NO_2	H	NO_2	H
Cl	H	NO_2	H	NO_2	H
Me	Cl	NO_2	H	NO_2	Cl
Cl	Cl	NO_2	H	NO_2	Cl
Me	H	NO_2	H	H	H
Cl	H	NO_2	H	H	H
Cl	H	OPh	H	H	H

original three in any subsequent correlation analysis.

PCA generates two pieces of information, the PC scores and the PC loadings for each component. The PC scores are the values each compound takes on this new descriptor (the projections of the compounds onto this new axis). The PC loadings tell the relation of each of the original descriptors to the new extracted component; it tells how important each of the original descriptors was in defining each component. Close examination of the PC loadings can sometimes allow the meaning of the component to be identified.

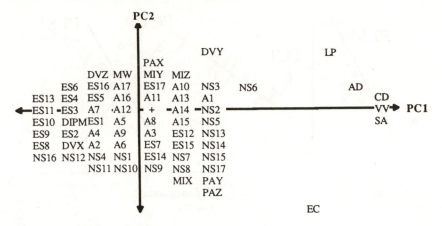

Figure 9: *Plot of the loadings of the 70 descriptors onto PC1 and PC2 for a set of 13 pyrethroid insecticides*

Ford and Livingstone used PCA/PCR methods in their study of a set of pyrethroid insecticides[18] (Table 5). The synthetic targets were chosen using cluster analysis considering log$P$, electronic field and resonance descriptors and MR, so that these properties were only weakly correlated and well spread across the property space. A descriptor set of 70 properties were calculated covering 51 atom specific parameters (partial atomic charges, electrophilic and nucleophilic superdelocalisabilities for the 19 core atoms) and 19 traditional QSAR descriptors including dipole moments and vectors, van der Waals radius, surface areas, moments of inertia, principal ellipsoid axes, log$P$ etc. The data set contains 19 whole molecule descriptors and 51 partial electronic descriptors which would dominate principal component extraction by their sheer numbers if not dealt with appropriately. We have calculated principal components after scaling the dataset in a blockwise fashion to give each type of descriptor a fair chance of contributing to the model.

Principal components analysis extracted four components which together described 83% of the information of the original 70 variables (PC1 described 36.1%, PC2, PC3, and PC4 described a further 23.7, 17.1, and 9.3% respectively). The loadings of the original variables upon PC1 and PC2 are shown in Figure 9. It can be seen that the whole molecule descriptors log$P$, apparent diameter, collision diameter, van der Waals volume, and surface area load heavily on the positive end of PC1. It appears that this component largely describes the overall bulk of the compounds. For PC2 the electron–electron repulsion energy and total energy load high and positive on PC2 whereas EC loads high and negative. These components can now be used in MLR.

6 PARTIAL LEAST SQUARES (PLS) ANALYSIS

The technique of Partial Least Squares can be considered as a hybrid between principal components analysis and multiple regression. Instead of extracting underlying components that best describe the *x*-block as in PCA in PLS they are

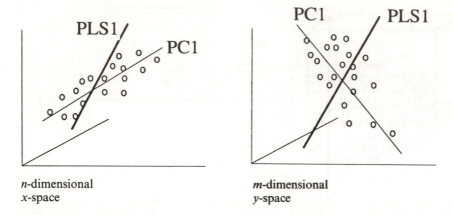

n-dimensional
x-space

m-dimensional
y-space

Figure 10: *3-D representation of the difference between PCA and PLS. Principal components of the x- and y-spaces are 'rotated' so as to maximise their intercorrelation*

extracted to summarise x and be as highly correlated with y as possible (or with the underlying components of the y-space if more than one y is included). The significance of the extracted components is generally not tested by traditional significance tests as in MLR.

In PLS, compounds of the training set are left out of the component extraction process, and the activities of the left out compounds are predicted by the model. In reality the model is recalculated a number of times, and at each step one or more compounds are left out, so that overall each compound is left out once. The errors between the predicted and observed values for the left out compounds are used to generate a prediction statistic, the PRESS value (Predicted Sum of Squares) to describe the predictiveness of the statistical model. This technique, known as cross-validation, is more powerful than traditional statistical approaches based on assumed distribution of errors and is inherently more useful to QSAR as the model is always tested on how well the model predicts. Figure 10 shows the conceptual difference between principal components analysis and partial least squares. Partial least squares is a very powerful statistical technique, and one on which CoMFA, one of the newest and the most powerful QSAR techniques, depends.

7 3-D QSAR METHODS

The CoMFA approach was developed by Cramer and co-workers,[19] is only available in the SYBYL suite of software, and is an example of what are now known as 3-D QSAR methods. The approach of CoMFA is intuitively different from all other approaches to QSAR and is based on the statistical analysis of the 3-D interaction fields. These are generated by measuring over a regular 3-D grid the interaction energy between a small probe atom or group and the drug targets.

Initially the 3-D structures of the training set of compounds are aligned based on common molecular features so as to occupy the same volume of space. The interaction energies of the small probe, in CoMFA usually a methyl group with

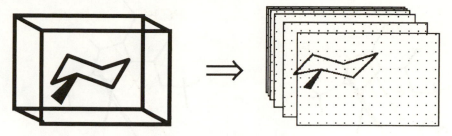

Figure 11: *The generation of interaction fields in CoMFA approach*

unit positive charge, is measured with each of the training set compounds at each grid co-ordinate in space (Figure 11).

The interaction energies at each GRID point in space become descriptors in a QSAR analysis. CoMFA normally considers the steric and electrostatic energies separately. It is possible to end up with a data table containing several hundred or even thousands of descriptors in the analysis. PLS is used to find correlations with these points in space and activity. The resulting regression equation relates the importance of each point in space in describing y and can be mapped back onto the 3-D structures generating 3-D steric and electrostatic regression maps. These maps represent regions in space around the overlayed molecules where it is favourable and unfavourable for the drugs to pick up on electrostatic and steric interactions with 'the receptor'.

CoMFA fields are the default 3-D fields in the CoMFA program, but other 3-D field sources can also be used, for example 3-D fields from the program GRID[20] which explicitly codes for hydrogen bonding as well as electrostatic and steric interactions or electrostatic isopotential maps. Also other more traditional QSAR descriptors can be included with these 3-D fields. Figure 12 shows the results from a 3-D QSAR analysis of 36 calcium channel agonists, varying in the 2-position of the phenyl ring as described previously.[21]

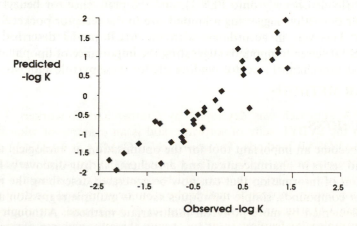

Figure 12: *Plot of observed $-\log K$ vs. predicted $-\log K$ from 36 compound GRID–PLS model, $r^2 = 0.86$*

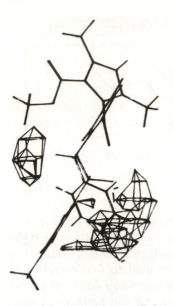
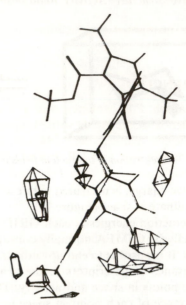

(a) positive regression coefficients   (b) negative regression coefficients

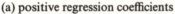

Figure 13: *Results of PLS analysis using whole molecule descriptors and GRID fields on the calcium channel agonists data-set. Regions of positive (a) and negative (b) regression coefficients displayed over the structures containing the benzyl substituent (a highly active compound) and the p-toluenesulphonyl substituent (a weakly active compound) from the calcium channel agonist data-set*

Fields from the GRID program were used because these include hydrogen bonding as well as steric and electrostatic interaction contributions to the overall interaction energy. Also whole molecule descriptors for log$P$ and MR were included. PLS analysis extracted four significant components, and the overall regression maps are shown in Figure 13. This suggested the importance of lipophilicity (loaded heavily onto PLS 1), and the preference for benzyl and its isosteres over phenethyl suggesting a limited size to the receptor pocket for these compounds. This was in accordance with the MLR model described earlier derived from far fewer compounds suggesting the importance of lipophilicity and size to the calcium channel receptor binding site for these pyrrole agonists.

8 CONCLUSIONS

QSAR has become an important tool for the optimisation of 'biological activity' in compound series in pharmaceutical and agrochemical drug discovery. Because of the amount of information that can now be generated describing the physical properties of compounds, simple techniques such as multiple regression are now being complemented by more powerful multivariate methods. Although mathematically these techniques are complicated conceptually they are not, and it is these concepts we have tried to clarify. A more detailed description of all the techniques mentioned can be found in the books of Manley[21] and Flury and Riedwyl.[22]

9 REFERENCES

1. C. Hansch, P.P. Maloney, and T. Fujita, Correlation of Biological Activity of Phenoxyacetic Acids with Hammett Substituent Constants and Partition Coefficients. *Nature*, 1962, **194**, 178.
2. A. Crum-Brown, and T.R. Frazer, *Trans. R. Soc. Edinburgh*, 1868, **25**, 151.
3. B.J. Richardson, *Medical Times and Gazette* 1868, **2**, 703.
4. C. Richet, *C.R. Seances Soc. Biol.* 1893, **9**, 775.
5. C.E. Overton, *Studien uber die Narkose, Jugleich ein Beitrag zue Allgemeinen Pharmakologie*, G. Fischer; Jena, 1901.
6. C.E. Overton, 'Studies of Narcosis', Chapman and Hall, London, Wood Library–Museum of Anaesthesiology, 1993.
7. H. Meyer, *Arch.F. Experim. Pathol. und Pharmakol.*,1899, **42**, 109.
8. A. Albert, S.D. Rubbo, R.J. Goldacre, M.E. Davey, and J.D. Stone, *Br. J. Exp. Pathol.* ,1945, **26**, 160.
9. L.P. Hammett, Physical Organic Chemistry; Reaction Rates, Equilibra and Mechanism, 2nd Edn., McGraw-Hill, New York, 1970.
10. R.W. Taft and I.C. Lewis, *J. Amer. Chem. Soc.*, 1959 **81**, 5343.
11. R.W. Taft, 'Steric Effects in Organic Chemistry', Wiley, New York, 1956, pp. 556.
12. C. Hansch and W.J. Dunn III, *J. Pharm. Sci.*, 1972, **61**, 1.
13. C. Hansch and J.M. Clayton, *J. Pharm. Sci.,* 1973, **62**, 1.
14. J.G. Topliss and R.O. Edwards, *J. Med. Chem.*, 1979, **22**, 1238.
15. A.J.G. Baxter, J. Dixon, F. Ince, C. N. Manners, and S. J. Teague, *J. Med. Chem.*, 1993, **36**, 2739.
16. W.J. Dunn, M.J. Greenberg, and S.S. Callejas, *J. Med. Chem.*, 1976, **19**, 1299.
17. C. Hansch, S.H. Unger, and A.B. Forsythe, *J. Med. Chem.*, 1973, **16**, 1217.
18. M.G. Ford and D.J. Livingstone, *Quant. Struct.-Act. Relat.*, 1990, **9**, 107.
19. R.D. Cramer, D.E. Patterson, and J.D. Bunce, *J. Amer. Chem. Soc.*, 1988, **110**, 5959.
20. P.J. Goodford, *J. Med. Chem.*, 1985, **28**, 849.
21. A. M. Davis, N. P. Gensmantel, E. Johannson, and D. P. Marriott, *J. Med. Chem.*, 1994, **37**, 963.
22. B.F.J. Manly, 'Multivariate Statistical Methods, A Primer', Chapman and Hall, London, 1986.
23. B. Flury and H. Riedwyl, 'Multivariate Statistics – A Practical Approach', Chapman and Hall, London, 1988.

CHAPTER 9

Considerations for the Use of Computational Chemistry Techniques by Medicinal Chemists

MIKE M. HANN

1 INTRODUCTION

Computational Chemistry has been defined by Tony Hopfinger, one of the early exponents of the subject, as 'the quantitative modelling of chemical behaviour on a computer by the formalisms of theoretical chemistry'.[1] Theoretical chemistry is that branch of chemistry based on finding theories to describe experimentally measured quantities. Computational chemistry is the implementation of algorithms on a computer to exploit these theories for the prediction of measurable and unmeasurable properties. The following subjects would all be considered to be relevant to computational chemistry: Quantum Mechanics, Molecular Mechanics, Molecular Dynamics, Conformational Analysis, Molecular Graphics, Databases of structure and sequences, Computer Aided Molecular Design (CAMD), Quantitative Structure Activity Relationships (QSAR). All these techniques are available to medicinal chemists to aid in the overall objective that medicinal chemists have – that is the discovery and development of a chemical lead into a drug candidate by optimisation of the required biological profile through alterations to its chemical structure. The consideration of, and possible use of, all available tools in this search is the hallmark of good medicinal chemistry. On this basis it seems very appropriate that the Canterbury Medicinal Chemistry Course has contained computational chemistry as part of its core teaching material for the last eight years.

The majority of chemists who are recruited into the pharmaceutical and agrochemical industries have a very strong background in synthetic organic chemistry. They are then expected to learn the skills of a medicinal chemist through 'on the job' training and attendance at workshops. Many synthetic organic chemists chose that branch of chemistry because they either enjoy the practical synthetic work, the challenge of synthetic ingenuity or perhaps were uncomfortable with the more mathematical aspects of other branches of chemistry. In order to make aspects of theoretical chemistry more available to such chemists we have had to wait for the availability of computers with graphical interfaces and appropriate software for them to be able to make use of these techniques. It is now clear that computational chemistry is accepted as a part of medicinal chemistry. Browsing through any recent copy of the *Journal of Medicinal Chemistry* will show the contribution that is now being made by

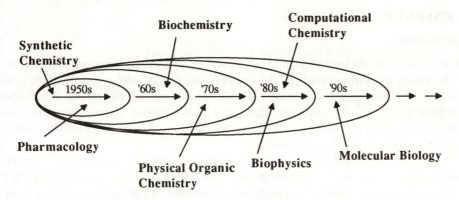

Figure 1: *The shifting and expanding ground of Medicinal Chemistry*

computational chemistry in medicinal chemistry projects. Figure 1 illustrates how the subject matter of medicinal chemistry has both shifted and expanded over the last few decades to become a truly interdisciplinary subject.

Synthetic organic chemistry is principally concerned with synthesising molecules and is therefore centred on intramolecular or covalent chemistry. On the other hand, as we learn more about drug–receptor interactions it is clear that it is intermolecular or non-covalent interactions which determine the activity of most drugs. Thus rates of dissolution, passage of molecules through membranes, and interaction of molecules with most receptors is principally governed by non-covalent forces. The use of theoretical techniques to assist in the understanding of these complex forces is one of the important roles that computational chemistry can play in a medicinal chemistry project. With this in mind, chemists who are specialists in making and breaking bonds and who want to learn more about intermolecular forces may want to add computational chemistry to their repertoire. Some will be happy to use it in a 'black box' manner while others will want to learn more of the underlying principles. Some may only feel comfortable if the work is done by an 'expert'. Whatever the need or preference, it is important that synthetic chemists learn some aspects of what computational chemistry can do in order for them to operate effectively as medicinal chemists. Even if they want an 'expert' to do the work they will need to know some of the jargon to be able to communicate effectively and know what questions to ask. If they want to use a black box approach they will still need to know the principles and be given suitable guidelines for usage. Additionally they will have to maintain a cautious scepticism for the results and ensure that they will always ask the question: *does it make sense* and *can I test the hypothesis through experimental work?*

With the above thoughts in mind, this chapter is written with the intention of giving medicinal chemists with little knowledge of computation chemistry some insight into the computational chemist's jargon and what it means.

2 ENERGY CALCULATIONS

Introduction

One of the most important techniques which underpins computational chemistry is the ability to perform energy calculations. The role of energy calculations is to quantify interactions inside and outside molecules which reflect molecular properties. To do this, both covalent and non-covalent interactions must be considered. However, before describing the techniques that are available, some general *caveats* should be considered.

Algorithms invariably have approximations with them (parameters, computational approximations *etc.*) which means that results of computational chemistry calculations should always be considered in the light of the approximations used. This is somewhat akin to ensuring that the errors in experimental measurements are not ignored. Another consideration is that accuracy and correctness should not be confused – computers will calculate incorrect answers as accurately as you want! A more subtle point is that some properties of molecules which can be calculated are not directly comparable to observable data; *e.g.* electrostatic potential fields cannot be observed. It is therefore important to ensure that testable hypotheses are constructed – and that they are tested! Finally, in these caveats, it is worth remembering that biological measurements usually reflect free energy changes while the majority of computational chemistry energy calculations have, until recently, calculated only enthalpies and ignored entropic contributions to the system. Similarly the possibility of solvent effects, either explicit or as continuum models, have only recently begun to be included in many calculations.

Quantum Mechanics

Quantum mechanics is one method by which we can calculate the energies of a system. Central to the technique is the solution to Schrödinger's equation, $H\psi = E\psi$, for the system being studied.[2] H is the Hamiltonian operator by which the energy E of the molecular wave function ψ is described and can be calculated. The equation is actually a set of differential equations with the solutions being a number of molecular orbitals ψ_j, each corresponding to a quantised energy, E_j. The majority of techniques used to solve this equation are based on the linear combination of atomic orbitals (LCAO) method: the molecular orbital description of the wave function ψ is replaced according to the equation $\psi_j = \Sigma_{ij}\phi$, where ψ_j are molecular orbitals, ϕ are atomic orbitals and c_{ij} are coefficients. The atomic orbitals themselves are often described by Slater type orbitals (STO) which are approximated by Gaussian functions – thus for example an STO-3G basis set has three Gaussian functions to describe each atomic orbital. The set of simultaneous differential equations which results from the application of these approximations is solved by iteration to self consistency of the coefficients. This means that the electron distribution in the orbitals defined by the basis set is such that the energy of the system defined by the nuclear positions is at a minimum. If variation of the nuclear positions is also allowed, then minimum energy geometries can be found.

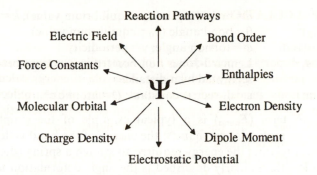

Figure 2: *Properties that can be derived from the wave function*

In order to speed up the calculations and/or to make them more tractable, further approximations can be made. These give rise to the so called semi-empirical calculations in which some of the computationally intense elements of the Hamiltonian are replaced by parameters which are based on experimental data. These parameters have been optimised to reproduce experimental geometries and heats of formation, *etc.* An example of such a program in common usage is MOPAC[3] and, using a modern workstation, a typical drug sized molecule can be geometry-optimised in just a few minutes. *Ab initio* calculations, in which no experimental data are incorporated, are much slower to run but with care give more correct results for energies and geometries. Examples of such programs in common usage are Gaussian,[4] GAMESS,[5] and CADPAC.[6] In addition to the geometry-optimised nuclear positions, all molecular orbital programs will give a description of the total wavefunction of the molecule, ψ. The accuracy of this wavefunction is dependent on the approximations used in the description of the Hamiltonian and also the degree of sophistication used in describing the atomic orbitals through the basis sets.

The total wavefunction can be used to gain access to all chemical properties – obviously the correctness of these properties also depends on the accuracy with which the wave function was calculated in the first place. Figure 2 illustrates some of the properties that can be derived from the wavefunction; again it should be remembered that not all of these are directly measurable.

Molecular Mechanics

In contrast to the complexity of quantum mechanics, the methods of molecular mechanics are conceptually easier to understand.[7] The energy of the system is described by partitioning it into different components which can be independently calculated. A typical molecular mechanics force field description is as follows:

$E_{str} = k(d - d_0)^2$ d = bond length (d_0 = equilibrium value); k = constant

$E_{angle} = k(\theta - \theta_0)^2$ θ = bond angle (θ_0 = equilibrium value)

$E_{tors} = k(1 + \cos(v\omega))$ ω = torsion angle; v = periodicity

$E_{vdw} = B/r^{12} - A/r^6$ Lennard-Jones non-bonded interactions between atoms separated by a distance r

$E_{elec} = Q_1 Q_2 / 4\pi\varepsilon\, r$ ε = dielectric constant; Q = atomic charge

The bond length term (E_{bond}) is a typical example of the simplicity of the description used in molecular mechanics; the energy of the bond is described by a Hooke's law term relating the energy required to stretch a spring (the bond) from its equilibrium length. Similarly described is the angle deformation term (E_{angle}). The torsional term (E_{tors}) is used to approximate conjugation effects which have no direct macroscopic equivalent because they reflect the electronic interactions which are only effectively treated quantum mechanically. The van der Waals non-bonded interactions (E_{vdw}) can be described by a Lennard-Jones 6–12 potential; the r^6 term is the attractive term and the r^{12} term the repulsive term. The electrostatic energy is described by a classical electrostatic term incorporating a macroscopic description of the dielectric constant.

Underlying all molecular mechanics calculations are the collection of terms such as force constants, strain-free angles and bond lengths, atomic polarisabilities, *etc.* which make up the force field description. Classically these parameters are derived from experimental measurements; *e.g.* bond lengths from *X*-ray crystallography, force constants from microwave and infrared spectroscopy. Often these are now supplemented by, or replaced by, numbers derived from quantum mechanical calculations. Whichever source is used for these parameters, the resulting energies which are calculated are highly dependent on the care that has gone into deriving the parameters and, possibly more important, their transferability between molecular systems. Fortunately for the current generation of molecular mechanics users there are many programs available which have extensive parameterisations for a wide range of molecular systems. Where parameters are missing, generalised parameters are often defaulted to and this, coupled with the ease with which such programs can now be used, means that it is vital to bear in mind the caveats discussed above. Examples of different force fields for molecular mechanics calculations are MM2,[8] AMBER,[9] CHARMM,[10] and CVFF.[11]

Analysis of Conformational Space

Until recently the most extensive use of molecular mechanics and quantum mechanics calculations was the derivation of minimum energy configurations of molecular systems by minimisation. The resulting molecular co-ordinates reflect molecular systems in which all kinetic energy has been removed from the system and therefore correspond to systems at 0 K. This not only gives bond lengths slightly shorter than would be observed at room temperature but means that there is no motion in the system. However, having derived an energy description of a molecular system it is possible to use molecular dynamics to study the time-dependent motional behaviour of the system. If the position of an atom is changed from its minimum energy position then a force will act on that atom. By using Newton's equations of motion this force can be translated into an acceleration and, by integrating over time steps, it is possible to study the change in velocities of the atoms and derive a simulation of the dynamic behaviour of the system. Critical to such simulations are the choice of starting points, the time steps for integration, the temperature, the method of equilibration, and, as ever, the force field. Such simulations might seem to be the panacea for molecular modellers in that they give the opportunity to simulate the molecular motion of complex systems thus giving access to configurational sampling from which entropic contributions to the free energy of the system can be derived. In theory this is true but such simulations are inherently limited by the time steps that can be taken.

In a molecular dynamics simulation based on a molecular mechanics force field, the length of time step that can be taken in the integration steps is limited to about 1 fs (10^{-15} s). Longer time steps than this exceed the periodicity of the vibrations of the highest frequency molecular vibrations (*i.e.* bonds to hydrogen atoms) and therefore destroy the partitioning of energy between vibrational modes. With time steps limited to 1 fs, most molecular simulations have, to date, been limited to hundreds of picoseconds and in some cases nanoseconds.

Table 1 gives time scales of representative and important molecular motions, from which it can be seen that simulations longer those currently available are needed to approach 'useful' time scales. As computers become faster, such simulations will become tractable in the future and the correlation of such long simulations with experimentally derived dynamic data will be an important impetus to further improving force fields.

Although molecular dynamics is currently an inappropriate technique for routinely studying the available conformational states of complex molecular systems, it can be used for small systems. An array of other techniques has also been developed to study the conformational flexibility of molecules.[12] Based on energy calculations, conformational analysis is one of the fundamental techniques that computational chemistry has to offer to medicinal chemists. The aim of conformational analysis is to find accessible conformations, and therefore shapes, of molecules under the conditions and assumptions of the methodology used to quantify the energy of the system.

Table 1: *Illustrative timescales for molecular motions*

Motion	Amplitude (Å)	Time scale
Atomic vibrations	0.01–0.1	fs–ps
Sugar repuckering	2	ps–ns
Protein sidechain torsional changes	5–10	ps–ns
Protein interior torsional changes	5–10	ms–s

Several different techniques have been developed for conformational analysis. The most rigorous entails an exhaustive search of conformational space by systematically varying the torsional angles of the single bonds within a molecule and calculating the energy at each state. Because most molecules of interest have several such bonds, the problem rapidly becomes a combinatorially explosive one. Thus for 6 bonds in a molecule, rotated at 30° at each step, there are $(360/30)^6 = ca.$ 3×10^6 conformations to be accessed; if 10 energy calculations are completed per second then the analysis will still take about 3 days; if energy minimisation is carried out at every conformation the required time will be many times longer.

In contrast, a knowledgeable chemist with a set of plastic models can estimate 'likely' conformations of a molecule in a much shorter time than this – essentially based on experience and observation. If this knowledge could be embedded within an algorithm, there is no need to carry out a computationally expensive energy calculation for obviously unfavourable conformations – for instance, certain combinations of torsional angles will always lead to some atoms overlapping. Such 'knowledge based' systems are now implemented in many conformational search programs and can dramatically improve the speed of conformational searching.[13,14,15] Even so, the systematic evaluation of conformational space can still be prohibitive and techniques which give representative conformations from the total space are often resorted to.

Representative conformations of a molecular system can be derived by a number of techniques. Distance geometry is a technique in which a matrix is built up which contains the upper and lower possible interatomic distances within the molecule.[6] A structure is generated (by a process called embedding) from a random selection of distances which are consistent with the bounds and the structure is then refined to minimise violations of the matrix bounds – additional structures can be found by selecting new random distances. Another method for finding representative structures which again includes a random element is the Metropolis Monte Carlo method. The conformation of an initially low-energy structure is changed by a defined amount and the energy of the new conformation is calculated. If the energy is lower than the initial energy the conformation is accepted or, if it is higher in energy, it will be accepted if the difference in energy ΔE satisfies the condition that a random number between 0 and 1 is less than $\exp(-\Delta E/kT)$.[17] This ensures that a wide range of conformations with a Boltzmann type distribution of energies is found. Ensembles so derived (and also those that come from extensive molecular dynamics calculations) can be used to derive entropic contributions to the free energy of the system. When explicit or continuum solvation models are also included in the description of the system, or the force field, then Monte Carlo of Molecular Dynamics calculations are the most sophisticated calculations currently available to molecular modellers. Quantum mechanics can also be used for such calculations but the length of time required for each energy evaluation is currently prohibitive for most systems of interest to medicinal chemists.

Many techniques have been developed for the analysis of conformations generated by the techniques discussed above. Visual inspection of the low-energy structures with 3D graphics devices is an important first step to gauge the scope of the results; in particular, the dynamic replay of the results of molecular

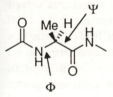

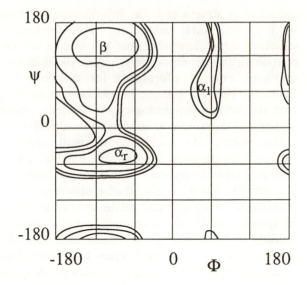

The contours 'enclose' regions of low energy conformations (i.e. β sheet and α helix)

Figure 3: *Example of an energy contour map for rotation about a backbone torsional angles of a peptide unit (Ramachandran plot)*

dynamics trajectories is a particularly striking way of trying to grasp the subtleties of the three-dimensional behaviour of molecules. Additionally conformations can be sorted or clustered by energetic and geometric considerations or the results plotted as the variation of energy with geometry. An example of the latter is the classic Ramachandran plot often used to describe the conformational states allowed for the backbone of a peptide unit but it is just as valid for any molecule (see Figure 3).

Another important technique, which was pioneered by Garland Marshall, is the Active Analogue Approach in which distances within different molecules are compared with the aim of trying to derive the pharmacophore responsible for the activity of a series of compounds.[18] Many variants of this technique have been developed which have been further enhanced by techniques such as Comparative Molecular Field Analysis (CoMFA) in which the steric and electrostatic environments are compared with a view to delineating the regions around the set of molecules which are favourable or unfavourable for interactions with the macromolecular receptor.[19]

3 DATABASES

All theoretical calculations must at some stage be related back to experiment, and large numbers of experimentally determined structures are available from the Cambridge database to aid in this – approximately 120 000 crystal structures can be searched for by substructure or geometric queries.[20] Another important collection of structures is the Brookhaven database of protein structures solved by *X*-ray and NMR techniques.[21] This database currently contains about 1100 structures which represent over 100 unique families of protein folds. While not containing any structural information, databases of protein sequence are also an important pool of information for molecular modellers interested in protein structure. This will become increasingly so as the size of these databases grows with the genome sequencing efforts currently underway and the need to try and understand the structural information embedded within the sequence.[22]

Databases of 3D co-ordinates of small organic molecules are also now being derived from the older 2D files that have traditionally been used as the registry systems within companies. 2D files just contain a description of molecular connectivity, but with the aid of a program like CONCORD[23] it is possible to generate a 3D co-ordinate set in an automated manner for large numbers of compounds. A database containing only one conformation of a molecule is unlikely to be representative of the intermolecular distances accessible to the molecule and therefore techniques have been developed which incorporate an assessment of the likely variance of such distances. One way this can be done is by computing all the likely distances within a molecule by pre-processing the molecules through a conformational analysis. The ranges of distances observed are stored in the database rather than the explicit conformations, as the latter would require enormous amounts of disk space. This is the method implemented with Chem-X.[13]

An alternative approach is to use knowledge from the 2D connection table to give likely upper and lower bounds for a distance of interest within a molecule and then to use fast conformational searching or template forcing techniques to check whether molecules that pass the initial bounds check can actually fit the desired 3D query. These techniques are implemented within the MACCS-3D CFS[24] and Tripos UNITY-3D[25] programs. The program COBRA[26] offers yet another method of automated conformational analysis by the construction of low-energy conformations from fragments and a knowledge base of acceptable joining rules.

4 *DE NOVO* LIGAND DESIGN

With the increasing availability of three-dimensional structures of proteins and other macromolecules relevant to drug discovery projects, there is a new generation of software tools being developed for the analysis of active sites of proteins and the *de novo* design of novel molecular structures to bind them. The program GRID is commonly used to help characterise a binding site.[27] Probe 'atoms' with the properties of, for example, carbonyl oxygens or amidic protons are moved around in the active site on a regular 3D grid and an energy of interaction of the probe with the protein is calculated at each point. When the results are contoured and displayed on a graphics device it is possible to pick out those regions where particular functional groups might be expected to bind. The minimum energy co-ordinate positions of the probes can then be used to search for equivalent positions of real atoms in databases of 3D structures of the type outlined above. Additional programs that have been developed to assist in these types of searches are DOCK[28] and CAVEAT.[29] Once a lead compound has been characterised in its binding mode by *X*-ray analysis then modifications to increase potency or to modify other properties can be contemplated. Programs such as LUDI[30] are designed to help in this process by searching through a database of 3D structures of small organic functional groups and ranking them in terms of their ability to increase binding when appended to the lead at particular points. A more fundamental approach to ligand design is to take, for instance, the GRID points and use a computer program to design from scratch compounds that might fit the steric and electrostatic requirements of the active site. To consider doing this in a truly exhaustive and objective manner is both beyond the scope of current computer power and the 'accuracy' of force fields to predict the correct binding energy. However, by restricting the scope of molecules considered by only using a limited set of building blocks and encoding, within the design algorithm, elements of knowledge about sensible things to try first, it is possible to develop programs which are certainly able to generate molecules with similarities to known inhibitors; the program SPROUT[31] is a good example of this type of approach. Although currently in their infancy, programs of this type are likely to become an important tool in the future for the medicinal chemist who is open minded to new ideas – even those that have come from a computer!

5 MOLECULAR GRAPHICS AND THE VISUALISATION OF MOLE-CULES

The current generation of UNIX workstations with high resolution and stereo display systems has done much to make the techniques discussed above more accessible to medicinal chemists and professional modellers alike. Stephen Hanessian, in a paper entitled 'The psychobiological basis of heuristic synthesis planning,[31] has discussed how the two hemispheres of the brain contribute to two important aspects of synthetic organic chemistry: synthesis planning and retrosynthetic analysis. The left hemisphere of the brain is associated with temporal, rational, and analytical processes which reflect the constructive planning of a synthesis. However, the right side is more involved with visual, spatial, and relational processes which are exactly those which appear to be essential for retrosynthetic analysis. Similarly, the role of molecular modelling in the thought processes of a medicinal chemist can be considered to be a combination of left and right side activities. To the left side would go the analytical results and data from a systematic and objective study of a problem while on the right side our 3D spatial capacity for thought would be fed by the visual and relational information that interactive molecular graphics presents. The productive combination of all these processes stimulates thought which, as Aristotle observed, is impossible without an image.

Computer graphics allow us to translate the results of complex calculations into readily assimilable images which help us to more easily interpret the data. It provides new ways of looking at data and challenging dogma. Who after all, knows what a molecule looks like? All our mental and macroscopic images of molecules are an interpretation within our macro world of events that we can not directly 'see' in the atomic world of molecules. Even with the advent of techniques such as Scanning Tunnelling Microscopy, which allows an atomic probe to 'feel' an individual molecule, we are not 'seeing' a molecule. We have to use false colour and visual conventions of molecular surfaces (*e.g.* CPK) to present the experimental data in our macro world. What computational chemistry and molecular graphics offer us is the opportunity to challenge the conventions and look for new ways of studying and presenting molecular systems. Further evolution of the molecular graphics paradigm to incorporate such techniques as Virtual Reality can only strengthen our links between the atomic and macroscopic world.[33]

However, despite the advantages that molecular graphics brings to the medicinal chemists there is again a caveat that must be discussed. Images can be very powerful and persuasive; the advertising industry has learnt that, even if we haven't. The term WYSIWIG (standing for What You See Is What You Get) was coined to describe word processing systems where, what you see on the screen is what you will get when it is printed – quite a novelty when such systems first appeared! A parody on this expression can be used to describe some misuses of molecular graphics: WYSI NONSENSE – What You See Is NOt Necessarily SciENcE. Just because a graphics picture looks visually compelling it does not mean that the data behind it are valid.

When the surrealist painter Magritte painted a picture of a pipe and wrote underneath it 'Ceci n'est pas une pipe' he was making the point that the picture was not a pipe but a picture of a pipe. However, at least he knew what a pipe looked like. As we do not really know what a molecule looks like the caption to Figure 4 has a very important message. Molecular graphics allow thought to be stimulated by images, but the ideas that arise must be explored through

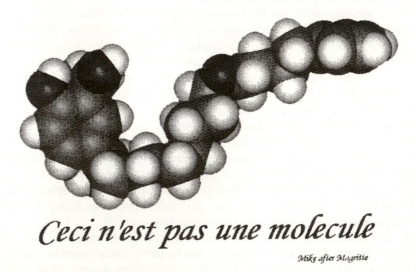

Ceci n'est pas une molecule

Mike after Magritte

Figure 4.   *This is not a molecule*

experiment. Do not expect graphics to give you the answer in black and white (or even colour)!

6 ACKNOWLEDGEMENTS

My thanks to the many colleagues who have contributed over several years to the ideas developed in this chapter.

7 REFERENCES

1. A.J. Hopfinger, *J. Med. Chem.*, 1985, **28**, 1133.
2. See for example C.A. Coulson, 'The Shape and Structure of Molecules', OUP, 1985; G. Richards, 'Quantum Pharmacology', Butterworths, 1983; A. Hinchliffe, 'Computational Quantum Chemistry' John Wiley and Sons, 1988.
3. J.P. Stewart, *J. Comp. Aided. Mol. Design,* 1990, **4**, 1.
4. W. Hehre, R. Ditchfield, L. Radom, and J.A. Pople, *J. Am. Chem. Soc.*, 1970, **92**, 4796.
5. M.F. Guest, GAMESS-UK, Computational Science Group, SERC, Daresbury Laboratory, Warrington, UK.
6. R.D. Amos and J.E. Rice, CADPAC 4.0, University of Cambridge, 1988.
7. See for example U. Buckert and N.L. Allinger, 'Molecular Mechanics', ACS, Washington, DC, 1982.
8. N. Allinger, *J. Am. Chem. Soc.*, 1977, **99**, 8127.
9. S.J. Weiner *et al.*, *J. Am. Chem. Soc.*, 1984, **106**, 765.
10. B.R. Brooks, *et al.*, *J. Comp. Chem.*, 1983, **4**, 187.
11. S. Lifson, A.T. Hagler, and P. Dauber, *J. Chem. Soc.*, 1979, **101**, 5111.
12. A.E. Howard and P.A. Kollman, *J. Am. Chem. Soc.*, 1988, **31**, 1669.
13. Chem-X developed and distributed by Chemical Design Ltd., Oxford, UK.
14. Sybyl developed and distributed by Tripos Associates, St. Louis, MO, USA.
15 F. Mohamadi, *et al.*, *J. Comp. Chem.*, 1990, **11**, 440.
16. (a) G. Crippen and T.F. Havel, 'Distance Geometry and Molecular Conformation', Research Studies Press, Wiley (1981); (b) I.D. Kuntz, *J. Amer. Chem. Soc.*, 1975, **97**, 4362.
17. N. Metropolis, *et al.*, *J. Chem. Phys.*, 1953, **21**, 1087; T. Noguti, N. Go, *Biopolymers*, 1985, **24**, 527.
18. G.R. Marshall *et al.*, in 'Computer-Assisted Drug Design', ACS Symposium Series 112, ACS, Washington, 1979, p. 205.
19. R.D. Cramer III, D.E. Patterson, and J.D. Bunce, *J. Am. Chem. Soc.*, 1988, **110**, 5959.
20. F.H. Allen *et al.*, *J. Chem. Info. Comp. Sci.*, 1991, **31**, 187.
21. F.C. Bernsein *et al.*, *J. Mol. Biol.*, 1977, **112**, 535.
22. See for example Program Manual for the Genetics Computer Group (GCG) Package, Version 7, April 1991, 575 Science Drive, Madison, Wisconsin, USA.

23. A. Rusinko III *et al.*, CONCORD, Univerisity of Texas at Austin, distributed by Tripos Associates, St. Louis, MO, 1987.
24. Maccs-3D-CFS developed and distributed by Molecular Design Ltd., San Leandro, CA, USA.
25 Sybyl-3DB/Unity developed and distributed by Tripos Associates, St. Louis, MO, USA.
26. A.R. Leach, K. Prout, and D.P. Dolata, *J. Comp. Aided Mol. Design*, 1990, **4**, 271.
27. P.J. Goodford, *J. Med. Chem.***28**, 849.
28. R.L. DesJarlais *et al.*, *J. Med. Chem.*1988, **31**, 722.
29. P.A. Bartlett *et al.*, in 'Molecular Recognition: Chemical and Biological Problems', ed. S.M. Roberts, Royal Society of Chemistry, London, 1989, p. 182.
30. H.-J. Bohm, *J. Comp. Aided Mol. Design*, 1992, **6**, 593.
31. V. Gillet *et al.*, *J. Comp. Aided Mol. Design*, 1993, **7**, 127.
32. S. Hanessian, J. Franco, and B. Larouche, *Pure & Appl. Chem.*, 1990, **62**, 1887.
33. R. Hubbard, *Chemical Design Automation News*, 1992, p. 34.

CHAPTER 10

'Patent Medicine'

BILL TYRRELL

1 INTRODUCTION

Perhaps more than ever before, patents (and other forms of intellectual property such as copyright and Trade Marks) are in the news! One only has to look at the business section of the *London Times* to appreciate that the fortunes of major companies are critically dependent on what patents they own and when their patents will expire or are likely to be successfully challenged in the courts. One only has to pick up a scientific publication like *Nature* to read about some new ethical problem the patent authorities are grappling with – for example whether to allow patents to be granted for genetically engineered (transgenic) animals. Yet, for all that, few people outside the patent profession have much idea of what patents really are – except perhaps a misguided opinion that they are boring! In my view (and, it seems, in the view of distinguished societies such as the Royal Society of Chemistry) ignorance of the patent system is something that chemists should seek to correct. In the pharmaceutical industry, in particular, it is vital that new medicines are adequately protected by patents so that companies can recover the huge R&D costs involved in developing new drugs. Before he or she has been long in the job, therefore, the medicinal chemist in industry – or in any institution carrying out research with a commercial objective – is bound to come into contact with a patent attorney.

It should not be forgotten that it can easily take £100–200 million in R&D investment to bring a drug containing a new chemical entity (NCE) to the market-place. If every NCE researched could be counted upon to be a 'blockbuster', pharmaceutical companies would be less uneasy about committing such massive resources. However, for each successful drug developed thousands of compounds and materials may be tried and discarded, sometimes in late stages of development. Even those drugs which do 'make it' may fail to generate an adequate return on investment. Unfortunately the situation is worsening: pharmaceutical R&D costs are escalating and new active substances must be safer and be more innovative to be successful. The number of NCEs launched onto the world market per year has **halved** in the last 20 years. Against this background it is hardly surprising that R&D based pharmaceutical companies are becoming even more dependent on effective patent protection to fend off copiers of successful drugs who spend little or no money on research of their own. To encourage investment in the development of new medicines strong patent protection is seen as absolutely essential.

It is therefore important that every medicinal chemist has a basic knowledge of

the patent system and understands how best to maximise (or how not to jeopardise) getting strong patent protection for his or her employer.

What follows is not a historical discourse about the potions popular in times gone by such as William Beer's Reanimating Vital Fluid, or Buffalo Bill's Buffalo's Pills ('a safe cure for empty pockets'), most of which in fact were **not** patented (although Beer's product was the subject of UK Patent No. 2667 in 1802). This is about patenting medicines today.

2 PATENTS IN THE WIDER CONTEXT OF INTELLECTUAL PROPERTY

Patents are an important part of a whole gamut of rights known as *Intellectual Property (IP) rights*. Just as you would not want anyone to steal your personal ('tangible') property, you would not want anyone to steal the fruits of your thought processes. Intellectual Property protection is intended to address precisely this point.

The most fundamental point about *Patents* is that they are granted for *inventions* (see further below). Other forms of IP include *Trade Marks*, intended to protect a word or logo associated with a particular product (TAGAMET and ZANTAC are examples) and *Registered Designs*, intended to protect the 'look' of a particular article which has eye appeal. Protection of patents, Trade Marks, and registered designs has in common the fact that appropriate applications have to be made to Government bodies. Two other important IP rights – *Copyright* and *Trade Secrets* – are automatic and do not need to be registered.[1] This sounds convenient, but to prove copyright infringement, for example, one has the difficult task of providing evidence that the work in question (literary or artistic) has actually been copied. In contrast, patents, Trade Marks and registered designs can be held to be infringed by the activities of an individual working independently who may be totally unaware of the relevant IP right. That is why it is important to carry out a search prior to any commercialisation of one's own to check that third party rights are not being infringed.

Patents and other forms of IP can be bought, sold, or leased in just the same way as tangible property like a house or a car, except that for IP rights one normally talks about 'assigning' or 'licensing'. Using patents to obtain royalty income or as bargaining chips in cross-licensing deals is an important part of modern business practice. A major difference between tangible property and intangible intellectual property, however, is that if someone steals (*i.e.* infringes) your IP rights that is (except in one or two countries) a civil 'tort'. The matter can therefore only be pursued through the civil, rather than the criminal, courts. But if copying becomes outright *counterfeiting* that **is** a criminal offence. Counterfeiting is becoming an increasingly serious problem, even in the pharmaceutical industry.[2]

In the R&D based pharmaceutical industry patents are the number one IP right. It is worth noting, though, that Trade Marks are also extremely important. Unlike patents, registered Trade Marks have no fixed 'life' and can potentially last for ever if kept in force by payment of renewal fees – assuming they do not come to grief in any other way.[3] Thus, even when a pharmaceutical product comes 'off-patent' and becomes 'generic', only the original manufacturer is entitled to use the Trade Mark (unless it has been assigned or licensed in the meanwhile).

Before concentrating exclusively on patents it is appropriate to finish this section by saying a word about trade secrets, sometimes referred to as proprietary **know-how**. This is another important aspect of IP which should always be considered as an alternative to patenting. The fundamental difference between patenting and maintaining an invention as a trade secret is that in the former case the invention is inevitably published, whereas with know-how the intention is to keep it deliberately a secret to steal a march on one's competitors. Opting for trade secret protection is an inherently risky business for several reasons, one being that there is no patent position to fall back on if a competitor independently makes the same finding. Trade secret protection is inappropriate, for example, for a novel compound since if the compound is eventually marketed the formula can rapidly be found and copied. On the other hand, it may well be advantageous to keep an invention a secret if a competitor is unlikely to discover a particular process 'trick', *e.g.* a way, found empirically, of increasing the yield of a key step by 10%. Know-how can of course be traded just like any other form of intellectual property. In fact it is not uncommon for agreements to relate to the licensing of both patents and know-how.

3 WHAT IS A PATENT?

The term 'patent' is short for 'Letters Patent', derived from the Latin *litterae patentes*, meaning 'open letters'. In the UK, the grant of a patent monopoly by open letter (*i.e.* a letter sealed 'open' so that all can read the contents without breaking the seal) goes back several hundreds of years. According to the Statute of Monopolies (1624) objectionable monopolies in commodities which had been previously granted by the Crown were abolished and monopolies were subsequently granted only for a limited number of activities, notably for inventions.[4] As the law relating to patents became refined it was established that a limited monopoly could only be granted for making **and disclosing** an invention. An open letter would be addressed by the monarch to the people in the realm so that everyone was made aware of the inventor's monopoly and of the invention. Although Letters Patent documents now look less impressive than they used to when sealing wax was used, the grant of a patent in the form of an open letter or certificate of grant from the monarch or state is still precisely what happens in most major countries today (see Figure 1).

I make no apologies for introducing a historical note because part of the fascination of patents is that they are steeped in history.[5] One of the first British patents relating to medicines was granted in 1698 for a method of making Epsom salts, starting a great tradition of invention. Well over 2 million UK patents in all fields have now been granted. In the USA patent law began just over 200 years ago and great names such as Bell, Edison, Morse, Colt, and Eastman have US patents to their credit. Even Abraham Lincoln was a patentee. The explosion of invention in 19th Century America led one observer to write in 1899 in a letter to

COMMONWEALTH OF AUSTRALIA   No. 517,098

LETTERS 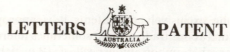 PATENT

(STANDARD PATENT)

𝕰𝖑𝖎𝖟𝖆𝖇𝖊𝖙𝖍 𝖙𝖍𝖊 𝕾𝖊𝖈𝖔𝖓𝖉, by the Grace of God Queen of Australia and Her other Realms and Territories, Head of the Commonwealth.

To all to whom these presents shall come Greeting:

WE DO, by these Letters Patent, give and grant to the person   whose name is specified hereunder Our Special Licence and the exclusive right, subject to the laws in force from time to time in Australia or a part of Australia, by itself, its agents and licensees, at all times during the term of these Letters Patent, to make, use, exercise and vend throughout Australia the invention the title of which is specified hereunder and being the invention that is fully defined in the claim or claims of the complete specification accepted in accordance with the *Patents Act* 1952 in such manner as it   thinks fit, so that it shall have and enjoy the whole profit and advantage accruing by reason of the invention during that term.

Name of Patentee   :   BEECHAM GROUP LIMITED

Address of Patentee   :   Beecham House, Great West Road, Brentford, Middlesex, England

Name of Actual Inventor   :   STUART ANTHONY HILL

Title of Invention: Pharmaceutical composition

Number of Complete Specification: 517,098

Term of Letters Patent: Sixteen years commencing on 11 May 1977

These Letters Patent have been granted on a Convention application. Particulars of the basic application   on which the Convention application is based are as follows:

Name of Convention Country in which basic application   filed: Great Britain

Date   of filing basic application   :   13 May 1976

Application number of basic application   :   19652/76

IN WITNESS whereof Our Commissioner of Patents has caused these Our Letters Patent to be dated as of the Eleventh   day of   May   , One thousand nine hundred and Seventy-seven   , and to be sealed with the seal of the Patent Office this   Twentieth   day of   November   , One thousand nine hundred and Eighty-one

C.H. FRIEMANN
Acting/ *Commissioner of Patents*

Figure 1: *An example of a 'Letters Patent' document*

the President: '*Everything that can be invented has been invented*'. Since then over 4 million US patents have been granted and inventive activity shows no sign of abating.

The point about **disclosing** the invention is an important one because the rationale for the patent system is not only to reward inventors but also to encourage the dissemination of inventions. This basic idea, accepted by most countries of the world, ensures that the patentee is rewarded, yet everyone will be free to practice the invention when the patent has expired. Mankind as a whole benefits and the march of progress goes ever onwards. This rationale is why patenting necessarily means publishing. It is also why a patent can be found invalid for what is known as 'insufficient disclosure', that is cheating on the system by giving an inadequate description of the invention (whether intentionally or not). It is clearly wrong for the inventor to be awarded a monopoly yet still effectively deny the public the chance to practice the invention when the patent has expired. Since patents are inevitably published and since they have fully to disclose the invention (see Section 5), they are an excellent source of technical information (as well as a way of knowing what your competitors are up to!). It is therefore important for the medicinal chemist to keep up with the patent literature (*e.g.* through Derwent Abstracts) as well as the scientific literature.

A modern day definition of a patent is as follows:

A **patent** is an **exclusive right** granted by the state for an **invention**, this right being subject to certain **restrictions**.

By the term **exclusive right** I mean that the patentee has the right to **exclude others** from commercially enjoying the patented invention without his, her, or (if the patentee is an organisation) its permission. Commercial enjoyment can include selling, manufacturing, using or stockpiling the patented invention, or even, in many countries, carrying out trials of a commercial nature on it (*e.g.* clinical trials to demonstrate efficacy).

Two things are worthy of special note at this point:

1. Carrying out non-commercial experiments using the patented product, process, or apparatus is permitted and is not an infringement.
2. While the patentee has a right to exclude others as explained above, it does **not mean to say he necessarily has the right to practice, commercially, his own invention himself!** This is a commonly misunderstood feature of the patent system which looks strange at first glance. However, as mentioned earlier, before commercialising an invention it is always necessary, whether a patentee or not, to check that there are not earlier filed, **broader patents** in existence which could potentially dominate one's activities.[6] Being unable to commercialise one's own invention because of a broader exclusive right of someone else is quite common in the pharmaceutical industry; an example of how this can arise is given in Section 5 under the discussion of 'selection inventions'.

Reverting to the modern definition of a patent (above), I have deliberately highlighted the words *invention* and *restrictions*. It is important to recognise that patents are only granted for certain types of inventions (those in the correct category, see Section 4 below, and those which satisfy the requirements for patentability, see Section 5). Furthermore, as noted already, a patent is only a *limited* monopoly (more accurately exclusive right), the most straightforward limitations being those of duration and geographic scope. These and other restrictions are discussed in Section 6.

4 WHAT CAN BE PATENTED?

In addition to satisfying the key criteria discussed in Section 5, an invention (as defined in the 'claims' of a patent specification) can only be patented if it is in the **correct category**, *i.e.* is not specifically excluded from being patentable. The inventions which are not patentable are listed below for general interest but most are not particularly relevant in the pharmaceutical industry.

Inventions specifically **excluded** from patentability include:

- Methods for treating the human body (*except in the USA*)
- Animal or plant varieties (*separate IP right available for plants; see footnote 1*)
- Computer software (*protectable by copyright*)
- The presentation of information (*and business methods*)
- Scientific laws or mathematical theories (*e.g. $E = mc^2$ is not patentable!*)
- Anything contrary to morality (*e.g. a method of forging banknotes; also footnote 7*)

In the pharmaceutical industry the following inventions relating to a new chemical compound can, in principle, be claimed in a patent:[8]

- Compound or class of compounds
- Formulation containing the compound or class of compounds
- Processes for making the above
- Intermediates involved in the processes
- The compound or class of compounds for use in therapy
- Method of treating humans or animals by administering an effective amount of the compound or class of compounds (**USA only**)
- The use of the compound or class of compounds in the manufacture of a medicament for the treatment of a particular disease (**Europe and certain other countries only; non-USA**).

Of the above, claims relating to final novel products ('compound claims') are by far the strongest since the compound (or class of compounds) will be covered regardless of the method of manufacture. Claims relating to chemical methods ('process claims') or intermediates are inherently weaker as it is frequently difficult to tell whether such claims are in fact being infringed by a competitor, especially in countries where the burden of proving infringement lies with the patentee (see Section 9 under politics). Analytical scientists are often called upon by patent attorneys to see whether they can find in a suspected infringing product a characteristic fingerprint, *i.e.* a tell-tale trace of an impurity which could only have arisen if the patented process or intermediate had been used.

It can be seen from the lists above that claims to methods of treating the human or animal body are excluded from patentability in Europe and in many other countries but are patentable in the USA. The rationale for the exclusion, as I understand it, is that doctors and vets, in carrying out their daily work, should not have to give any thought to possible patent infringement. This possibility does not seem to be of concern in the USA where it is appreciated that the whole point of having a method of treatment claim in a patent is not in order be able to sue physicians (hardly a sound policy for a pharmaceutical company) but to be able to sue the manufacturer of the drug under a doctrine of indirect (or contributory) infringement.

The method of treatment claim particularly comes into its own when one is dealing with a new medical use for a **known** substance. In such a case the compound *per se* cannot be patented (because it is not novel; see Section 5). Unfortunately straightforward method of treatment claims are unpatentable in Europe and getting round this problem led to an interesting chapter in patent law in the mid 1980s which I cannot go into here. Suffice it to say that a solution was found, employing the convoluted wording of the so-called 'Swiss claim',[9] that is to claim: 'The use of [known compound X] in the manufacture of a medicament for the treatment of [particular disease Y]'. A masterpiece of patent drafting!

It is particularly important for medicinal chemists to appreciate that new uses for known compounds are patentable. One often encounters a situation where a drug developed for one utility turns out to be of benefit in a different condition entirely. A particularly interesting situation can arise when a patent is obtained by company A for a new use of a company B's drug! This is a good example of how patents operate to exclude others from using an invention and how cross-licensing can lead to a win–win situation for both companies (see further under selection inventions; section 5).

5 REQUIREMENTS FOR PATENTABILITY

Besides being in the right category an invention, to be patentable, must fulfil several other important requirements – in most countries. I say 'in most countries' because as the reader has probably by now realised patent law can vary considerably from one country to another. Getting to grips with foreign law and dealing with overseas agents is another interesting facet of patent work!

The basic requirements for patentability are that an invention is:

(a) useful (the jargon in Europe is 'capable of industrial application');
(b) novel;
(c) not obvious (*i.e.* involves an 'inventive step'); and
(d) adequately described (for the reasons given in Section 3).

I will say a word about each of these requirements.

Utility

A key point to bear in mind is that an invention need not be earth-shattering to be patentable. Not every invention ranks with the preparation of the first semi-synthetic penicillin or the development of the hovercraft. Quite mundane inventions can be patented as long as there is, arguably, some use for them. This can be seen from my collection of humorous patents (yes, there are such things) where patents have been granted for 'a pat on the back apparatus' (US Patent Number 4 608 967) or even for 'improvements in automobiles driven from the back seat' (UK Patent Specification Number 1 394 639). While speaking in a lighter vein, I should point out that the latter patent is one of 150 or more zany inventions by the great A.P. Pedrick, a former examiner in the British Patent Office, whose patent applications were waved through because they were simply harmless fun. Perhaps his greatest work was entitled: 'Photon push–pull radiation detector for use in chromatically selective cat flap control and 1,000 megaton, earth-orbital peace keeping bomb' (UK Patent Specification 1 426 698).

From the above it can be seen that satisfying the utility requirement is rarely a problem. However in Europe the exclusion from patentability of methods of treating the human or animal body (see Section 4) was formally made on the grounds that such methods are incapable of industrial application. A similar criticism has been levelled at patent applications directed to perpetual motion machines. On a more topical note, doubt has been expressed about the patentability of partial gene sequences in the USA (and Europe) in the absence of any known utility.[10]

Novelty

Novelty and inventive step (discussed below) are always judged in relation to the 'prior art' which may be any disclosure the patentee has made or may be written or oral disclosures made by others.

Most countries of the world operate an 'absolute novelty' system, meaning that any disclosure of an invention, anywhere in the world, before the priority date (see Section 7 below) of a relevant patent application can be potentially damaging. The reason for this is to be found in the basic rationale for the patent system: it is not fair for a person to obtain a monopoly on an invention the public are already aware of. There are exceptions to this philosophy. Of particular note is the USA which operates a 'grace period' of one year during which a patent application can still be filed following disclosure of one's own invention. Some countries still operate a 'local novelty' system. However since one normally wants to obtain a world-wide patent position for an important pharmaceutical invention the golden rule is: **do not disclose your invention, except in confidence to colleagues, before a patent application has been filed**. If you publish, or otherwise disclose the invention – even verbally – you run the very real risk that any subsequent patent which is applied for or obtained will be invalid for lack of novelty (or alternatively, in the light of the disclosure, will be invalid for obviousness; see below). There are numerous instances of where this rule has not

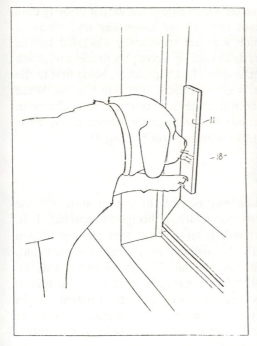

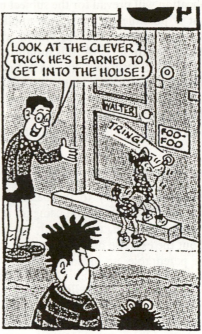

Figure 2: *Front page of patent application*
relating to entry signal for pets

© D. C. Thomson & Co. Ltd.
Figure 3: *Alleged prior art shown in 'Beano'*
comic
(Reproduced by kind permission of the
publishers)

been followed and the chance to obtain valuable patent protection has been lost. A frequently cited example is the work of Kohler and Milstein on monoclonal antibodies, published in 1975. The seminal work of Cohen and Boyer on genetic engineering was also published before patent filings were made and as a result only US patents were obtained.

It is understandable that scientists are anxious to publish their work and patent departments are sometimes unpopular for appearing to be obstructive. I hope that the above adequately explains why!

On a lighter note, the applicant for UK Patent Number 2 117 179 must have been surprised when one of the citations made by the Patent Office against his invention (a pet-operated entry signal system) was a 1981 issue of the *Beano* depicting what appeared to be a similar device (Figures 2 and 3)! This illustrates the point that any potentially relevant documents can be considered in assessing novelty and inventive step.

A special type of novelty objection can arise, even in the absence of a public disclosure, if two parties have filed a patent application in the same territory for essentially the same invention at about the same time so that one is not published when the other is filed. In such a case of 'conflicting applications' national rules again apply and the situation can become complex. In **Europe**, the earlier filed application will prevail for the subject matter which enjoys the earlier priority date but it is possible that the later applicant can salvage something and obtain a (narrower) patent on an invention which was not specifically disclosed by the earlier party. In the USA, this situation is dealt with by a complex procedure, much beloved of US attorneys, known as 'interference'. In US practice, being first to the Patent Office, although highly desirable, is not as critical as it is in Europe. What counts is showing that one was first to conceive the invention and was diligent in 'reducing it to practice'. It is possible that interference practice will disappear in the USA if ongoing 'patent harmonisation' talks bear fruit (see Section 9).

Inventive Step

It would be contrary to the basic philosophy behind the patent system if the public were prevented from using an invention which, although not specifically in the public domain, could easily be arrived at from what was already known without the exercise of any inventive skill. Accordingly most countries insist that, to be patentable, an invention should not be **obvious**. This raises two questions: *obvious over what?* and *obvious to whom?* Almost certainly more has been said in the courts on the subject of obviousness than on any other facet of patent law. In contrast to novelty (it is usually pretty clear whether an invention is novel or whether it is not) determination of whether an invention is obvious is frankly a matter of opinion. Opinions can differ widely!

Case law over the years, however, has led to some helpful guidelines. As regards the question: *obvious over what?* the answer is *from all relevant prior art*, that is any disclosure, anywhere in the world, in any language, which is directly relevant to (*i.e.* is in the same field as) the claimed invention. A 'conflicting' patent application (see under Novelty above), not published when a later patent application was filed, cannot be cited against the later application on the grounds of obviousness.

As regards the question: *obvious to whom?*, the courts have established over the years the patent equivalent of 'the man on the Clapham omnibus'. This is the famous 'person skilled in the art', who while being assumed to have an encyclopaedic knowledge of all the world literature in his or her specialist field, is credited with absolutely no inventive flair! As Lord Reid put it:

> *'To whom must the invention be obvious? It is not disputed that the hypothetical addressee is a skilled technician who is well acquainted with workshop technique and who has carefully read the relevant literature. He is supposed to have an unlimited capacity to assimilate the contents of, it may be, scores of specifications but to be incapable of a scintilla of invention.'*

It can be seen that being called a person skilled in the art is not as complimentary as it would at first sight appear!

In deciding whether a claimed invention is obvious or not care must be taken to avoid looking at the invention with the benefit of hindsight.[11] Once one knows what the invention is, it is all too easy to put together an argument as to why the skilled person could have arrived at the invention by combining the teaching of this document and that. The correct approach is to put oneself in the shoes of the person skilled in the art (this can include a team of people) at the priority date of the invention. The European Patent Office likes to identify the closest prior art and to work from there. Documents hinting at technical prejudices, teaching away from the invention, are helpful in rebutting the obviousness arguments that Patent Examiners frequently introduce to test the applicant. So too are unexpected and surprising results, such as improved biological activity over prior art compounds. Scientists will frequently be asked to submit such results to their patent department, often in the form of an expert declaration, to bolster the arguments that are being advanced in support of non-obviousness.

At this point it is convenient to mention that a particular type of patent, often encountered in the pharmaceutical industry, is the 'selection patent', based on a 'selection invention'. Rebutting an allegation of obviousness by submission of scientific data is the norm in this situation. A selection patent is not distinguishable on its face from any other sort of patent: it is simply an ordinary patent claiming a preferred sub-species selected from a genus in a broader, earlier disclosure. The earlier case can belong to a third party or, as is more usually the case, to the applicant for the selection patent.

Selection inventions are common because the policy of most pharmaceutical companies working in a competitive area is to file as early as possible, claiming the invention as broadly as possible, even though only a few examples may by that time have been prepared. As the work is refined particulary good results will often be found for a particular class of compounds within the broad scope of the earlier patent filing but not specifically disclosed within it. This is the time for the Patent Department to file an application directed to the sub-class which has been identified, the primary objective being to obtain a longer patent term for the preferred compound(s) than is afforded by the earlier case. Patent Office Examiners will object that the class of compounds has been selected arbitrarily from the earlier case (usually by then published prior art), without any inventive skill, and a patent should not be granted. If it can be shown, however, that the identified compounds have advantageous properties this is a very good argument against obviousness.

In the following situation imagine that two companies A and B are working on a series of 1,2-benzisothiazol-3-ones (I) with a 2-position side-chain R.

(I)   R = C_{1-10} alkyl

(II)   R = n-octyl

Company A files first and claims R = 1–10 alkyl on the strength of having made the methyl, n-propyl, and n-decyl compounds, shown to be active as platelet aggregation inhibitors.[12] After the publication of A's patent application, B carries out research and finds that the n-octyl derivative (II) is, surprisingly, 10 times more active than the adjacent homologues. In those circumstances I would expect B, after submitting technical data, to obtain a selection patent (in for example Europe or the USA) directed to the n-octyl compound, even in the light of A's disclosure.

This example also provides a nice illustration of my earlier comment that having a patent of your own does not automatically give you the right to commercialise the invention disclosed. If A and B both obtain patents in a certain country and the n-octyl derivative is the preferred commercial product, B cannot market it in that country without a licence from A because the preferred compound – albeit that B has patented it – falls within the broad generic scope of A's patent. Similarly A cannot market the preferred compound because it falls within the scope of B's patent. Because of the exclusive right conferred by a patent there is an impasse and neither company can market the preferred product! A good way out of this situation (short of trying to get one or other patents revoked) is for each company to cross-license the other.

Sufficiency of Disclosure

The reason it is necessary to give an adequate ('sufficient') description of an invention has already been mentioned (see Section 3). Insufficiency is not often a problem in chemical inventions but the author is aware of one patent which was revoked because the process described was allegedly shown not to work. The European Patent Office has also taken a strict approach when it comes to identifying the source of one's starting materials. The medicinal chemist can clearly help the patent attorney in this respect by providing a thorough 'write-up' of experimental work such that the skilled person can easily repeat it, albeit with a permissible amount of trial and error.

There is no requirement in most countries for a patent application to describe the best way of carrying out the invention. However it is important to be aware that that is not true in the USA where there is a statutory requirement fully to disclose the best method or best compound known to the applicant at the time of filing (the **'best mode'** requirement). Failure to disclose best mode can seriously jeopardise the validity of a US patent. The medicinal chemist should be alive to this when submitting patent examples.

Providing a sufficient description of an invention can be a problem in the biotechnology field where one may find it impossible to put into words how reproducibly to obtain a particular micro-organism, especially if the micro-organism has been isolated from a natural source such as a soil sample. It is not permissible to append an Ordinance Survey map to the patent specification with 'X' marking the spot where the micro-organism was dug up! That is no guarantee that the skilled person will be able to obtain exactly the same thing again. In this situation it is normal to deposit the micro-organism in a culture collection to ensure that the sufficiency requirement is satisfied. The skilled person, wishing to reproduce the invention, can then go to the culture collection to obtain a sample of the micro-organism. In some countries it is possible to withold release of a valuable micro-organism to a competitor until a patent has granted.

6 PATENT RESTRICTIONS

Geographic Constraints

The position is simple: if one wishes to have patent protection in a particular territory, one has to file a patent application in that territory. A UK patent is no good against an infringer operating in Japan and *vice versa*. Accordingly a decision has to be taken fairly early about geographical breadth of filing. A company cannot foreign file a patent application in just Europe and the USA and then decide a couple of years later that it wants a filing in Australia also. By that time (even assuming no other disclosure) the European patent application will have been published and the invention sought to be patented in Australia will lack novelty. An exception to this is that in certain territories, *e.g.* in Hong Kong (at present), later filings can be made based on the registration of a granted patent which is effective in another country (commonly the UK).

Important pharmaceutical inventions are naturally filed very widely, often *via* the 'PCT route' explained in Section 7, to cut down on initial costs and paperwork. Since there is no such thing as a 'world patent' patent attorneys inevitably have to instruct foreign associates on how to deal with local Patent Office objections in many interesting countries. In addition, differences in national laws frequently result in the eventual scope of protection obtained differing from one country to another.

Patent Term

The maximum term of a patent is normally 20 years from the date of *application in* many countries. There are however notable exceptions: the term of a US patent is 17 years from the date of *grant*. Some countries discriminate against the patenting of pharmaceuticals in the belief that local industry will suffer or prices will rise. Several Latin American and Asian countries, for example, have laws giving less than a 20 year term. These considerations obviously affect the value of patents in such countries.

In practically all countries a patent must be kept in force by payment of regular (usually annual) renewal fees. Most large companies employ specialist firms to ensure that annuities are paid on time.

In special circumstances it is possible to obtain an extension of patent term. For example in New Zealand (at present) and certain other countries it is possible to apply for patent term extension on the basis of inadequate remuneration. An unusual ground for extension of patent term is 'war loss' – currently applicable, I understand, in Slovenia.

One type of 'patent term extension' deserves special mention in a pharmaceutical context. That is the extended period of legal protection which is available in certain countries to compensate for the length of time it takes to satisfy the relevant Regulatory Authorities of a drug's safety and efficacy. This is vitally important in the pharmaceutical industry because by the time a drug gets on to the market as much as 12 years of patent protection may already have elapsed, giving only 8 years of **effective patent term** absent an extension. The US led the way in this initiative by passing the Patent Term Restoration Act of 1984 and since then several other countries, notably Japan, Korea, France, and Italy (at a national level) and the European Community as a whole have introduced their own versions of the same system.

In the EC the rules were hammered out only after great political argument and are complex. In essence, a Supplementary Protection Certificate (SPC) can be applied for in qualifying member states, affording a further period of legal protection for the authorised product. The term of an SPC can be up to 5 years beyond the expiry date of a relevant patent but must not exceed 15 years from the date of obtaining the first marketing authorisation in an EC Member State.

Scope of Claims

In my view, that part of a patent specification called 'the claims' has, more than anything else, given patent documents a bad reputation as being impossible to read. The claims are the numbered paragraphs at the back of the specification which are intended to set out the scope of protection.

I was once told about the Gunning 'Fog Index' which is a way of assessing the readability of a piece of writing. The steps for the calculation are given in footnote 13. A score of 7 or 8 means that a piece of writing is standard; 9 to 11 is fairly difficult and 17 or above is very difficult (I have not dared work out the Fog Index score for this chapter!).

Consider now the following claim 1 in UK Patent 2 027 681 to a corkscrew many people have in their homes (it covers the Hallen 'self-pulling' corkscrew; Figure 4).

According to my calculations this has a Gunning Fog Index of well over 80!

One reason patent claims are so turgid is that they are written as just one sentence, apparently for 'legal certainty'. They are also **not** full of elegant variation: once a spade has been called a spade it must continue, for the avoidance of doubt, to be called a spade.

Difficult as they often are to understand, patent claims fulfil a vital function in staking out the metes and bounds of a patented invention. The claims should as precisely as possible indicate what is intended to be covered. An assessment of patentability (see Section 5) can then be made and third parties will know with a reasonable degree of certainty whether or not their commercial activities will constitute patent infringement.

Whilst patent claims are drafted in an attempt to obtain legal precision some ambiguities are inevitable. In a celebrated patent case known as Catnic a claim to a door lintel used the word 'vertically'. The question was whether an alleged infringing product with a back plate a few degrees off the vertical fell within the scope of Catnic's claims. The matter was eventually appealed from the Patents Court (part of the Chancery Division of the High Court) via the Court of Appeal

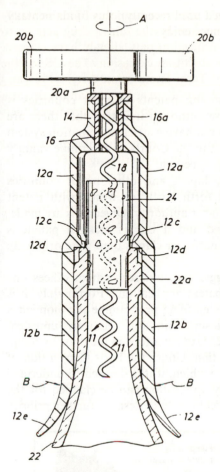

"Apparatus for extracting a cork from a bottle comprising:
a corkscrew comprising a helical body and an outer layer of a friction-reducing material;
guide means receiving said corkscrew and permitting longitudinal and rotative movement of said corkscrew;
bottle engaging means connected to said guide means for positioning said guide means and said corkscrew in general coaxial alignment with the neck of the bottle, said bottle engaging means including stop means for limiting downward (as hereinbefore defined) movement of said guide means with respect to said bottle;
spacer means interconnecting said guide means and said bottle-engaging means and spacing said guide means upwardly (as hereinbefore defined) from said bottle engaging means, said spacer means defining an opening of receipt of said cork as it emerges from said bottle;
and abutment means carried by said corkscrew for limiting downward (as hereinbefore defined) movement of said corkscrew with respect to said guide means;
said corkscrew being a length such that when said abutment means are engaged to so limit downward (as hereinbefore defined) movement of said corkscrew, said corkscrew extends into said cork-receiving opening whereby said cork may move threadedly upwardly (as hereinbefore defined) on said corkscrew as said corkscrew is rotated to withdraw said cork from said bottle."

Figure 4: *Claim 1 in UK Patent 2 027 681*

to five learned Law Lords in the House of Lords who held there **was** infringement. Lord Diplock, giving his judgment, delivered the immortal lines:

'A patent specification should be given a purposive construction rather than a purely literal one derived from applying to it the kind of meticulous verbal analysis in which lawyers are too often tempted by their training to indulge.'

The conclusion is that in modern UK law claims do have a certain (albeit small) degree of elasticity and should not be read absolutely literally. The same is broadly true in the USA where, if there is not literal infringement, infringement may nevertheless be found under the 'doctrine of equivalents'.

Putting aside the legal niceties, a more critical consideration for pharmaceutical patents is what **type** of claim is going to be allowed. The strength of product, rather than process, claims has already been mentioned (Section 4), yet in some countries it is an unfortunate fact that for pharmaceutical inventions only process claims are allowed (or have only been allowed until recently); this fundamentally restricts the scope of protection that the patentee enjoys.

7 HOW ARE PATENTS OBTAINED?

I hope that by now it is clear that obtaining patents in most countries is emphatically not a rubber stamping exercise, although it is true that there are some countries (*e.g.* South Africa) which do not have a strict examination system and will grant patents 'on the nod', leaving it to the Courts to determine validity in any post-grant challenge or infringement proceeding.

Obtaining patents in Europe, the USA, Japan, and other major countries nearly always involves a tough back and forth battle of words with patent examiners and occasionally an appeal to a higher authority. Objections are made, responses are filed, amendments are agreed and if one is lucky a patent is eventually granted, often with considerably narrower claims than were originally filed.

Before embarking on this tortuous struggle with overseas patent offices one must first of course make the appropriate patent applications. Fortunately, it is not necessary to carry out an expensive foreign filing programme the moment a medicinal chemist turns up with a promising, but still relatively untested, invention. In the UK, it is possible, for just £25, to get a foot in the door by filing, at the UK Patent Office,[14] a **priority application**. Under the Paris Convention of 1883 there then follows a 12 month period in which, if it is decided to undertake foreign filings, the filing date of the priority application can be claimed for the subject matter disclosed in the priority application. If so desired, further priority

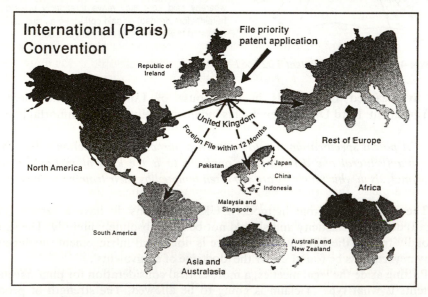

Figure 5: *Foreign filing: the Paris Convention enables priority to be claimed (within 12 months) from an earlier filed domestic (e.g. UK) application*

applications disclosing further information can be filed throughout the 'convention year' and cognated together at the foreign filing stage.

Establishing one or more **priority dates** by making a local filing is a very common practice. In most countries it is also necessary to satisfy regulations regarding national security. In the UK these regulations state that a patent application cannot be foreign filed unless a specification describing the invention has first been lodged at the UK Patent Office for a certain period of time (or specific clearance has been obtained). This rule exists in case the patent specification really does describe an earth-orbital 1000 megaton bomb or other useful military inventions we would not wish to disclose to foreign powers!

If a decision is taken to foreign file an application, based on the priority application(s), one must decide in which countries the application is to be filed. Prior to 1978 foreign filing involved a vast amount of paperwork because a national application had to be separately made in each country chosen. The position has now simplified somewhat thanks to two international agreements: the European Patent Convention (EPC) and the Patent Cooperation Treaty (PCT).

The **EPC** enables a single application to be filed at the European Patent Office (head office in Munich but a receiving branch also at the Hague), designating as many EPC Member States as desired.[15] The application is examined by the European Patent Office (EPO) and if granted the resulting European Patent becomes effective in the designated states as though it were a national patent. Although this approach suffers from the drawback that one has all one's eggs in one basket, it does have significant advantages over filing separate national applications (which nevertheless is still possible).

The **PCT** provides an optional, but convenient, way of initiating national filings in numerous different foreign countries by means of a single application which can be filed in English. The PCT system is somewhat complicated but rapidly growing in popularity and over 50 member states can now be designated. The PCT, or 'international', application stays as a single entity in the initial stages of its life and is published as such 18 months from the earliest priority date. Up to this point only the initial filing costs will have been incurred (less than £2000 for designating over 50 countries is good value). It is after that point that life becomes expensive if the application is going to be pursued. At 20 or 30 months from priority (according to the applicant's choice) the application can be converted into numerous national applications, for which the payment of further filing fees will be required, together with a translation where appropriate. In this 'national phase' the original PCT application is a thing of the past and national applications are prosecuted in the usual way. A filing at the European Patent Office can, if desired, be made *via* the PCT route. Unfortunately there are still some important countries which are not member states of the PCT (*e.g.* Mexico). For these, national filings in an appropriate language still have to be made.

When a foreign filing is made it is not usually known with absolute certainty exactly what is in the prior art. Some nasty surprises may be in store and an invention may already have been disclosed by someone else. To check on this point, Patent Offices in the countries in which the application has been filed (or the EPO or PCT Search Divisions as appropriate) will carry out a search and provide the applicant with a search report indicating the perceived relevance of the cited documents. The applicant can then decide whether to spend more money pursuing the application. Although search reports are generally quite good they can never be assumed to be totally comprehensive. It is quite conceivable, therefore, that when a patent is granted (or even before it is granted) competitors who have an interest in opposing the patent will produce additional prior art documents which were not considered by the patent examiner and allege that the patent is invalid. Revocation of granted patents is discussed further in Section 8.

Incidentally, in most countries the applicant is not required to disclose relevant prior art to the patent examiner but the USA is a notable exception. Any potentially relevant prior art of which the applicant is aware **must** be made part of a US information disclosure statement. This is another area where good communication between medicinal chemist and patent attorney is essential.

Finally a word about inventorship since to obtain a patent it is essential to designate one or more inventors. It is up to the patent attorney to ensure that inventorship has been correctly determined and this is often a difficult task. Only those who actually made the invention are entitled to be named as inventors and their names appear on the front of the published patent specification. Apart from the kudos associated with that, there is little else to which an inventor is normally entitled. If the invention was carried out in the normal course of one's duties the invention belongs to one's employer. There are complex provisions, at least in the UK Patents Act, for an inventor to be rewarded if the patent subsequently proves to be of 'outstanding benefit' but these provisions will only apply in exceptional circumstances and the few attempts to invoke them have generally met with failure. Being an inventor in the pharmaceutical industry is unfortunately not a way to get rich quick!

8 THE POWER OF PATENTS

'The only thing that keeps us alive is our brilliance.
The only thing protecting our brilliance is our patents.'

So said Edwin H. Land, the inventor of the 'instant' (Polaroid) camera. This statement was made before Polaroid reportedly collected some $986 million in damages from Kodak in the US litigation relating to such cameras; no doubt he would endorse his remark even more emphatically today!

The Polaroid case is a good – if extreme – example of the ultimate power of patents. That is, the power to apply to the court for an order awarding damages on past sales, delivery up of infringing articles to the patentee and an injunction against further copying. Litigation is always a long and expensive process (especially in the USA) and the outcome is never certain. That is because in most countries an almost automatic consequence of bringing an infringement action against a third party is that the validity of the patent will be thoroughly tested. The alleged infringer, by way of defence, will counterclaim for revocation saying that the patent is worthless. The patent literature is full of cases where arguments for invalidity have succeeded and, instead of the patentee obtaining an injunction, the patent has been revoked. A recent and much publicised example in the pharmaceutical field was the Genentech v Wellcome litigation in the UK relating to tissue plasminogen activator (t-PA).

Where there is a blatant case of infringement, it is obviously frustrating for the patentee to have to wait – perhaps for years – for the slow wheels of justice to turn before an injunction is awarded. In the meantime the infringer's activities could cause irreparable harm. To overcome this problem it is possible, if one does not delay, to apply for an **interlocutory injunction**, pending a full trial. The idea is that rapid court proceedings take place, not to examine infringement and validity in depth, but to determine whether the patentee has an arguable case. Following well established legal precedent[16] the court ultimately has to determine the 'balance of convenience' in deciding whether or not to grant an injunction, *i.e.* decide who would suffer the most harm if the injunction were wrongly given and in fact the other party succeeded at full trial.

One point about patent litigation which should be borne in mind by medicinal chemists is that in many countries (*e.g.* UK and USA) 'discovery' of documents is involved. That is to say that each side has to power to inspect any documents in their opponents' possession which have a bearing on the case. Patent attorneys and lawyers can usually claim 'legal privilege' for their written opinions, making them immune from discovery and allowing them to express candidly their views on infringement and validity. The same is not true for medicinal chemists who should avoid expressing their own view of a particular patent or paraphrasing their patent adviser's opinions in their own words. In the trawl through filing cabinets that discovery inevitably involves it can be embarrassing to find injudiciously worded memoranda by one's own scientists, stating, for example, that Smith's results made it obvious to prepare the n-octyl compound. Almost certainly the Patent Attorney will have spent years of his or her life arguing that Smith's results did not make it obvious to prepare the n-octyl compound! My advice would be to review each memorandum you write on the basis that it might one day be discovered in patent litigation.

Although patent enforcement is the ultimate threat, full scale litigation is often avoided by out of court settlements or deals between the parties. In particular it is common for patents to be licensed (exclusively or non-exclusively), perhaps in exchange for up-front money, milestone payments, and royalty income. Patents are also frequently used as bargaining chips in a cross-licensing arrangement.

If it is not practicable to make a deal, what can be done to attack a problematical third party patent? Applying for national revocation of the patent is sometimes one option if convincing arguments can be put forward as to why the patent should never have been granted in the first place. Better, under the European Patent Convention (see Section 7), a granted patent can be opposed at the European Patent Office within 9 months of its grant. The decision of the EPO Opposition Division can be further appealed to the EPO Technical Board of Appeal. If the European patent is successfully revoked it can be nipped in the bud before finally becoming effective in each of the designated States. Attack and defence of European Patents at the EPO is common and gives European Patent Attorneys a chance to practice advocacy skills.

9 PATENTS AND POLITICS

Patents are a political issue!

We have already touched in this chapter on the different attitudes various countries adopt to patents, particularly to patenting medicines. Some countries believe in no patent protection at all for pharmaceuticals (*e.g.* Brazil at the time of writing, although it is hoped that the law will soon change); some have only a short patent term; some insist on process-only claims (this was even true until recently in Austria, Greece and Spain); and some do not have reversal of the burden of proving infringement (see Section 4). Numerous industry groups, for example INTERPAT and the ABPI, are constantly lobbying to improve patent protection for pharmaceuticals. Furthermore Trade Related Intellectual Property Rights (TRIPS) are an important part of the GATT agreement. The USA has even employed or threatened trade sanctions under the Special Provisions of the US Trade Act to force recalcitrant countries to take steps to improve their patent laws. All these efforts, it seems, are slowly succeeding. For example, the strength of patent law in Eastern Europe and in parts of Latin America has improved considerably in recent years.

Within the European Community there are also, under the Treaty of Rome, well-established principles of Competition Law to prevent practices which may affect trade between Member States (in the USA there is similarly 'anti-trust' law). These considerations frequently have a bearing on patent matters, for example what can or cannot be agreed between parties in patents and know-how agreements.

Political disputes about patents have, in fact, been going on for centuries and show no sign of abating. Currently, Supplementary Protection Certificates which had to be fought for so hard in the EC are under attack by the Spanish Government who want them abolished on the grounds that they were agreed unconstitutionally! There is uncertainty about the effect of the Biodiversity Treaty (signed by 157 countries in Rio in 1992) on intellectual property rights. There is a row in Europe over a draft Directive on Biotechnology patenting and whether, on ethical grounds, transgenic animals should be patentable. There are grave doubts whether the USA, Europe, and Japan will ever agree to harmonise their patent systems. And so it goes on. You can be sure that patents will continue to be a political issue for a long time to come. But that, after all, is part of their fascination.

10 CONCLUSION

When I attended the RSC Medicinal Chemistry School in Bradford in 1978, having then had some four years experience as a research chemist in the pharmaceutical industry (Beecham, many years pre-merger), I did not expect one day to be addressing the same school on the subject of patents!

In those days, if I considered patents at all, I am sure I thought they were very dull things indeed: turgid documents – not like a decent scientific paper – full of verbiose phrases like 'the invention provides...', 'the man skilled in the art', 'as hereinabove described', and dotted here and there with numerous 'preferably's, 'suitably's and 'aptly's.

Nine years into my second career I have radically changed my views. The great secret that fortunately few people are aware of is that the patent profession[17] is like none other in the amazing variety of subject matter it offers and the interest it provides. Patent cases, as reported in Court proceedings, are literally stranger than fiction and make compulsive reading, as do other intellectual property cases.[18]

I do not expect the reader to believe this for one minute. But I hope that, having read this chapter, you will have formed the view that the patent system (as hereinabove defined) is not as bad as you thought. That it makes sense, even. Most important of all I hope you will see the value in medicinal chemists knowing something about the subject. Because the more patent-aware you are the easier it will be for you to recognise an invention and to work more effectively with your patent attorney to achieve strong intellectual property protection. And that – apart from a reference to some sources of further information[19] – is the bottom line.

11 FOOTNOTES AND REFERENCES

1. There are other IP rights which are of little interest in the pharmaceutical industry but which are of potential value in other industries, for example plant variety protection and unregistered design rights.
2. See: T. Masland, and R. Marshall, 'The Pill Pirates', *Newsweek*, 5th November 1990, p. 18 ff.
3. One way in which a registered Trade Mark can be lost is if the word passes into the language as generic and no longer distinguishes the product for which the mark was granted. Examples of Trade Marks which have been struck off the Register for this reason include aspirin, linoleum, and gramophone.
4. Originally the term of a patent was 14 years, that being the time it would take to train two generations of apprentices to carry out the invention.
5. The patent system began even earlier than the 17th century. In Venice a patent law was passed in 1474.
6. In the UK and in many other countries one has a statutory right to continue a commercial act done or seriously contemplated before the filing date of a relevant third party patent. The act may be continued after the grant of the patent without infringement.
7. The whole question of patenting and ethics is at present being studied by the European Patent Office, mainly as a result of the furore over the patenting of the 'oncomouse', a transgenic mouse specifically engineered to have within

its genetic make-up a cancer-forming gene (and therefore useful as an animal model in cancer research). The mouse was deemed not to be an animal variety as such and in granting the patent in 1992 the invention was held by the EPO not to be contrary to morality. The patent is now under opposition. A corresponding US patent was granted in 1988 and a further three US patents on transgenic animals were granted in December 1992.

8. Obviously I have not specifically covered all the possibilities that can be encountered. If the main invention is a novel protein made by recombinant DNA techniques, for example, it is possible to claim a variety of 'biotech intermediates', *e.g.* DNA sequences, vectors containing such sequences, and hosts containing the vectors. Patenting in the biotechnology field is a somewhat specialised topic largely outside the scope of this chapter.

9. For those interested in reading more about the landmark 'second medical indication' decision by the European Patent Office Enlarged Board of Appeal, see case Gr 05/83, Official Journal of the European Patent Office 3/1985, pages 64–66. This will be kept in your in-house patent department or is available at the address shown in reference 19. To complicate the issue further there is also a 'first medical use' decision (Decision T 128/82; OJEPO 4/1984, pages 164 – 172) which addressed the question of how to claim the first **medical** use for a known compound. In such a case a claim reading: '[known compound X] for use in therapy' is allowable.

10. For further information on the so-called 'NIH patent controversy', see *Bio/Technology* 9: 1310 (1991). The issue of patenting partial gene sequences spread from the USA to Europe where the MRC followed a similar policy to the NIH as a defensive measure [see *Bio/Technology* 10: 956 (1992)]. *Note added in proof: the NIH and MRC abandoned their patent applications in early 1994.*

11. John Milton pointed to the dangers of hindsight analysis in Paradise Lost (Book VI)! As he put it (spelling updated):
    'The invention all admired and each how he to be the inventor missed.
    So easy it seemed, once found, which yet unfound, most would have thought impossible!'

12. For a detailed study of the effects of substituted 1,2-benzisothiazol-3-ones on blood platelets see K.H. Baggaley, P.D. English, L.J.A. Jennings, B. Morgan, B. Nunn, and A.W.R. Tyrrell, *J. Med. Chem.*, 1985, **28**, 1661.

13. R. Gunning, 'More Effective Writing in Business and Industry' (Industrial Education International, 1962), pages 2 to 15. The steps for the calculation of the Fog Index are as follows:
    (a) Find the average number of words per sentence. Use a sample at least 100 words long. Divide the total number of words by the number of sentences. This gives you the average length of each sentence.
    (b) Count the number of words of three syllables or more per 100 words. Do not count: (1) words which are capitalised; (2) combinations of short easy words; (3) verbs that are made 3 syllables by adding 'ed' or 'es'.
    (c) Add the two factors above together and multiply by 0.4. This will give you the Fog Index. It corresponds roughly with the number of years of

schooling a person would require to read a passage with ease and understanding.

14. The UK Patent Office is now based at Newport in Wales. There is still a receiving office in London for patent applications to be hand-filed.

15. There are currently 17 member states of the European Patent Convention, namely: Austria, Belgium, Denmark, France, Germany, Greece, Ireland, Italy, Liechtenstein, Luxembourg, Netherlands, Monaco, Portugal, Spain, Sweden, Switzerland, and UK. Liechtenstein and Switzerland are covered in just one designation.

16. See American Cyanamid *vs* Ethicon (1974), a case relating to surgical sutures.

17. The patent profession seems to be growing in popularity but is still a small one. In the UK there are only about 1300 Fellows of the Chartered Institute of Patent Agents. In Europe at large there are approximately 5500 European Patent Attorneys of which most are British, German, or French. At the last count there were just three in Monaco!

18. More outlandish intellectual property cases include *Carson vs Here's Johnny Portable Toilets Inc* and *Dallas Cowboy Cheerleaders Inc vs Pussycat Cinema Ltd*. Stranger than fiction cases of bygone years include *Baird vs Moule's Patent Earth Closet Co. Ltd.* (1876) and *United States vs Eleven and a quarter dozen Packages of Article labeled in part Mrs Moffat's shoo fly powder for drunkenness* (1941)!

19. For further reading see, for example:
R.J. Pidgeon, *Chem. Br.*, 1993, **29**, 489.
'A Practical Guide to Patent Law' 2nd Ed., Brian C. Reid (Sweet and Maxwell, 1993); Various UK Patent Office Publications, *e.g.* 'Patent Protection' (1992) and 'What is Intellectual Property' (1993). For details of publications and services available from the Patent Office, contact The Patent Office, Cardiff Road, Newport, Gwent NP9 1RH. Telephone 0633-813535.
When in London, the place to look at patents, both British and foreign, is the British Library at 25, Southampton Buildings.

Those interested in a career in the patent profession should consult the Chartered Institute of Patent Agents, Staple Inn Buildings, High Holborn, London WC1V 7PZ (telephone 071 405 9450).

Molecular Biology – A New Route to Drug Discovery

JANET E. CAREY

This chapter is intended to give a brief overview of gene cloning at a basic level and a taste of some of its many applications within the pharmaceutical industry.

1 DNA STRUCTURE

The information required to build and subsequently direct the day to day housekeeping processes of a cell is carried within deoxyribonucleic acid or DNA. It is built up of four deoxynucleotides containing the bases adenine (A), thymine

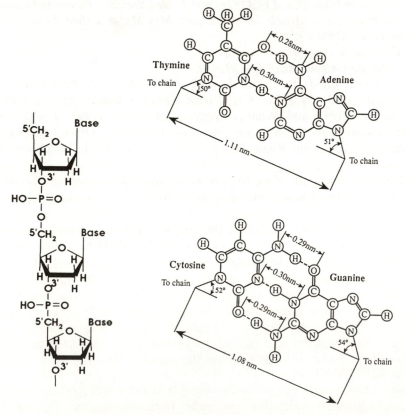

Figure 1: *Deoxyribose/phosphate backbone and hydrogen bonding between bases*

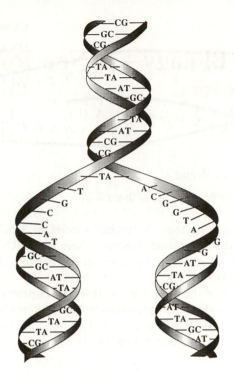

Figure 2: *DNA double helix undergoing replication*

(T), guanine (G), and cytidine (C). These are linked together into a string which has a deoxyribose/phosphate backbone from which the bases protrude. Each chain of bases has a complementary partner in which A pairs with T and G pairs with C *via* hydrogen bonds (Figure 1).

The two chains are then coiled into the familiar double helix structure first described by Watson and Crick in 1953. The complementarity of the strands forms the basis of the replication mechanism. As the cell prepares to divide the two DNA strands separate, incoming bases are matched to the exposed single strand and incorporated enzymatically into the growing replicate daughter strands (Figure 2).

Contiguous stretches of nucleotides form structures known as GENES and, in general, a single gene directs the production of one protein. The information held within the DNA is converted into protein structures *via* another nucleic acid intermediate called messenger ribonucleic acid or mRNA. It is very similar in structure to DNA except that it is single stranded, has a ribose/phosphate backbone, and contains uracil (U) residues rather than thymine. The DNA is enzymatically copied into mRNA within the nucleus. This process is known as TRANSCRIPTION (Figure 3).

Within each gene only one of the two strands of DNA will be transcribed into RNA although which strand this is may vary from gene to gene. The mRNA is transported out of the nucleus into the cytoplasm of the cell where it is

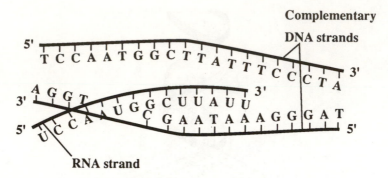

Figure 3: *Transcription of DNA to form an RNA copy*

TRANSLATED into a protein. A further species of RNA called transfer or tRNA is utilised in the translation process. These small RNA molecules form a characteristic clover leaf structure by base pairing between different parts of the single strand (Figure 4).

The bottom portion of the molecule has three bases protruding (an anticodon) which match up with three complementary bases in the mRNA molecule (a codon) and the top carries an amino acid. The four different bases can form a total of 64 possible three base combinations. As there are only twenty-two amino

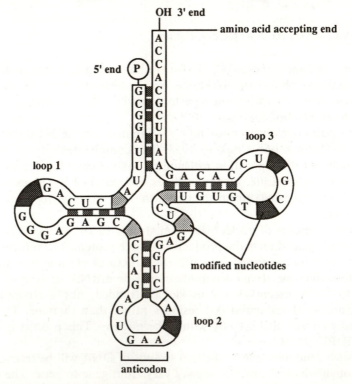

Figure 4: *Representation of a tRNA molecule*

acids, most are specified by more than one codon. The relationship between codons and amino acids is referred to as the GENETIC CODE and is highly conserved across different organisms.

The Genetic Code

A	R	N	D	C	Q	E	G	H	I
Ala	Arg	Asn	Asp	Cys	Gln	Glu	Gly	His	Ile
5' GCA	CGA	AAC	GAC	UGC	CAA	GAA	GGA	CAC	AUA
C	C	U	U	U	G	G	C	U	C
G	G						G		U
U	U						U		
	or								
	AGA								
	G								

L	K	M	F	P	S	T	W	Y	V
Leu	Lys	Met	Phe	Pro	Ser	The	Trp	Tyr	Val
CUA	AAA	AUG	UUC	CCA	UCA	ACA	UGG	UAC	GUA 3'
C	G		U	C	C	C		U	C
G				G	G	G			G
U				U	U	U			U
or					or				
UUA					AGC				
G					U				

Translation occurs on a structure called a ribosome which 'flattens' out the mRNA and presents it as a template for the incoming tRNA molecules carrying amino acids. As each tRNA matches itself to a group of three bases, its amino acid is added to the growing protein chain (Figure 5).

The signals required to start and stop transcription and subsequently direct translation are carried within the DNA sequence as motifs which are recognised by the enzymes which direct the processes.

2 WHAT DETERMINES THE DIFFERENCES BETWEEN CELL TYPES?

A newly fertilised ovum has the ability to produce proteins from its full repertoire of genes – it is TOTIPOTENT. As the single cell divides to form an embryo the component cells become more specialised as they begin to be committed to the formation of specific tissues. These changes are effected by closing down parts of the genome and only expressing the limited range of proteins characteristic of that cell type. All the necessary on/off switches which control this narrowing down process are carried within the DNA itself.

In summary:

• The information required to produce proteins is contained within DNA as a series of nucleotide triplets called codons.
• The DNA in a gene contains all the information required to make a protein.

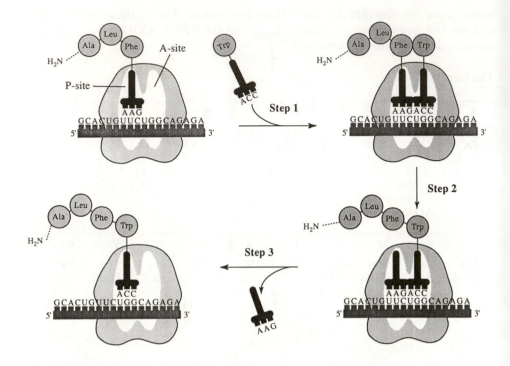

Figure 5: *Translation of a mRNA molecule at the ribosome to form a protein*

- Protein is produced using an intermediate nucleic acid – mRNA.
- Each cell type produces a unique repertoire of proteins and hence contains the corresponding repertoire of mRNAs.

3 GENE CLONING – PROPAGATION OF GENETIC MATERIAL IN ALTERNATIVE HOST SYSTEMS

When we set out to clone a gene coding for a particular protein the first task is to identify either a tissue or cell line which produces that protein. The tissue is then disrupted and the mRNA isolated. This is then copied using enzymes – initially into single-stranded and then into double-stranded copy or cDNA. These cDNA molecules are incorporated into carrying vectors or PLASMIDS which carry antibiotic selection markers and can be introduced into an alternative host system, such as bacteria, for replication. It is possible to screen this pool of bacteria (each of which will carry a replica of a single mRNA which was expressed in the original starting material) and select CLONES of bacteria carrying the gene of interest (Figure 6).

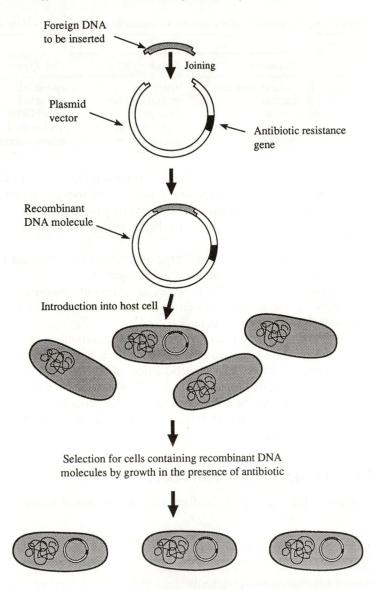

Foreign DNA
to be inserted

Joining

Plasmid
vector

Antibiotic resistance
gene

Recombinant
DNA molecule

Introduction into host cell

Selection for cells containing recombinant DNA
molecules by growth in the presence of antibiotic

Figure 6: *Diagramatic representation of the cloning process*

4 EXPRESSION OF CLONED GENES

In general terms we are not interested in the cloned genes per se but rather more
in the proteins encoded by them. There are a number of different cell systems
commonly used to produce recombinant proteins which all have disadvantages as
well as advantages.

Prokaryotic (bacterial) systems are suitable for production of prokaryotic
proteins or a limited number of eukaryotic (mammalian) proteins. The limitation

Table 1: *Some examples of tissue culture cell lines commonly used to express cloned genes*

| Name | Origin | | |
	Organism	Tissue	Cell Type
CHO	chinese hamster	ovary	epithelial
HeLa	human	cervical cancer	epithelial
NIH3T3	mouse	embryo	fibroblast
HEK293	human	embryonic kidney	unclassified
SH-SY-5Y	human	neuroblastoma	neurally derived

occurs because bacteria are usually unable to form disulphide bridges often found in eukaryotic proteins and are therefore unable to introduce the elements of tertiary structure conferred by them. Any eukaryotic proteins produced in such a system may have to be isolated from the bacteria and refolded *in vitro* under stringent conditions.

Yeast is a good system for producing large quantities of protein, but it tends to be over glycosylated which may ultimately affect function.

Baculovirus grown in insect cells provides an excellent system for producing secreted proteins on a rapid large batch basis particularly for use in the initial evaluation phase for novel protein agents.

Eukaryotic tissue culture systems are ideal for the production of proteins with complex tertiary structure which can either be secreted or membrane bound and are often the system of choice for the production of clinical grade material. The disadvantage of this type of expression is that development of a stable high level expression cell line can often be a very time consuming process.

Some examples of tissue culture cell lines commonly used to express cloned genes are shown in Table 1.

5 USES OF CLONED HUMAN PROTEINS

The remainder of the chapter will address the uses of cloned human proteins in three ways:

- As therapeutic agents in their own right.
- As screening tools to aid in chemical SAR.
- As structure/function mapping tools.

Use of Proteins as Therapeutic Agents Exemplified by the Development of Novel Thrombolytics.

Myocardial infarction is a major cause of death and morbidity in the western world. It is caused by the formation of a blockage in any of the major coronary arteries which in turn interrupts the blood flow and therefore the supply of oxygen to the heart muscle. This results in permanent damage to the oxygen-starved region and a consequent reduction in heart function. Blood clots usually form in vessels which are already partially occluded by atherosclerotic plaque – a matrix of a protein called fibrin forms which then traps platelets and cells within it. The body has a very finely balanced system to clear small build-ups of fibrin. An inactive protein, plasminogen, is cleaved to its active form plasmin by agents known as plasminogen activators. Plasmin in turn breaks down fibrin into soluble fibrin derived products.

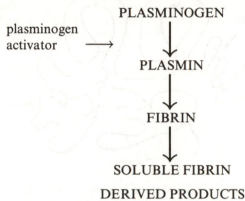

This chain of enzymic reactions has to be very highly regulated to prevent the breakdown of beneficial clots, for example those blocking holes in damaged vessel walls. This regulation prevents potentially damaging internal bleeding and is achieved partly by maintaining very low circulating levels of endogenous plasminogen activators. One of the most potent naturally occurring plasminogen activators is a 527 amino acid protein called tissue plasminogen activator or tPA. It binds to fibrin with very high specificity, is very potent but is cleared from the bloodstream rapidly by the liver ($t_{1/2} < 2$ mins).

The human form of the enzyme was cloned by Genentech and marketed as a thrombolytic agent for the treatment of heart attack. The major drawback for its use as a therapeutic agent was the short half-life which meant that the route of administration was continuous i.v. infusion. This treatment could not be started until the patient reached hospital – wasting vital time. Our remit was to produce a thrombolytic agent with high potency, high specificity, and a long half-life in the body.

The tPA protein contains a number of recognisable domains (Figure 7). Within the A chain are a fibronectin finger (F), a growth factor domain (G), and two kringles (K1 and K2): the latter are thought to be involved in binding to fibrin. The B chain of the enzyme contains the active site.

It is possible to dissect out the regions of the gene which encode these domains using enzymes which recognise specific sequences in the DNA and effect cleavage at that point. Enzymes are selected which recognise flanking sequences of the region to be removed, the DNA is cut, and the remaining portions are then stuck back together. If this altered piece of DNA is introduced into a tissue culture cell line it will direct the production of a correspondingly altered or mutated protein. We constructed a range of mutant genes with various domains of the protein removed, *e.g.*

tPA

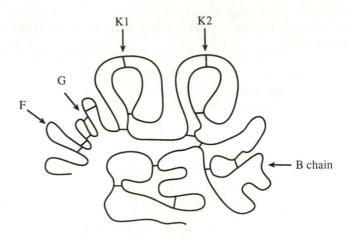

Figure 7: *Diagramatic representation of tissue plasminogen activator protein, tPA*

where tPA = FGK1K2B   mutant 1 = FK1K2B
                                                     2 = GK1K2B
                                                     3 = FGK2B
                                                     4 = FGK1B

The mutant with the growth factor domain removed (FK1K2B) showed altered clearance properties with an increase in half-life to approximately 12 minutes. This may have been because we have removed the liver recognition site from the protein or because the new mutant protein is folded in such a way that it is disrupted or hidden.[1]

A further line of investigation involved the production of hybrid protein molecules. The protein plasminogen (the inactive precursor at the head of the physiological fibrinolytic cascade) has a very high affinity for fibrin which is thought to be associated with five kringle structures within its A chain. This A chain was linked biochemically to the B chain of the tPA in an attempt to remove the liver recognition site from t-PA but retain fibrin binding activity.

The small amount of hybrid protein produced in this way showed potential as a thrombolytic agent but could not be produced in sufficient quantities for full scale evaluation. To overcome this problem the genes for plasminogen and tPA were cloned and the portion of the plasminogen gene encoding the A chain was cut out and spliced to the portion of the t-PA gene carrying the B chain (Figure 8). The hybrid gene coding sequence was introduced into tissue culture cells which synthesised the novel protein at high level.

Pharmacological testing revealed the hybrid to be an excellent thrombolytic agent. The half life in the body was around 90 minutes, it showed greater potency in a clot lysis model than tPA, and it spared plasma fibrinogen levels indicating that it had a high degree of clot specificity. The three desired properties for an

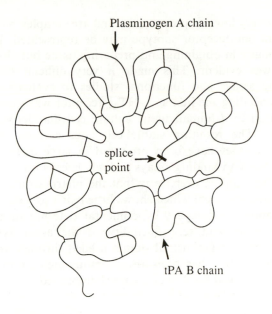

Figure 8: *Diagramatic representation of a hybrid protein formed from the t-PA A chain and the plasminogen B chain*

injectable thrombolytic – long half life, potency and specificity had been achieved in this genetically engineered molecule.[2]

Its eventual role in the front line treatment of myocardial infarction would require further evaluation *in vivo* and large-scale clinical trials.

Proteins as Screening Tools

Our understanding of human metabolism and disease processes is increasing at a very rapid rate and, as knowledge accumulates, the requirement for specificity in the drugs we design is correspondingly increased. In no field is this currently more apparent than that of the superfamily of seven transmembrane domain G protein coupled receptors. There are a large number of subtypes of receptor, many of which are implicated in specific disease areas. For example various serotonin receptors are thought to be involved in anxiety, panic, depression, and migraine. The implication of the existence of so many closely related receptors for the medicinal chemist is the possibility of developing highly specific therapeutic agents.

Molecular biology is not only adding extra layers of complexity to the area by the seemingly endless discovery of novel receptors but is also contributing to the drug discovery process by providing cloned genes for use in screens to aid chemical SAR studies.

A recent example of this is illustrated by the serotonin 5-HT$_{2C}$ receptor. This was thought to represent a novel target for which there were no selective agonists or antagonists. Pharmacologists were working with rodent and porcine brain tissue which have a very low receptor density and are complex biological systems in which more than one receptor subtype may be represented. In addition not only was there difficulty in obtaining and preparing tissue but also high batch to batch variability was evident. This made it very difficult to perform both radioligand binding assays and functional studies to evaluate novel chemical entities. The gene encoding the human 5-HT$_{2C}$ receptor was isolated from brain tissue and transferred to a human tissue culture cell line derived from human embryonic kidney.[3] The resulting stable cell lines carrying human 5-HT$_{2C}$ receptors on their surfaces have been produced in large quantities to provide membranes for radioligand binding assays and whole cells for functional studies. The end point of this cloning exercise is that the pharmacologists are working with a simple human test system which shows little batch to batch variation. This has reduced the number of repeat experimental determinations required by increasing the reliability and reproducibility of the assay system and also decreased the number of experimental points needed through improved signal/noise ratio. Ultimately there has been an enormous increase in throughput of compounds and the chemical SAR data are much improved.

Genetically Engineered Proteins as Structure/Function Mapping Tools

Medicinal chemists are increasingly using molecular modelling by complex computer algorithms as a means of designing chemical entities to perform specific functions. This is particularly true in areas where agonists/antagonists are being designed to interact with protein molecules or cellular receptors.

Molecular biologists have the ability to alter or mutate any amino acid within a protein. I will use two literature examples to show how such techniques can be used to examine the role of particular amino acids or domains within a protein.

The literature examples both refer to studies on seven transmembrane domain G coupled receptors where it is predicted that the seven membrane spanning 'barrels' form a cylinder which provides a pocket in which ligands are bound. By comparing structures within this protein family it is possible to postulate which amino acids might be important in the binding process.

The first example is a piece of work by Hartig *et al.*[4] which shows how the alteration of a single amino acid within a protein can radically affect its function. The group were studying the rat and human 5-HT$_{2A}$ receptors which are 92% identical at the amino acid level but show very different binding to the ligand mesulergine, which has an approximately 50-fold greater affinity for the rat receptor than for its human counterpart. Comparison of the protein sequences within the transmembrane domains show only three amino acid differences between the two proteins.

Two of these represent conservative changes (one non-polar amino acid being substituted for another). The third amino acid difference in transmembrane domain 5, where the rat receptor contains a non-polar alanine and the human receptor a polar serine, was potentially of more interest as this represented a region implicated by molecular modelling as being important in ligand binding in adrenergic receptors (Table 2).

Table 2: *Comparison of 5-HT$_2$ receptor sequence in transmembrane 5*

	S	F	V	S	F	F	I	P	L
h5-HT$_2$ (Normal Human)	TCT	TTT	GTG	TCA	TTT	TTC	ATT	CCC	TTA
	S	F	V	A	F	F	I	P	L
h5-HT$_2$mu (Mutant Human)	TCT	TTT	GTG	GCA	TTT	TTC	ATT	CCC	TTA
	S	F	V	A	F	F	I	P	L
r5-HT$_2$ (Normal Rat)	TCT	TTT	GTG	GCA	TTT	TTC	ATC	CCC	CTA

A gene was constructed which encoded a mutant human protein where the relevant serine residue in transmembrane domain 5 was altered to an alanine, in line with the structure of the rat receptor. The mutant gene was introduced into a eukaryotic cell line and the binding affinity of mesulergine determined. The mutated human receptor showed an increased affinity for mesulergine which was comparable with the native rat 5-HT$_{2A}$ receptor indicating that a single amino acid substitution can radically affect the pharmacology of a seven transmembrane receptor.

The second example of a mutagenesis study is provided by the work of Frielle *et al.*[5] This group was attempting to determine which transmembrane domains in the β_1 and β_2 adrenergic receptors are important in agonist/antagonist binding. The β_1 and β_2 adrenergic receptors have a 71% amino acid homology over the important seven transmembrane domain regions. They are however pharmacologically distinct with respect to both agonists and antagonists. The agonists isoproteronol, norepinephrine, and epinephrine show a different rank order of affinities for the two receptors:

β_1 receptor isoproteronol > norepinephrine = epinephrine
β_2 receptor isopreteronol > epinephrine > norepinephrine

There are distinct selective antagonists for both receptors. β_1 is antagonised by betaxolol and β_2 is antagonised by ICI 118551. A series of hybrid molecules was constructed by starting with the gene for the β_1 receptor and progressively exchanging domains with the β_2 receptor, *e.g.*:

If A B C D E F G represent the transmembrane domains of the β_1 receptor and a b c d e f g their β_2 counterparts the hybrid series of molecules would be represented by:

A B C D E F G
a B C D E F G
a b C D E F G
a b c D E F G and so on through to
a b c d e f g

The pharmacology of the spliced receptors was assessed using both agonists and antagonists. Exchange of the first three transmembrane domains had no effect on the rank order of agonist binding affinities. Addition of transmembrane domain 4 caused a dramatic conversion of the hybrid toward a β_2-like profile. The further addition of transmembrane domains 5, 6, and 7 did not result in further significant changes indicating that the amino acids within transmembrane domain 4 are strongly implicated in agonist binding.

The situation with regard to the specific antagonists is not so clear cut; the addition of successive domains contributes to a gradual change in the binding profiles with transmembrane domains 3, 5, and 7 showing the greatest influence.

Experiments such as these show what an important part molecular biology has to play in the design of chemical entities either as a means of testing hypotheses developed using molecular modelling or by guiding the chemist toward the important target areas of protein molecules.

Genetic engineering is an area of science which has shown exponential growth over the last twenty years and the level of understanding it provides of the structure of protein targets should greatly aid the drug development process. For this to happen medicinal chemists must feel free to access and use the information generated by molecular biologists and this can only occur when a basic understanding of the processes involved is achieved. This chapter and the lecture from which it was derived may hopefully go some way to giving you a start on the learning curve. For further general background reading I can recommend 'Molecular Biology of the Cell' by Bruce Alberts *et al.* published by Garland Publishing Inc. This is an easily understandable textbook with excellent illustrations.

6 REFERENCES

1. M. J. Browne *et al.*, *J. Biol. Chem.*, 1988, **263**, 1599.
2. J. H. Robinson *et al.*, *Circulation*, 1992, **86**, 548.
3. J.E. Carey *et al.*, Proceedings of the Second NIMH conference on Molecular Neurobiology, Keystone, Colorado, 1992.
4. P. Hartig *et al.*, *FEBS Lett.*, 1992, **307**, 324.
5. T. Frielle *et al.*, *Proc. Natl. Acad. Sci.*, 1988, **85**, 9494.

CHAPTER 12

Devising a Research Strategy

COLIN W. GREENGRASS

1 INTRODUCTION

Most of the chapters in this book have focused on the scientific and operational aspects of research as applied directly to a programme of medicinal chemical research. However, before experimental work commences, a strategy is needed to ensure that research is focused on an area of significant medical need and commercial opportunity, and to expedite the progress of research. Therefore, some broader aspects of the drug discovery process should be considered, and efforts should be made to assess whether there are aspects of the programme which are likely to be especially challenging. In this chapter I would like to take the opportunity to draw together some of the themes which have been discussed more fully during the book, and suggest how they may be taken into account as a research programme is developed. First of all, though, I would like to consider some broader aspects of a research programme, beginning with selection of a disease target.

2 DECIDING ON AN AREA FOR RESEARCH

In the early days of the pharmaceutical industry, there were many therapeutic opportunities which were successfully exploited and provided the medicines on which today's industry was founded. In the areas of antibiotics and psycho-trophics, for example, it was possible to produce breakthrough remedies for conditions which were not previously treatable. By contrast, in the 1990s, whilst there are still many serious disease challenges, we must also recognise that acceptable therapies are available for many conditions. Therefore, one task facing the pharmaceutical industry is to provide new agents which have clear advantages over existing therapy.[1] This might arise, for example, by virtue of increased selectivity for a particular biological mechanism. Alternatively, it may be possible to provide a new dosage form which results in a particular advantage to the patient. Fortunately, advances in pharmacology, pharmacokinetics and drug metabolism, molecular biology, and formulation science make such objectives realistic.

In choosing a target for industrial pharmaceutical research, it is essential to bear in mind that the resulting product must be commercially viable. Assuming the project is successful, about ten years are likely to elapse before an agent can be marketed. Therefore, careful evaluation of the opportunity is essential before any new project is commenced. Those proposing a new research project should consider the medical need, commercial opportunity, current therapy, and competitor activity. These factors can be thought of as a summary of the need for a new or improved therapy. Thus, evaluation of the opportunity should include a consideration of the following:

- severity of the condition: is it self limiting – life threatening?
- current therapy: is the level of satisfaction high or low?
- patient numbers
- duration of the proposed therapy: acute or chronic?
- will the new drug permit a novel approach to the management of the disease?

Information on these topics can be gathered in various ways, though care is often needed when interpreting raw data. Epidemiological studies may be consulted to provide information about the number of individuals affected, for example by analysis of patient visits to medical practitioners or by the number of work days lost through illness. However, such data can be potentially misleading and should be interpreted with care. Allergic rhinitis, for example, has a high incidence though not all sufferers will pay visits to their medical practitioners. For many, it is a relatively mild and self-limiting condition which is controlled by OTC products, and dosing convenience plays a significant role in their selection. In contrast, despite its high profile, AIDS affects a relatively small, though still increasing, number of individuals. However, since AIDS is invariably fatal, the medical need to develop an effective treatment is very high. Thus efficacy, rather than dosing convenience, would be the criterion for prescribing a novel anti-HIV product. In some cases, there may be a desire for improved therapy which is not reflected in practitioner visits, since it is not generally thought that an effective prescription medicine is available. This provides an opportunity to produce a new therapeutic approach, perhaps an oral remedy for an indication which previously has been treated topically. Oral treatment of vaginal candidiasis by fluconazole is a recent example of this. Thus the medical opportunity should be considered both in the context of numbers affected, the severity and duration of the condition, and the degree of satisfaction with currently available therapy.

It is likely that, at the project selection stage, the feasibility of running a successful clinical development programme will also be considered. Although this assessment would normally be carried out by members of the clinical group who would be responsible for trials, the medicinal chemist should be aware that a simple demonstration of efficacy and safety is unlikely to be sufficient for approval of most potential therapies. Usually it will be necessary to show some advantage compared with existing therapy. This is likely to be difficult in situations where there is a high degree of satisfaction with existing therapy, where a particularly long course of treatment is needed or where recruitment of patients is likely to be a problem. For example, clinical efficacy would be straightforward to demonstrate for an oral antibiotic which is intended for the community market, but showing an advantage over available agents would be much more resource intensive, since current therapy is generally effective.

Finally, it is worthwhile to consider whether there are special needs such as gaps in your corporate portfolio, or special situations which argue for a particular therapeutic area. Thus, a particular case might be made to develop a follow-on product with improved properties for an agent which is nearing the end of its patent life.

It is wise for the scientists who are proposing a new project to consider the foregoing factors, even if the formal review of the opportunity is conducted by a specialist group, since this will enable them to reject approaches which are obviously flawed and concentrate on the most worthwhile opportunities which are likely to attract support and maximum resources. Such an analysis, if thoughtfully conducted, could be a significant factor in determining the clinical objective for the project. It will highlight those features of current therapy which should be retained, and underscore those which require improvement. In this way, the target profile can be defined, and this could have a direct bearing on the selection of a biological mechanism which will become the strategy for the project. Thus, if current therapy is effective and well tolerated, but has the disadvantage of an inconvenient dosing regime, then it may be sufficient to pursue agents of the same therapeutic class and seek improvements to pharmacokinetics, perhaps through a pro-drug or formulation.

Some examples of this are BW 245U87, a pro-drug of acyclovir which is in advanced trials at Burroughs Wellcome, and Procardia XL (TM, marketed by Pfizer) a once-daily formulation of the short acting calcium channel blocker, nifedipine. Alternatively, it might be recognised that optimum agents of a particular mechanistic class have been identified, and that the next therapeutic advance will require an alternative pharmacological approach. This belief lies behind the battle for the anti-ulcer market being waged by the H_2 antagonists such as ranitidine (Glaxo), and the proton pump inhibitors such as omeprazole (Astra). Thus, an important issue for the pharmacologist and medicinal chemist is to decide whether to seek improvements within an existing drug class, or to follow a novel mechanistic approach.

3 SCREEN SEQUENCES

New projects can be divided into those which have lead structures on which to base the design of novel analogues, and those which do not. In this section, I will focus on the former category but I will return to the latter class in the section 'Finding A Lead'.

It is obvious, but worth stating for emphasis, that the screening cascade must reflect the properties you are seeking. Assuming synthesis is ongoing there must be primary screens available which have sufficient capacity to enable an acceptable rate of progress, and are capable of discriminating between compounds which are worthy of further investigation and those which are not. Thus potency and/or selectivity at a given receptor or enzyme may be primary selection criteria. Choice of an *in vitro* screen is helpful in most cases in ensuring that new compounds act by the chosen mechanism and meet minimum levels of potency and selectivity. If selectivity is paramount, then the variability of the screen should be small compared with the degree of selectivity sought. If it is not, then the relevance of small differences of selectivity must be questionable, and results obtained from screens run on different days will be difficult to compare. In many areas there will be more detailed *in vitro* assays, but it is important that these primary selection screens are followed up with meaningful *in vivo* animal models. These should be designed to confirm the relevance of compounds found active in *in vitro* assays. At this secondary level, it is again helpful to have the capacity to evaluate a significant number of analogues so that rapid turn-round is achieved to guide chemistry. Typically these screens might provide data on *in vivo* potency, dose response, duration of action, and pharmacokinetics. At the third level, there is a place for a more complex efficacy model, though this might be reserved for compounds of substantial interest. In some areas it is impractical or impossible to employ an efficacy model and compounds may be advanced to the clinic on the basis of animal pharmacology and pharmacokinetics. However, although advances in the study of transgenic animals may enable the development of animal models of diseases which exclusively affect humans, their use must be approached cautiously and with thoughtful choice of controls to validate their use.

So far I have barely mentioned medicinal chemistry. This has been deliberate since I wished to highlight the fact that synthesis should not commence until systems are in place to evaluate test compounds. However, it is now timely to turn to lead identification and optimisation.

4 FINDING A LEAD

What is a lead? I suggest that a rather rigid definition should be used so that the term 'lead' is used to identify those prototype structures which are of substantial interest. Thus, a lead structure should fulfil several requirements. It should meet potency and selectivity criteria *in vitro*. It must have a structure which is suitable for chemical modifications designed to optimise properties. Ideally, it should offer the potential for *in vivo* activity. Finally, it is helpful if it has a molecular weight similar to the target range. Overall, it should be an advance over previously examined compounds, and 'lead' the project towards a development candidate.

In many new projects, there will be known compounds to help identify lead structures. The medicinal chemist must use his knowledge and experience to identify those structural features which contribute to their profiles. Various computational techniques are most helpful here to recognise areas of high binding potential – such as H-bonding sites, which contribute to selectivity, and hydrophobic areas, which contribute to potency. The 'goodness of fit' of a ligand can be estimated by docking into a molecular model or empirically by means of an 'Andrews' calculation.[2] A similar approach can be used to identify, and avoid, functionalities which introduce undesirable activity, thereby increasing the selectivity for a particular target mechanism. Thus, it is possible to consider all compounds which are known to have some activity of the type sought and, on the basis of this knowledge, propose novel targets for synthesis. I would describe this as an evolutionary approach to finding a lead. Those compounds which provide a recognisable advance over their progenitors become project leads. Typically, each lead constitutes a milestone in a research project. In the classical discovery of cimetidine, several milestone compounds can be recognised. Indeed, two of these, burimamide and metiamide, were themselves potential drugs and were advanced to clinical trials. However, these two compounds were subsequently withdrawn from development and, with the benefit of hindsight, they can be considered as leads which were exploited eventually to afford cimetidine.[3]

4-methylhistamine	– selective for H_2 receptor
guanylhistamine	– partial agonist at H_2 receptor
burimamide	– suboptimal potency, toxic
metiamide	– potent H_2 antagonist, but toxic
cimetidine	– first marketed H_2 antagonist

Sometimes a project may be established for which there are no known chemical starting points, and a lead must be sought by a screening approach. Following a period in the 1980s when random screening was unfashionable and rational drug design was in vogue, a more empirical approach to the identification of a novel chemical starting point is now receiving revived interest. This resurgence of interest is encouraged by improvements in screening technology, which make it possible to screen very large numbers of compounds using automated systems, together with advances in pharmacology and molecular biology which have allowed a more precise definition of pharmacological targets, and provided purified receptors and enzymes. Thus, it is now possible to screen large compound files against single biological targets, often using recombinant human enzymes or receptors, and hence empirically find new chemical starting points for chemical modification. Such screens do not depend on a knowledge of enzyme or receptor structure.

Both the evolutionary and the empirical approach to finding a lead can be exemplified with examples from the HIV area. By inspection of the sequence of the HIV-1 genome, it was suggested that a proteinase might be encoded near the 5′ terminus of the *pol* open reading frame.[4] Subsequently, it was possible to map the proteinase to a 99 amino acid coding region which included the sequence Asp.Thr.Gly, which is characteristic of an aspartyl proteinase. However, the aspartyl proteinases which had been studied up to that time contained two such sequences. Therefore, on the basis of this and other evidence, it was proposed that the HIV-1 proteinase comprised two identical 99 amino acid domains. This knowledge allowed the analogy to be drawn that the HIV-1 proteinase is related to renin, and this proposal has been crucial to the rapid progress made in this area. Research programmes in many companies had been successful in the design of potent inhibitors of renin, based on transition state analogies. This knowledge was therefore employed to design peptidic analogue inhibitors of HIV-1 proteinase, and rapid initial progress was made by numerous companies in the design of novel inhibitors of this important target. However, since all were designed using the same principles, many of the compounds had related structures and a particular concern for research workers in such a competitive area is that they could be entering a patent race. Therefore, if compounds are being 'rationally' designed on the basis of well known data it is particularly important for the chemists to seek prototypes which have 'less obvious' structures; indeed it may be worthwhile to tackle more difficult chemistry in order

Ro 31-8959

to identify a proprietary series. In this respect the Roche group were particularly successful and Ro 31–8959, which is currently in clinical trials, is a member of a structural series which appears to be exclusive to that company.[5]

In contrast, an empirical screening approach to anti-HIV drugs, pursued at several companies, has identified several distinct series of compounds which inhibit HIV reverse transcriptase and act by binding at an allosteric inhibitory site,[6] see below.

All are structurally quite distinct from the active site-directed nucleosides, such as AZT. This suggests a method by which lead structures of unprecedented structure can sometimes be identified and provides a strategy by which leads from a unique structural series may be found. It should be mentioned that development of resistant strains of HIV is rapid in laboratory tests using these allosteric inhibitors, and the clinical relevance of this is currently being assessed. Nevertheless, this illustration of the concept of finding novel leads by empirical screening remains valid.

A second example of lead generation by an empirical screening approach comes from work on inhibitors of the HIV gene-regulatory protein, tat. The role of this protein had been characterised, but there were no data on which to base the rational design of specific antagonists. However, the lead structure, Ro 5–

AZT   Nevirapine   U–85,961

E-BPU   R-82,913   L-697,661

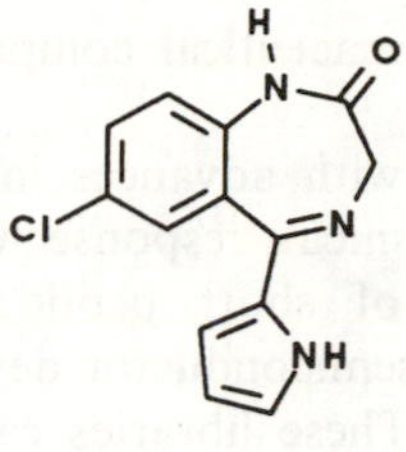

Ro 5-3335

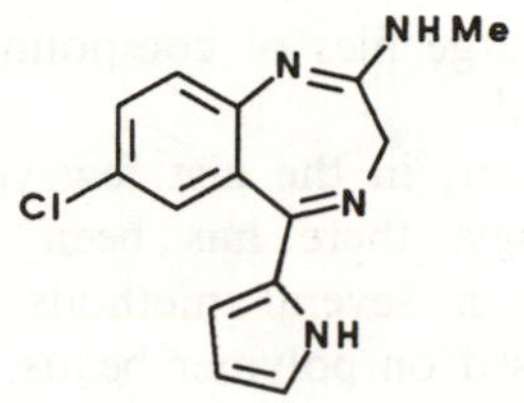

Ro 24-7429

3335, was identified and subsequently optimised as Ro 24–7429.[7] This illustrated that there continues to be a role for screening approaches towards inhibitors of valid biological mechanisms which are not well defined chemically.

The foregoing are examples of the increasing success in development of non-peptide ligands for peptidic receptors. Three further examples are worth comment. The Merck CCK antagonist, MK 329,[8] which was based on asperlicin, and two substance P antagonists, CP 96,345 (Pfizer),[9] which was based on a screening lead, and RP 67,580 (Rhône Poulenc).[10] Although the two substance P-inhibitory lead structures are quite distinct, it is interesting to note that they possess some shared structural features: an example of dissimilarity with a common theme. Certainly, one would feel secure that there would be no interference between the patent claims of these two series.

Thus advances in technology and robotics have enabled dramatic advances to be made in high throughput screening: what was once the preserve of the microbiologist seeking novel antibiotics from microorganisms has now become a viable source of unique prototypes for pharmacological and enzyme inhibitory approaches. Until relatively recently, such automated screens have been fuelled

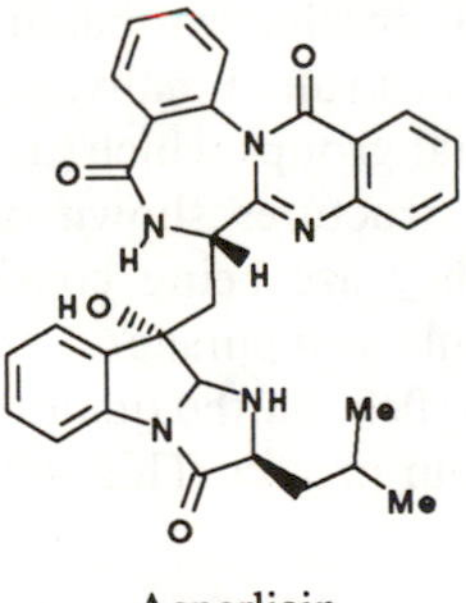

Asperlicin

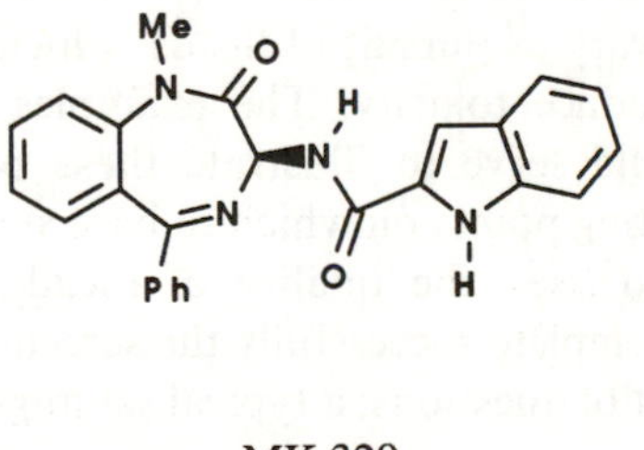

MK 329

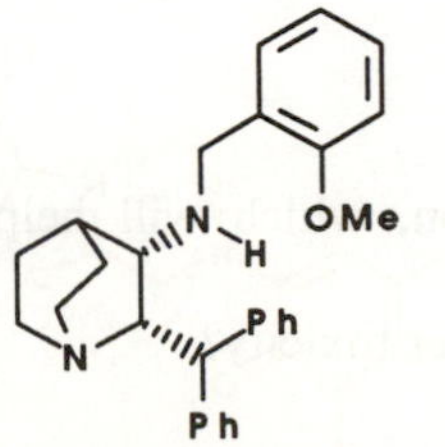

CP-96,345

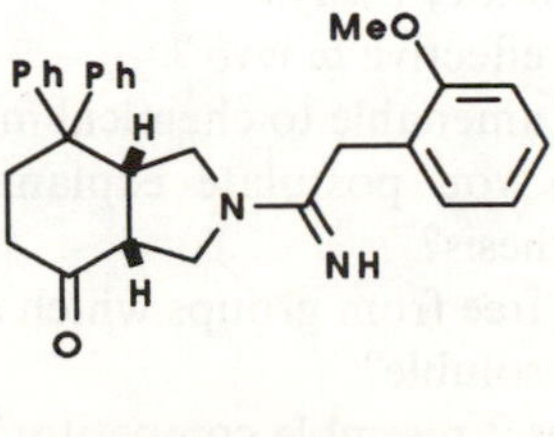

RP-67,580

by the large files of compounds which major pharmaceutical companies have generated.

However, in the last few years, and in parallel with advances in screening technology, there has been a broadly-based chemical response which has resulted in several methods by which libraries of short peptides can be synthesised on polymer beads, or pins, or even on semiconductor devices, such that they can be screened in automated assays.[11] These libraries can thus be used to define peptides which bind at peptide receptors. The challenge which now faces the medicinal chemist working in these areas is to transform these peptide prototypes into non-peptide leads which are a basis for novel drug candidates.

In discussing all of the above approaches, there is an underlying theme, namely that a good lead is capable of chemical modification in a relatively straightforward manner. So how can the 'quality' of a lead be assessed?

5 HOW CAN THE QUALITY OF A LEAD BE ASSESSED?

Initially, I would like to suggest some chemical criteria of quality. Firstly, it should possess structural features which make it amenable to chemical modification either directly or indirectly. Penicillin G was recognised as a lead par excellence when the technology became available to expose the amino group, and thereby afford 6-aminopenicillanic acid. Today this approach is as valid as ever, and the chemist should seek 'handles', either present or masked, which can be used to facilitate the synthesis of analogues.

Secondly, an attractive lead should not, in general, depend on chemically reactive groups to provide its activity: alkylating or acylating agents do not usually make good leads! The special case of mechanism-based enzyme inactivators is, however, an important exception to this rule. Finally, you should be wary of pursuit of 'leads' which contain functional groups which are likely to introduce toxicity. The examples of hypothetical structures shown on p. 187 should serve to illustrate these points. Imagine they are being considered as starting points on which to base synthesis; which would you pursue?

To assess the 'quality' of a lead it is necessary to reflect on the qualities needed to complete successfully the screening sequence of your project. This will generate a list of questions; a typical set might be as follows:

- Does it have the desired potency and selectivity in ligand binding or enzyme inhibitory assays?
- Is it effective *in vivo* ?
- Is it amenable to chemical modification?
- Can you postulate explanations for its action, which will help to guide synthesis?
- Is it free from groups which are likely to engender toxicity?
- Is it soluble?
- Does it resemble competitor's compounds?

– simple structure
– obvious disconnections
– soluble

– chirality readily accessible

– alkylating agent
– hydrolysed to *p*-hydroxyaniline

– difficult chirality, may epimerise
– sulphonic acid: oral absorption issues?

Generally some actives will be found in an empirical screening approach which will rank as 'good' leads, whilst others will be questionable. One particularly controversial area relates to compounds which 'look toxic'. By this I mean those compounds which contain groups which occur frequently in compounds known to be toxic. The rules are not strict, but it is possible to suggest some guidelines, and identify some of the groups which are likely to bring problems. That is, by inspection one can make predictions about some of the likely properties of certain compounds. Certain functional groups are more likely than others to produce toxicity. Nitroaromatics, thioureas, and azo compounds are some examples. Naturally, it is possible to find examples of each which are not toxic: but if they are included in your synthetic compounds then you increase the risk of producing a toxic agent. Other groups which usually should be avoided are reactive species such as alkylating agents including Michael acceptors. If the only lead available has such functionality, and you decide that it must be followed up, then a primary objective should be to replace it with a more acceptable bioisostere at the first opportunity.

Other structural features can be identified which are likely to produce a certain pharmacokinetic profile, for example lipophilic carboxylic acids with high molecular weight are likely to be rapidly excreted in the bile: not a good starting point if you are seeking a long duration serum half-life.

Overall, I would emphasise that many criteria are involved in assessing the quality of a lead. You should follow the best leads available and, as first priority, seek improved analogues in which the limiting properties have been overcome. However, if no improvements are evident after examination of a realistic number of analogues, reconsider the quality of the lead and be prepared to move to an alternative structural theme.

6 SUMMARY

In this overview I have outlined some of the strategic issues in project selection and also some aspects of lead identification and follow up. Naturally there are many other aspects involved in running a research programme. The chapters on pharmacokinetics and the case histories should give further examples of the relevance of pharmacokinetic and pharmacological half-lives, and also some indications as to the decisive factors in clinical studies.

It is important that the medicinal chemist is mindful of all such factors, but it is also important that he maintains his knowledge and interest in synthesis and also is prepared to follow hunches: for it is primarily by the imaginative design of new prototypes that unique chemical entities will be found.

7 REFERENCES

1. For a recent survey of the R & D strategy favoured by 49 leading companies see *J. Pharm. Med.*, 1993, **2**, 139.
2. P.R. Andrews, D.J. Craig, and J.L. Martin, *J. Med. Chem.*, 1984, **27**, 1648.
3. D.G. Cooper *et al.*, in 'Comprehensive Medicinal Chemistry', Vol. 3, ed. C. Hansch, P.G. Sammes, and J.C. Emmett, Pergamon Press, Oxford, pp. 323–421.
4. For a review see: T.L. Blundell *et al.*, *TiBS*, 1990, **15**, 425.
5. N.A. Roberts *et al.*, *Science*, 1990, **248**, 358.
6. R. Pauwels *et al.*, *Nature*, 1990, **343**, 470; V.J. Merluzzi *et al.*, *Science*, 1990, **250**, 1411; M. Baba *et al.*, *Proc. Natl. Acad. Sci. USA*, 1991, **88**, 2356; M.E. Goldman *et al.*, *ibid.*, 1991, **88**, 6863; D.L. Romero, *et al.*, *ibid.*, 1991, **88**, 8806.
7. S. Tam *et al.*, in 'Recent Advances in the Chemistry of Anti-infective Agents', ed. P.H. Bentley and R. Ponsford, Special Publication No. 119, The Royal Society of Chemistry, Cambridge, 1993, p. 314. See also *Inpharma*, 1993, 6th March, pp. 5.
8. B.E. Evans *et al.*, *Proc. Natl. Acad. Sci. USA*, 1986, **83**, 4918.
9. R.M. Snider *et al.*, *Science*, 1991, **251**, 435.
10. C. Garret *et al.*, *Proc. Natl. Acad. Sci. USA*, 1991, **88**, 10208.
11. Bioorganic and Medicinal Chemistry Letters, Symposia-in-Print No. 4, ed. M.R. Pavia, T.K. Sawyer, and W.H. Moos, *BioMed. Chem. Lett.*, 1993, **3**, pp. 381–478.

CHAPTER 13

Past Approaches to Discovering New Drugs as Medicines

C. ROBIN GANELLIN, FRS

1 INTRODUCTION

New medicines are mainly developed by the modern pharmaceutical industry where also most of the new drugs have been discovered. To put the present situation into context it is helpful to recall some of the main approaches to drug discovery which have been taken in the relatively recent past. For excellent accounts of many examples of drug discovery, see Sneader[1] and Bindra and Lednicer[2]. Broadly speaking, there are four main sources for new drug leads. These are:

- Natural products
- Existing drugs
- Screens
- Physiological transmitters

2 DRUGS DERIVED FROM NATURAL PRODUCTS

Natural products provide the oldest source for new medicines. Natural selection during evolution, and competition between the species, has produced powerful biologically active natural products which can serve as chemical leads. For example, moulds and bacteria produce substances that prevent other organisms from growing in their vicinity, *e.g.* penicillin. The discovery of penicillin gave rise to the concept of seeking naturally occurring antibiotics and to its further development by microbiologists who argued that bacteria which cause infections in humans do not survive for long in soil because they are destroyed by other soil-inhabiting microbes. Extensive soil screening research programmes have led to many antibiotics which have provided some very potent life-saving drugs, *e.g.* streptomycin, chloramphenicol, chlortetracycline, and erythromycin.

Microbial fermentation products may also provide leads to other types of drug when combined with a suitable screen. A classic example is that of the novel cholecystokinin (CCK) antagonist, obtained from *Aspergillus alliaceus* fermentation broths which served as the starting point for scientists at Merck Sharp and Dohme to develop very specific and potent nonpeptide antagonists at CCK-A and CCK-B receptors respectively.[3] Screening against the binding of $[^{125}I]$CCK-33 to a membrane preparation from rat pancreas furnished a substance,

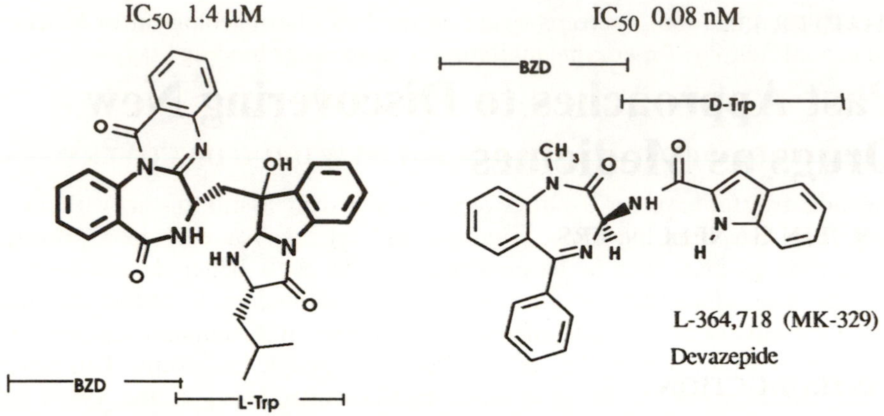

IC$_{50}$ 1.4 µM   IC$_{50}$ 0.08 nM

L-364,718 (MK-329)

Devazepide

Figure 1:   *Asperlicin, a natural product lead from Aspergillus alliaceus, was the starting point for designing potent non-peptide inhibitors at CCK-A receptors.[3] Two substructures were noticed, a benzodiazepine (BZD) and a tryptophan-derived group (L-Trp)*

Asperlicin, which had IC$_{50}$ = 1.4 µM; its structure was determined and served as a lead (Figure 1). Structure–activity exploration led to a very potent synthetic inhibitor (MK-329, devazepide), having IC$_{50}$ = 0.008 nM, *i.e.* over 10 000 fold increase in potency; a non-peptide antagonist of a peptide. Fermentation broths contain hundreds, if not thousands, of chemicals and are a potentially rich source of novel enzyme inhibitors and receptor blockers.

Venoms and toxins are used by animals as protection or to paralyse their prey; some are extremely potent, requiring only minute doses, *e.g.* tetrodotoxin (from puffer fish) which blocks sodium channels, charybdotoxin (from scorpion venom) which blocks Ca-activated potassium channels, α-bungarotoxin (from snake venom) which combines with acetylcholine receptors, and batroxobin (from the venom of a pit viper) which is a thrombin-like enzyme. They have served as starting points for investigation of ion channels, hormone receptors, or enzymes. Recent subjects for study include frogs, spiders, and sponges. Indeed, marine life offers a vast untapped resource for future investigation.[4]

Another fruitful means for identifying pharmacologically active natural products has been the folk law remedies, which are mainly plant products. Alkaloids such as atropine and hyoscine (from plants of the Solanaceae family known to the ancient Greeks), morphine (from the opium poppy known in ancient Egypt), and reserpine (from *Rauwolfia serpentina*, the snakeroot popular in India as a herbal remedy), and non-nitrogenous natural products such as salicylates, *e.g.* salicin from the willow tree (genus *Salix*, botanical sources known to Hippocrates), and the glycosides, *e.g.* digitoxin and digoxin in digitalis from the foxglove (in folk use in England for centuries).

Natural products continue to provide a fruitful source of drug leads. A recent example is the anticancer drug, taxol, isolated from the pacific yew tree. Testing the natural products has become much more efficient now that the procedure can be coupled with robotic screens based on modern pharmacological or biochemical procedures, *e.g.* for enzyme inhibitors or in receptor binding assays.

3 EXISTING DRUGS AS A SOURCE FOR NEW DRUG DISCOVERY

The most fruitful basis for the discovery of a new drug is still to start with an old drug. This has been the most common and reliable route to new products. Existing drugs may need to be improved, *e.g.* to get a better dosage form, to improve drug absorption or duration, to increase potency to reduce the daily dose, or to avoid certain side effects. For example antihistamines discovered in the 1940s, used for treating hay fever, often make people feel sleepy. This has led to the development of the new antihistamines introduced in the 1980s (*e.g.* terfenadine, astemizole, mequitazine) which have a much lower tendency to cause sedation.

Sometimes it is possible to exploit a side effect. A discovery usually starts with astute observation during pharmacological studies in animals or from clinical investigation in patients. Sulphonamide diuretics were discovered in the 1950s following an observation involving sulphanilamide (Figure 2), *i.e.* *p*-aminobenzenesulphonamide (the first antibacterial sulphonamide, see later). Sulphanilamide was found to cause alkaline diuresis in patients who had been given massive doses and this was later shown[5] to be due to inhibition of the enzyme, carbonic anhydrase. The lead was eventually used by chemists at Sharp and Dohme to make other benzene sulphonamides and this led to chlorothiazide (1957; Figure 2) the first of many thiazides which rapidly replaced the mercurial drugs as diuretics.

The phenothiazine tranquillisers resulted from an astute observation of the effects of the antihistamine promethazine[6]. Antihistamines were being studied by Laborit, a French Navy surgeon, for possibly preventing surgical shock since they partially block the vasodilator action of histamine. Promethazine seemed to be better than the others, but it had unusual effects on the central nervous system (CNS). Rhône-Poulenc (the manufacturers) became interested and, since promethazine is a phenothiazine, other phenothiazines were tested to enhance the CNS depressant effects in the (mistaken) belief that this would improve the utility in surgical shock; this led to the identification of chlorpromazine (Figure 3). When tested on patients undergoing surgery they seemed relaxed and unconcerned. The drug was therefore tried on a manic patient (1952) and the dramatic

Sulphanilamide   Chlorothiazide

Figure 2: *Sulphanilamide, an antibacterial drug, was the lead to chlorothiazide and the start of the new diuretics*

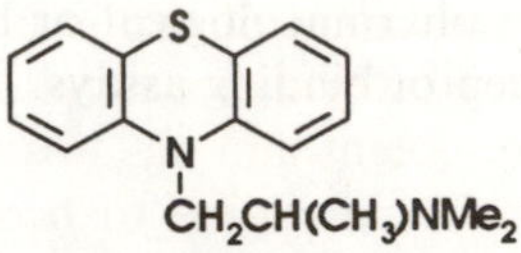

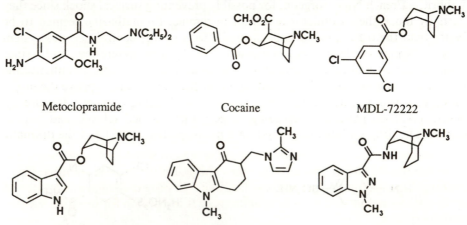

Figure 3: *The antihistamine promethazine, which provided a lead to chlorpromazine giving rise to the revolution in psychiatric medicine*

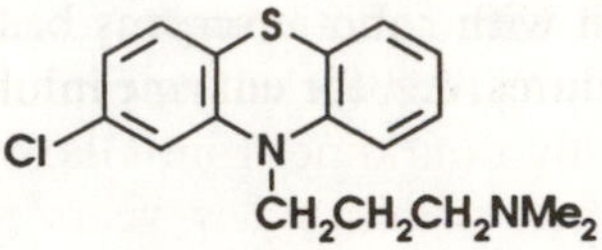

results led to chlorpromazine being used for the treatment of schizophrenia which transformed psychiatric medicine.

A much more recent example is metoclopramide (Figure 4), an antagonist of dopamine receptors, which was found to be useful in patients as an anti-emetic. More potent dopamine antagonists were not so effective, so that it was realised that the compounds were acting by another mechanism. It was shown[8] that metoclopramide and cocaine analogues were also antagonists of a subtype of 5-hydroxytryptamine (5-HT) receptors, then known as 5-HT(M). Further structure–activity studies led to a 3,5-dichlorobenzoate, MDL 72222, which was 40 times more potent than metoclopramide. Subsequently, chemists at Sandoz replaced the benzene ring by indole to give ICS 205-930 (tropisetron) which has a $pA_2 = 10.6$. Later, the receptor was defined as 5-HT$_3$ and work at Beecham and Glaxo led to the development of the new potent anti-emetics granisetron[9] and ondansetron.

Many new products arise which may only represent minor improvements. These are the so-called 'Me-Too' products. It is hard to predict the success of a 'Me-Too' product but some have become the product of choice, replacing the original lead product or at least having a wider usage, *e.g.* the drug cimetidine,

Metoclopramide   Cocaine   MDL-72222

Tropisetron (ICS 205-930)   Ondansetron (GR 38032)   Granisetron (BRL 43694)

Figure 4: *Metoclopramide, a dopamine antagonist, was later shown to act at 5-hydroxytryptamine 5-HT$_3$ receptors and provided the lead for the development of potent anti-emetic drugs tropisetron and granisetron*

from Smith Kline and French, revolutionised the treatment of peptic ulcers and for a while was the best selling prescription drug in the world; it was followed five years later by ranitidine from Glaxo which is more potent and has less effect on liver enzymes; within a few years ranitidine outsold cimetidine to become the number one product.

Historically, 'Me-Too' drugs have provided the main route whereby a particular type of drug action has been optimised in terms both of selectivity (to avoid side effects) and application (for a particular patient population). Eventually, to realise the full potential of a new 'Me-Too' drug and to reveal its advantages, it is necessary to market it in order to gain access to a sufficiently wide patient population. Unfortunately, this can lead to the proliferation of products and it can take many years for clinicians to determine the most suitable drug treatment.

4 USING DISEASE MODELS AS SCREENS FOR NEW DRUG LEADS

The screening approach with natural products for new antibiotics, receptor blockers, and enzyme inhibitors has also been used with synthetic chemicals. The idea has been to test large numbers of compounds on a relatively simple system to reveal the required activity. This has been a third main source of new drugs. The background for this approach lies in the dyestuffs industry. Paul Ehrlich discovered that synthetic dyes were absorbed differentially into tissues and that they could kill parasites and bacteria without affecting mammalian cells. From this work came Salvarsan in 1910, an arsenic compound for treating syphilis.[10] Several large chemical companies followed up this discovery by establishing their own research programmes seeking drugs against venereal diseases and initiated their own systematic examination of hundreds of synthetic chemicals.

In 1931 Gerhard Domagk, working for I.G. Farbenindustrie, turned to screening sulphonamide derivatives of azo dyes and discovered Prontosil Rubrum (red), published in 1935, the first truly effective chemotherapeutic agent for any generalised bacterial infection. This activity was shown to be due to sulphanilamide (Figure 2) and this led to the development of the sulphonamide class of antibacterials.[11]

The success of these discoveries in chemotherapy dominated the research approach in the pharmaceutical industry for many years and screens were also established for non-infectious diseases, *e.g.* for anti-convulsants (useful in epilepsy), analgesics (in the hope of being non addictive), anti-hypertensives, anti-inflammatories, anti-ulcer agents, *etc.* There is, however, a fundamental distinction between the anti-infective screens, and the screens which seek a treatment for a 'metabolically-based' disease. In the anti-infective screens (antibacterial, antifungal, antihelmintic, antiprotozoal, antiviral) a drug is sought which is lethal to the pathogen, but leaves the host unharmed. It is a search for selective toxicity between species.

By contrast, in the metabolically-based diseases, *e.g.* allergy, asthma, cancer, duodenal ulcers, epilepsy, the cause is often unknown, and we seek selectivity within the same being. In these latter situations, an animal model was used as a screening test, in which a clinical condition was induced in a laboratory animal such as a rabbit or rat, and compounds were tested to see whether they would alleviate it. Such models often simulate the disease by presenting similar symptoms, but may be misleading if the underlying causes are quite different; the procedure then throws up false leads, *e.g.* compounds that protect the laboratory animal, but when tested clinically are found not to be active in man. Nevertheless, notable successes have been achieved, *e.g.* non-steroidal ant-inflammatory drugs were discovered by screening in animals in which various forms of inflammation had been artificially induced.

The potassium channel opening class of drug, exemplified by cromakalim, was discovered by testing compounds in the spontaneously hypertensive rat. The compounds were found to reduce blood pressure through vasodilation (relaxing the smooth muscle of blood vessels) and later the mechanism was shown to involve the efflux of potassium ions.

5 PHYSIOLOGICAL MECHANISMS: THE MODERN 'RATIONAL APPROACH' TO DRUG DESIGN

With the advent of greater understanding of a physiological mechanism and with the use of modern technological developments it has become possible to take a more mechanistic approach to research and start from a rationally argued hypothesis to design drugs. Progress depends largely upon the current state of understanding of physiology in relation to diseases. This is the modern 'rational approach' to drug design which is becoming increasingly important with the development of information in cell biochemistry and cell biology, especially where this is understood at the molecular level. Indeed, there has been such a revolution in our ability to define new biological targets in a highly specific manner that the problem has now become one of the selection, *i.e.* which target next? The combination of radioligand binding, receptor cloning and laboratory robotics now makes it possible to screen thousands of compounds per week for blocking action at a specific site.

Modern drug discovery requires very close collaboration between chemists and biologists and a truly 'rational approach' requires several essential ingredients for success:

- evidence of a physiological basis for understanding a disease, so that one may hypothesise that a drug with a particular action should be therapeutically beneficial;
- an explicit chemical starting point;
- bioassay systems which measure the desired drug activity in the laboratory;
- a test which measures the activity of the drug in humans that can be related to a potential therapeutic treatment.

One may broadly discern five main sites for drug action:

1. *Enzymes* – where new molecules are made in tissues (the basis of metabolic activity);

2. *Receptors* – where circulating messengers, *e.g.* biogenic amines and peptides, act to alter cellular activity;
3. *Transport systems* – that selectively permit access through membranes into and out of cells, *e.g.* ion channels and transporter molecules;
4. *Cell replication and protein synthesis* – controlled by DNA and RNA;
5. *Storage sites* – where molecules are kept in an inactive form for subsequent release and re-uptake, *e.g.* mast cells, blood platelets, neurones.

The body is controlled by chemical messengers (physiological mediators) through an extraordinarily complex communication system. Each messenger has specific functions and is recognised at a specialised site where it acts. In disease,

Table 1: *Marketed drugs resulting from the search for useful antimetabolites as enzyme inhibitors of nucleic acid metabolic pathways*[12]

Drug		Year of synthesis	Use
	6-Thioguanine	1950	antileukemic
	6-Mercaptopurine	1951	immunosuppressive
	Azathioprine	1957	immunosuppressive
	Allopurinol	1956	antihyperuricemic
	Diaveridine	1949	coccidiostat
	Trimethoprim	1956	antibacterial, antiprotozoal
	Pyrimethamine	1950	antimalarial

something has got out of balance, and in drug therapy the aim is to redress that balance. Thus, enzymes have active sites which specifically recognise the appropriate substrates which they can process and it is possible to design enzyme inhibitors, using the chemistry of the substrate as a starting point. Hitchings describes[12] how in the 1940s at Burroughs Wellcome their proposed research effort was based on the exploration of the enzymes and metabolic pathways of nucleic acid anabolism... 'It was our thought that metabolites which were analogues of purine and pyrimidine bases could be used as probes of metabolic events, and that the findings could be used to design more specific antimetabolites which eventually might show sufficient selectivity to be useful in chemotherapy'. The research was outstandingly successful and led to such antimetabolite drugs as 6-mercaptopurine, azathioprine, pyrimethamine, trimethoprim, and allopurinol (Table 1). Antimetabolites are structural analogues of intermediates (substrates or coenzymes) in the physiologically occurring metabolic pathways. They act by inhibiting a particular enzyme and so may block the biosynthesis of a physiologically important substance.

If the enzymic activity can be adequately assayed, it may be possible to characterise the active site. For example, in the renin–angiotensin system, renin which is synthesised by the kidneys is secreted into the blood and acts on angiotensinogen which is transformed into a decapeptide angiotensin-I, H_2N-Asp.Arg.Val.Tyr.Ile.His.Pro.Phe.His.Leu-OH (Figure 5). The latter is acted upon by the angiotensin converting enzyme (ACE), an exopeptidase which cleaves off the terminal dipeptide fragment H_2N-His.Leu-OH to give the octapeptide angiotensin-II which is a very powerful vasoconstrictor which raises blood pressure.

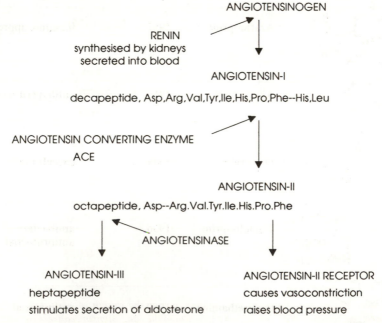

Figure 5: *The renin–angiotensin system*

The enzyme ACE was characterised as a metalloenzyme containing zinc at the active site. Following a natural product lead, namely that an extract from the venom of a South American pit viper, *Bothrops jararaca*, was found to inhibit ACE, and that a pentapeptide in the extract (pyroGlu.Lys.Trp.Ala.Pro-OH) was also an inhibitor, researchers at Squibb showed that derivatives of Ala.Pro-OH had some (albeit weak) inhibitory activity. They replaced amino by a second carboxyl, extended the chain length (Figure 6), and subsequently replaced the CO_2H by SH, reasoning that this should co-ordinate more effectively to Zn. This led to captopril, an inhibitor of ACE for treating hypertension by a new mechanism which is a very successful medicine. This has become a classic example of drug design.[13]

Substrate specificity may be studied using small peptides as probes which may then be converted into potent inhibitors, as was effected in the design of the enkephalinase inhibitor, thiorphan. Enkephalinase is a dipeptide hydrolase which specifically cleaves the Gly–Phe bond in the opioid enkephalin (Figure 7); hence an inhibitor might be an analgesic.

Llorens *et al.*[14] screened commercially available dipeptides looking for an inhibitor of enkephalinase activity in mouse brain (striatum) and then chose the best inhibitors as leads. The structure–activity studies suggested the presence of a hydrophobic binding pocket in the enzyme and they selected phenylalanylglycine (Phe.Gly.OH which had an IC_{50} of 1 μM) and incorporated a group to bind to

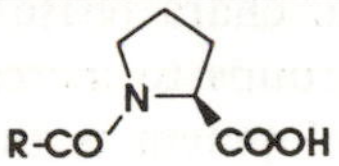 $\begin{array}{c} \text{R-CO} \diagdown \text{N} \diagup \text{COOH} \end{array}$	Inhibition of ACE from rat lung
R	**IC_{50} (μM)**
$HOOC(CH_2)_n$- n = 1	2600
n = 2	330
n = 3	70
n = 4	>4000
$\begin{array}{c} \overset{CH_3}{\vert} \\ HOOCCH_2CH_2CH- \end{array}$	4.9
$\begin{array}{c} HOOCCH_2CH_2CH- \\ \underset{\vert}{} \\ CH_3 \end{array}$	950
$HS.CH_2CH_2$-	0.20
$\begin{array}{c} \overset{CH_3}{\vert} \\ HS.CH_2CH- \end{array}$ SQ 14225 Captopril	0.023

Figure 6: *Some critical structure-activity findings during the design of captopril, the first antihypertensive drug to act by blocking the angiotensin converting enzyme (ACE).[13b]*

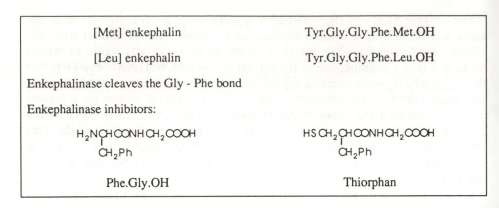

Figure 7:   *Enkephalin and enkephalinase inhibitors, Phe.Gly.OH (the dipeptide lead) and thiorphan*

Zn. By analogy with captopril, they included a thiol group to give thiorphan (Figure 7) and obtained an increase in potency of 1000-fold (K_i = 2 nM).

The work of Llorens *et al.* suggests an important approach which may have a wider application, namely the use of dipeptides and small oligopeptides to characterise binding to the enzymatic active site of peptidases. In future, when a new peptidase is isolated, it should be possible to characterise its binding site using dipeptides, and then incorporate suitable groups to increase affinity and stability to give inhibitors. Indeed a further development is the suggestion to establish dipeptide libraries for screening purposes (*e.g.* reference 15). The idea is to characterise an active site when seeking to design an enzyme antagonist (or peptide receptor antagonist) by using selected dipeptides and dipeptide derivatives. These are selected to span a range of physicochemical properties such as pK_a, hydrogen-bonding characteristics, lipophilicity, and shape. Looking further into the future, as the structures of enzymes become known, one would hope to design inhibitors using knowledge of the molecular structure of the active site.

Many different substances circulate as chemical messengers and combine with their own receptors, *e.g.* amino-acids, biogenic amines, peptides, prostaglandins, purines, steroids. They are remarkably specific since the messengers are not normally recognised by other receptors, *i.e.* the receptors discriminate between different messengers.

For biogenic amines, peptides and purines it has been possible to differentiate between sites for the same messenger, suggesting different subpopulations of receptors. Biogenic amine receptors, in particular, have been differentiated into many well characterised sub-classes (Table 2). These receptor sub-classes provide scope for introducing selectivity of drug action by modifying the chemical structure of the amine transmitter.[16,17] If the receptors are being over stimulated we can seek to design an antagonist to block the receptor using the chemistry of the natural messenger as a lead.[18,19]

Table 2: *Biogenic amines and their receptors*

Amine	Structure	Receptors
Acetyl choline	$CH_3CO.O.CH_2CH_2N^+Me_3$	nicotinic: muscle, neuronal muscarinic: M_1, M_2, M_3, M_4, M_5
Dopamine		D_1,D_2,D_3,D_4,D_5
Noradrenaline, R = H Adrenaline, R = CH_3		α_{1A-1D}, α_{2A-2C} β_1, β_2, β_3
Serotonin (5-Hydroxytryptamine)		5-HT_{1A-1F}, 5-HT_{2A-2C}, 5-HT_3, 5-HT_4, 5-HT_{5A-5B}, 5-HT_6, 5-HT_7
Histamine		H_1, H_2, H_3

In the past three decades biogenic amines have been extraordinarily fruitful starting points for new drug discovery . There are many potential sites for drug intervention to affect biogenic amine action especially in their role as neurotransmitters (Figure 8). In addition to blocking post-synaptic receptors (R_1, R_2 etc.), there are presynaptic autoreceptors which may modulate transmitter release or synthesis, storage sites and reuptake transporter proteins which modulate free transmitter concentration, and enzymes which can be blocked to alter the rate of transmitter turnover, *e.g.* inhibit biosynthesis to deplete the transmitter or inhibit metabolism to prolong its existence. Furthermore, the amine receptor is usually coupled to an amplification system such as a second messenger enzyme (protein kinase) or an ion channel, so that its influence may be modified by drug interference with the transducing mechanism.

Undoubtedly, some of the best examples of rational drug design have used the chemical structure of the natural transmitter (*i.e.* the biogenic amine) as a template. Thus selective agonists for post-synaptic receptors have been made for adrenergic β-receptors *e.g.* salbutamol,[20] dobutamine,[21] and xamoterol,[22] and 5-hydroxytryptamine receptors, *e.g.* sumatriptan[23] by the modification and addition of appropriate substituents to the biogenic amine structure (Figure 9).

Antagonists for biogenic amine receptors have been designed by retaining a partial structure of the amine (for receptor recognition), removing a key chemical feature required for receptor activation, and incorporating additional groups to

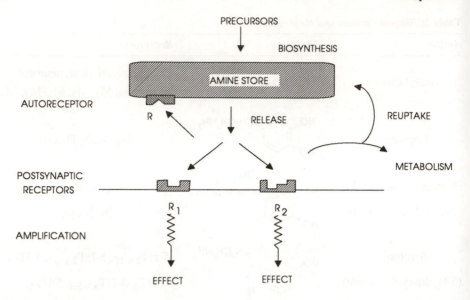

Figure 8: *Biogenic amine transmission can be modified by drug intervention at various stages and sites using enzyme inhibitors or receptor blockers or stimulants. Drugs may also affect amine release or uptake*

increase the binding affinity between drug and receptor,[19] *e.g.* pronethalol[24] for adrenergic β-receptors and burimamide[25] for histamine H_2-receptors (Figure 9).

Enzymes and receptors are highly specialised sites with a very high degree of selectivity and so provide very good opportunities for drug design. Since the key to a successful drug lies in its selectivity of action, the rational approach has been especially effective in modern drug discovery when based on enzymes or hormone receptors. Black, Elion, and Hitchings shared the Nobel Prize for Physiology or Medicine in 1988 for their pioneering work leading to the discoveries of adrenergic β-blockers, histamine H_2-antagonists, and antimetabolite enzyme inhibitors. This approach has now entered our general scientific consciousness but at the time it was highly imaginative and very speculative.

The past three decades have seen some notable drug design successes based on the approach of using as leads enzymes and substrates (Table 3), or receptors for biogenic amines (Table 4). With the development of biochemistry and cell biology has come a greater understanding of cellular mechanisms and control and many of the drugs discovered serendipitously or by screening procedures of the past three decades have subsequently been shown to act by interfering with particular mechanisms; some examples are shown in Table 5. Such examples have provided a further stimulus to develop agents rationally, from mechanistic considerations.

Thus there is a strong interplay between drug discovery and retrospective rationalisation. A semiempirical discovery of a useful drug provides the stimulus for deeper probing into how and why it works and thus to a deeper understanding of what underlies the disease. This in turn may give rise to new concepts and new discoveries.

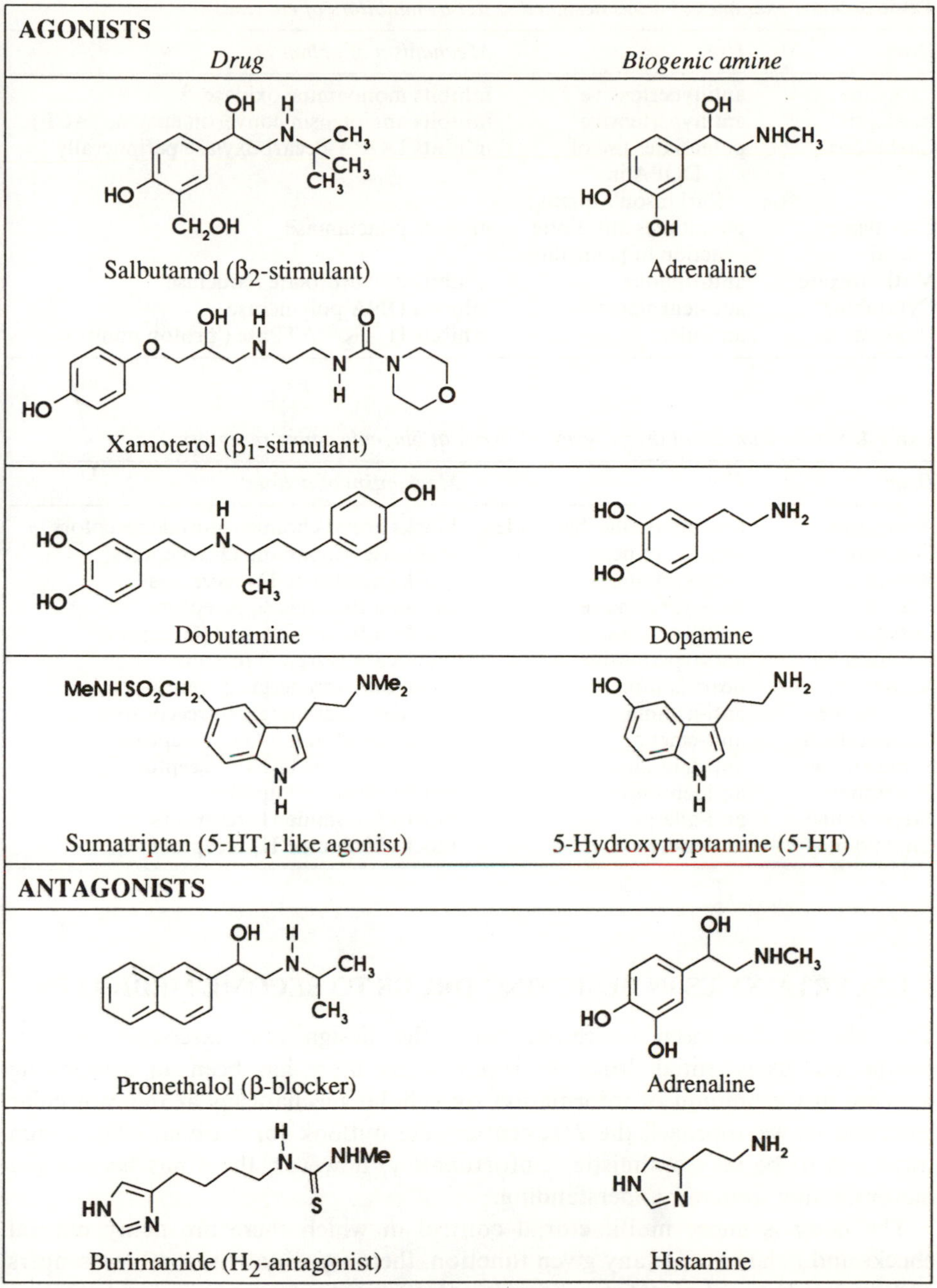

AGONISTS

Drug	*Biogenic amine*

Salbutamol (β_2-stimulant)

Adrenaline

Xamoterol (β_1-stimulant)

Dobutamine

Dopamine

Sumatriptan (5-HT$_1$-like agonist)

5-Hydroxytryptamine (5-HT)

ANTAGONISTS

Pronethalol (β-blocker)

Adrenaline

Burimamide (H$_2$-antagonist)

Histamine

Figure 9: *Chemical structures of some agonists and antagonists at biogenic amine receptors where the design was based on the amine structure as a template*

Table 3: *Some examples of drugs designed to act as inhibitors of enzymes*

Drug	Use	Mechanism of action
Pargyline	antihypertensive	inhibits monoamine oxidase-B
Enalapril	antihypertensive	inhibits angiotensin convertin enzyme (ACE)
Carbidopa	potentiates use of L-DOPA in Parkinson's disease	inhibits DOPA-decarboxylase peripherally
Clavulanic acid	potentiates antibiotic action of penicillins	inhibits β-lactamase
Methotrexate	anti-tumour	inhibits dihydrofolate reductase
Cytarabine	anti-leukaemia	inhibits DNA polymerase
Omeprazole	anti-ulcer	inhibits H^+/K^+ ATPase ('proton pump')

Table 4. *Some examples of drugs designed to act at biogenic amine receptors.*

Drug	Use	Mechanism of action
Atracurium	neuromuscular blockade	blocks acetyl choline nicotinic receptors
Fenoldopam	congestive heart failure	stimulates dopamine D_1 receptors
Butaclamol	antipsychotic	blocks dopamine D_2 receptors
Prazosin	antihypertensive	blocks adrenergic α_1 receptors
Labetolol	antihypertensive	blocks adrenergic α and β receptors
Propranolol	antihypertensive	blocks adrenergic β receptors
Xamoterol	heart failure	stimulates adrenergic β_1 receptors
Terbutaline	anti-asthma	stimulates adrenergic β_2 receptors
Ondansetron	anti-emetic	blocks serotonin 5-HT_3 receptors
Sumatriptan	anti-migraine	stimulates '5-HT_1-like' receptors
Fluoxetine	antidepressant	blocks serotonin uptake
Mepyramine	anti-allergy	blocks histamine H_1 receptors
Cimetidine	anti-ulcer	blocks histamine H_2 receptors

6 UNCERTAINTIES IN DESIGNING DRUGS TO BECOME MEDICINES

This chapter has been concerned with the design and discovery of new compounds as potential drugs. In recent years there has been an astounding increase in the amount of information on cellular mechanisms at the molecular level and as we approach the 21st century the outlook for rational drug design turns out to be very optimistic. Unfortunately, however, there has been a key factor missing from our understanding.

The body is under multifactorial control in which there are many natural checks and balances. For any given function, there are usually several messengers and several types of receptor. There are also amplification systems, modulating systems, feed-back inhibitory mechanisms, various ion fluxes, and so on. Blockade of one pathway by drug action may lead to another pathway taking over. The consequence is that one cannot know at the start of a research programme that designing a drug to act on a particular receptor or enzyme will necessarily provide treatment for a given medical condition, even though it is

Table 5: *Some examples of old drugs and new mechanisms*

Drug	Use	Mechanism of action
Aspirin	anti-inflammatory	inhibits the enzyme prostaglandin synthetase
Theophylline	anti-asthma (bronchodilator)	inhibits the enzyme phosphodiesterase
Atropine	mydriatic (dilates pupil of the eye)	blocks the muscarinic receptors for acetyl choline
Pirenzepine	anti-ulcer	selectively blocks acetyl choline muscarinic M_1 receptors on the acid-secreting cell in the stomach
Haloperidol	neuroleptic	blocks the receptors for dopamine in the brain
Chlordiazepoxide	anxiolytic	binds allosterically to the receptors for GABA (γ-aminobutyric acid) and opens the channels for the transport of Cl^- in brain neurones
Tolbutamide	hypoglycaemic	blocks the transport of K^+ through its channels in the insulin-secreting β cell of the pancreas
Nicorandil	vasodilator	stimulates K^+ transport through its channels in vascular smooth muscle
Nifedipine	coronary vasodilator used to treat angina	blocks the channels for transport of Ca^{2+} in vascular smooth muscle
Aminacrine	antibacterial	intercalates into the DNA of bacterial nucleus to inhibit growth
Cromoglycate	anti-asthma	prevents histamine release from its storage sites in mast cells in the lung

known to be involved in the physiological controlling mechanisms. Indeed, there are now many examples of nicely designed 'drugs' which are still looking for a suitable disease to treat.

Enzymes and receptors are ubiquitous and occur in many different tissue systems. Blocking them at a tissue site involved in a disease may be therapeutically effective but blockade concurrently in other tissue sites (not involved in the disease) may be undesirable.

Complications also arise during drug design because a drug has to be administered and find its way to the desired site of action. In contrast, the natural messenger may be generated or stored close to its required site of action. After it has acted, the natural transmitter is removed by specific enzymes or re-uptake mechanisms, whereas a drug has to be disposed of by being excreted. Thus one has to balance the desired pharmacology with the biochemical needs to achieve drug access and elimination. In altering the chemistry of a drug to achieve adequate biodisposition one may inadvertently introduce other pharmacological properties, thereby reducing the selectivity of action. Furthermore, differences often occur between species. The relative importance of a particular physiological mechanism in the laboratory test animal may not be the same as in the human.

Finally, to become a therapeutically useful medicine, a drug must be relatively safe to use. Side effects have to be tolerable and toxicity has to be minimal. It is not possible to obtain total selectivity but the separation between therapeutic dose and side effect dose must be sufficiently wide to permit reasonable use. In the past it has been extremely difficult to predict safety during the drug design stage, and many drugs have failed only after they have been studied during the very costly and time-consuming phase of drug development.

For the above reasons, there is still a strong element of speculation in drug design, and a considerable uncertainty in achieving success, and only a small proportion of drug discoveries are destined to become useful therapeutic agents. It takes many years to invent and develop a new drug; typically 10–15 years. Today's new research programmes are unlikely to reach fruition and become medicines until we have entered the next century! There is no doubt, however, that new drug discovery will continue to be an exciting challenge in which the role of the medicinal chemist will become less empirical and even more intellectually demanding.

7 REFERENCES

1. W. Sneader, 'Drug Discovery: the evolution of modern medicines', Wiley, Chichester, 1985.
2. 'Chronicles of Drug Discovery', 1 *et seq.*, ed. J.S. Bindra and D. Lednicer, J. Wiley, New York, 1982.
3. R.S.L. Chang V.J. Lotti, R,L. Monaghan, J. Birnbaum, E.O. Stapley, M.A. Goetz, G. Albers-Schönberg, A.A. Patchett, J.M. Liesch, O.D. Hensens, and J.P. Springer, *Science*, 1985, **230**, 177.
4. 'Marine Toxins: Origin, Structure and Molecular Pharmacology', S. Hall and G. Strichartz, ed. ACS Symposium Series 418, American Chemical Society, Washington DC, 1990.
5. W.B. Schwartz, *New Engl. J. Med.*, 1949, **240**, 173.
6. H. Laborit, *Presse Med.*, 1954, **62**, 359.
7. R.J. Gralla, L.M. Itri, S.E. Pisko, A.E. Squillante, D.P. Kelsen, D.W. Braun, L.A. Bordin, J.J. Braun, and C.W. Young, *New Engl. J. Med.*, 1981, **305**, 905.
8. J.R. Fozard and A.T.M. Mobarok Ali, *Eur. J. Pharmacol.*, 1981, **49**, 109.
9. J. Bermudez, C.S. Fake, G.F. Joiner, K.A. Joiner, F.D. King, W.D. Miner, and G.J. Sanger, *J. Med. Chem.*, 1990, **33**, 1924.
10. A. Burger, *Chem. Eng. News*, 1954, **32**, 4172.
11. F.L. Rose, *Chem. Ind.*, 1964, 858.
12. G.H. Hitchings, *TiPS*, 1980, **1**, 167.
13a. M.A. Ondetti, B. Rubin, and D.W. Cushman, *Science*, 1977, **196**, 441.
13b. D.W. Cushman, H.S. Cheung, E.F. Sabo, and M.A. Ondetti, *Biochem.*, 1977, **16**, 5484.
14. C. Llorens, G. Gacel, J.P. Swerts, R. Perdrisot, M.C. Fournie-Zaluski, J.C. Schwartz, and B.P. Roques, *Biochem. Biophys. Res. Commun.*, 1980, **96**, 1710.
15. D.C. Horwell, W. Howson, G.S. Ratcliffe, and D.C. Rees, *BioMed. Chem. Letts.*, 1993, **3**, 799.
16. D. Jack, *Pharm. J.*, 1976, 229.
17. D. Jack, *Br. J. Clin. Pharm.*, 1991, **31**, 501.

18. J.W. Black, *Pharm. J.*, 1976, **217**, 303.
19. J. Black, *Science*, 1989, **245**, 486.
20. D. Hartley, D. Jack, L. Lunts, and A.C.H. Ritchie, *Nature (London)*, 1968, **219**, 861.
21. R.R. Tuttle and J. Mills, *Circ. Res.*, 1975, **36**, 185.
22. J.J. Barlow, B.G. Main, and H.M. Snow, *J. Med. Chem.*, 1981, **24**, 315.
23. R.T. Brittain, D. Butina, I.H. Coates, W. Feniuk, P.P.A. Humphrey, D. Jack, A.W. Oxford, and M.J. Perrin, *Br. J. Pharmacol.*, 1987, **92,** (suppl.) 618P.
24. J.W. Black and J.S. Stephenson, *Lancet*, 1962, **2**, 311.
25. J.W. Black, W.A.M. Duncan, G.J. Durant, C.R. Ganellin, and M.E. Parsons, *Nature (London)*, 1972, **236**, 385.

CHAPTER 14

Bioisosteres, Conformational Restriction, and Pro-drugs – Case History: An Example of a Conformational Restriction Approach

FRANK D. KING

1 INTRODUCTION

The primary role of the medicinal chemist in a research project team within the pharmaceutical industry is to assist in the identification of a target lead compound and then convert that compound into a potential development candidate for eventual marketing as a drug. The lead compound can come from a number of sources, for example cross screening, a natural substrate or receptor mediator, an already marketed drug or competitor compound, or finally a structure designed from *ab initio* considerations of the receptor or enzyme. By definition, the lead compound does not normally satisfy the requirement for development due to some shortcoming in its properties. This could be, for example, a lack of specificity, low potency, metabolic or chemical instability, acute toxicity, poor bioavailability, unsatisfactory solubility, or even simply lack of novelty, precluding the possibility of patent protection, or a combination of these factors.

Faced with this challenge, the medicinal chemist has to devise a research strategy to achieve this objective in the shortest possible time. Initial approaches that can be taken can be loosely categorised into 'non-rational' and 'rational'. In the 'non-rational', all simple, readily accessible variations of the lead compound are made based on simple chemistry with little or no regard to biological activity. This approach, though intellectually unattractive, can be very successful provided that a large number and variety of compounds can be both prepared and tested in a very short period of time. A large amount of retrospective SAR knowledge can be built up very quickly which can be subsequently used for more rational approaches. In addition, the 'art' of medicinal chemistry is still such that this approach frequently throws up new exciting leads which no rational approach would ever have identified! The ultimate extreme of this is the concept of 'combinatorial libraries' where large numbers of compounds are rapidly prepared and tested as mixtures.

Alternatively, or in addition, 'rational' approaches can be adopted at an early stage. These approaches are particularly applicable to series of analogues which are difficult to synthesise and/or difficult to evaluate. One may adopt one or more approaches making the maximum possible use of SAR aids available. Some of these SAR aids have been covered in earlier QSAR and computational methodology chapters, but the experienced practitioner will frequently supplement these with more 'intuitive' approaches based on selective transformations of the molecule to probe the mechanism of binding and activation/inhibition. Thus, functionalities within the lead compound could be rationally altered based on hypotheses of, say, intermolecular binding or intramolecular conformation, and the results from like-for-like and like-for-non-like changes analysed and used for future target identification.

Three of the standard methodologies that the medicinal chemist can use as 'rational' approaches to lead optimisation form the basis of this chapter. These are bioisosteric replacement, conformational restriction, and pro-drug formation. The first topic has been covered in detail in a number of excellent reviews,[1,2] and therefore I shall only briefly touch on it here. Conformational restriction as a methodology for lead optimisation has been less comprehensively covered, and therefore I will examine this in more detail. The pro-drug approach is normally employed for optimisation of non-pharmacologically related properties such as pharmacokinetics, oral bioavailability, brain penetration *etc.* In the last section of the chapter I shall describe some of the work we, and others, have done using a conformational restriction approach to a weak, non-selective lead compound, metoclopramide, and as a result have identified potent and selective dopamine, 5-HT$_3$ and 5-HT$_4$ receptor antagonists and 5-HT$_4$ receptor agonists.

2 BIOISOSTERIC REPLACEMENT

Isosteres are substituents or groups which have the same size or volume. Bioisosteres, however, are substituents or groups that do not necessarily have the same size or volume, but have a similarity in chemical or physical properties which produce broadly similar biological properties. It is therefore unlikely that bioisosterism will produce marked increases in potency; however significant changes in selectivity, toxicity, and metabolic stability could be expected. Traditionally bioisosteres have been classified into two groups, *classical isosteres* which have approximately the same size, shape, and outer electronic configuration (Table 1) and *non-classical bioisosteres* which do not have the same number of atoms and do not fit the steric and electronic rules of the classical isososteres, but do produce similar biological activity (Table 2).

In general, *classical isosteric* replacement is *like-for-like* in terms of number of atoms, valency, degree of unsaturation, and aromaticity and only becomes a *bioisosteric* replacement if biological activity is retained. *Non-classical bioisosterism* retains activity by the retention of other properties such as pK_a, electrostatic potentials, HOMOs and LUMOs *etc.* for which modern computational analysis methodology can aid in rationalisation.

Table 1: *Classical isosteres which may function as bioisosteres*

Univalent atoms and groups	Bivalent
A. -CH$_3$; -NH$_2$; -OH; -F; -Cl	A. -CH$_2$-; -NH-; -O-; -S-; -Se-
B. -Cl; -PH$_2$; -SH	B. -COCH$_2$-; -CONH-; -COO-; -COS-
C. -Br; -i-Pr	**Trivalent** **Tetravalent**
D. -I; -t-Bu	A. -CH=; -N= A. >C<; >Si<
	B. -P=; -As= B. =C=; =N$^+$=; =P$^+$=

Ring equivalents
A. -CH=CH-; -S-   (*e.g.* benzene, thiophene)
B. -CH=; -N=   (*e.g.* benzene, pyridine)
C. -O-; -S-; -CH$_2$-; -NH-   (*e.g.* tetrahydrofuran, tetrahydrothiophene,
                                          cyclopentane, pyrrolidine)

Table 2: *Non-classical bioisosteres*

CARBONYL GROUP

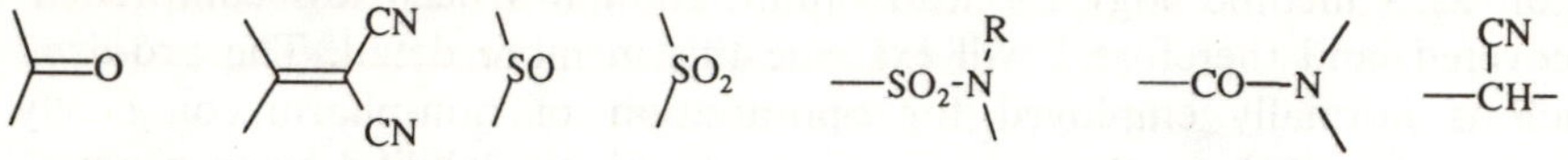

CARBOXYLIC ACID GROUP

COOH	SO$_2$NHR	SO$_3$H
CONHCN	CONHOH	
PO(OH)OEt	PO(OH)NH$_2$	

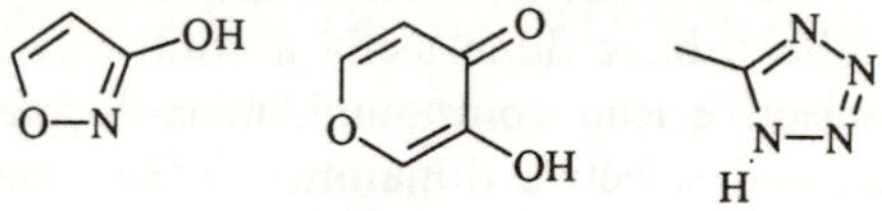

CARBOXYLIC ESTER GROUP

-COO-

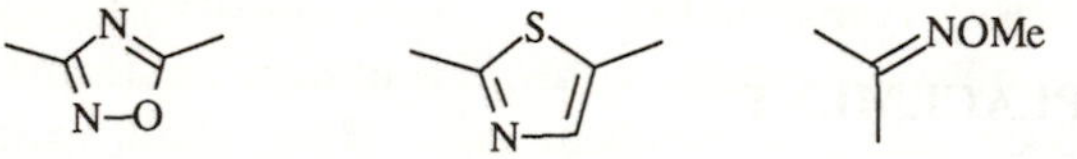

CARBOXYLIC AMIDE GROUP (IN PEPTIDES)
-CONH-   -CONMe-   -CSNH-   -CH$_2$NH-   -NHCO-   >C=C<   -CH$_2$S-

HYDROXY GROUP
-OH   -NHCOR   -NHSO$_2$R   -CH$_2$OH   -NHCONH$_2$ -NHCN   -CH(CN)$_2$

CATECHOL

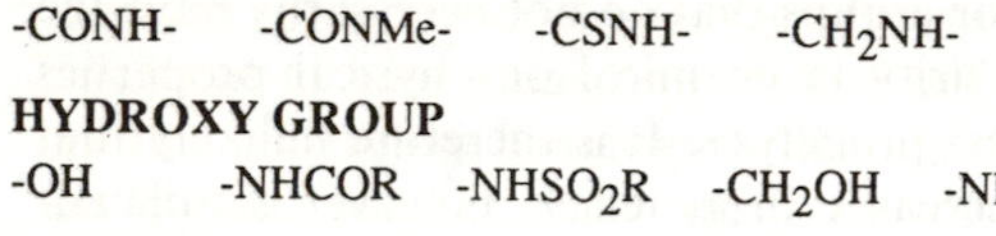

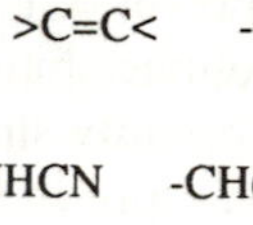

HALOGEN
HALOGEN   CF$_3$ CN   NCN$_2$ C(CN)$_3$

THIOUREA
NHC(=S)NH$_2$ NHC(=NCN)NH$_2$ NHC(=CHNO$_2$)NH$_2$

When considering any approach to lead optimisation, alteration of one part of the molecule almost always affects more than just one property. Isosteric and bioisosteric replacements are no exception and this should always be considered when analysing the result of such replacements. For example a simple CH_2 to O to S series of replacements can alter size, shape, electronic distribution, water or lipid solubility, pK_a, metabolism, or hydrogen bonding capacity, all with unpredictable effects upon biological activity. In addition isosteric and bioisosteric replacement can give very useful information regarding the key interacting functionalities of the compound with the enzyme or receptor. For example if the primary interaction of a secondary amide is as a hydrogen bonding acceptor, replacement of the amide by ester, ketone, or tertiary amide may retain potency. However, if the primary interaction involves NH as a hydrogen bond donor, all these changes will probably result in reduced potency. Similarly if the amide group is non-interactive, simply a spacer, then many isosteric replacements frequently used for peptide bond stabilisation, for example $-CH_2NH-$, $-CH_2S-$, $-CH=CH-$ or even $-CH_2CH_2-$, may retain activity. A more detailed discussion of this topic is beyond the scope of this chapter, but the reader is directed to the excellent reviews by Thornber[1] and Lipinski[2] where numerous examples of successful isosteric and bioisosteric replacements are listed.

3 CONFORMATIONAL RESTRICTION

In contrast to bioisosterism, which is intended to retain biological activity by replacement of either binding or non-binding functionalities, conformational restriction retains all the key binding functionalities intact, but seeks to fix their relative positions in the 'active' conformation.

There are many examples of highly conformationally restrained natural products which have been used as medicaments. Two such examples are morphine, which contains the key side chain binding functionalities of enkephalin, and the penicillins, which mimic the acyl-D-Ala-D-Ala of the bacterial cell wall peptidoglycan. Indeed one of the earlier approaches used in medicinal chemistry was to take highly conformationally restrained polycyclic natural products, and by simplification identify novel systems which retained many of the properties of the complex natural product, but were synthetically more amenable. The benzomorphan and piperidine analgesics are such examples derived from morphine.

However, many leads that are identified are small, flexible molecules or peptides which exist in many conformations. In these instances, conformational restriction can be a very powerful tool for lead optimisation to achieve the ultimate objective of identifying a potential drug. Conformational restriction can be achieved in a number of ways; by simple introduction of a methyl group which sterically restricts free bond rotation, by use of intramolecular hydrogen bonds, by introduction of unsaturation which fixes the relative positions of the terminal and geminal substituents due to the non-rotatability of a double bond, or by cyclisation, which fixes the relative position of the substituents either exocyclic or within the ring.

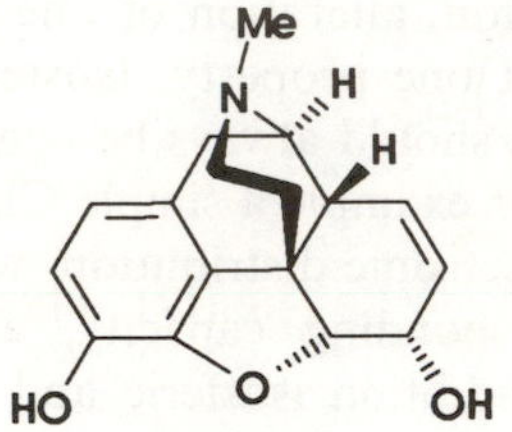

MORPHINE

Tyr - Gly - Gly - Phe - Leu/Met

ENKEPHALINS

PENICILLINS

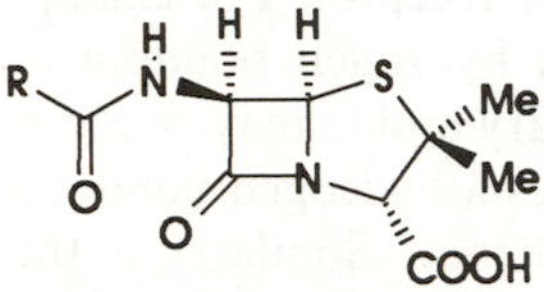

acyl - D - Ala - D - Ala -

in cell wall peptidoglycan

Expectations achievable from a conformational restriction approach are:

- increase in receptor/enzyme selectivity
- increase in receptor/enzyme affinity
- better definition of the 'pharmacophore'
- improved chemical/metabolic stabilisation
- reduced intrinsic activity of agonists
- mimicry of the tertiary structure of proteins
- identification of novel, original structural types

Each of these expectations will be treated in more detail.

Increase in Receptor/Enzyme Selectivity

The binding affinity of a drug depends upon how effectively it interacts with the side chain functionalities of the protein which make up the active site of the receptor or enzyme. Different enzymes and receptors contain different arrangements of these functionalities and even small differences in peptide sequence, for example a single amino acid difference between the rodent 5-HT_{1B} and human $5\text{-HT}_{1D\beta}$ receptor, can have major implications on binding affinities. Small molecules or peptides, which have a high degree of flexibility and which contain the key functionalities for interaction with common amino-acid residues on proteins, can often interact with more than one protein, and hence show a lack of selectivity. Clearly if one can fix the spatial arrangement of the binding functionalities so that they only interact well with one protein structure, then selective binding to that protein will be achieved. The third section of this chapter will exemplify this in practice in more detail. However, another example from our laboratories was derived from mianserin, which contains the functionalities of two aromatic rings and a basic centre, common to a large number of G-protein receptor mediators. Mianserin has high affinity for a number of receptors and is an antagonist at 5-HT_2, α_1 and histamine H_1 receptors. By further conforma-

mianserin

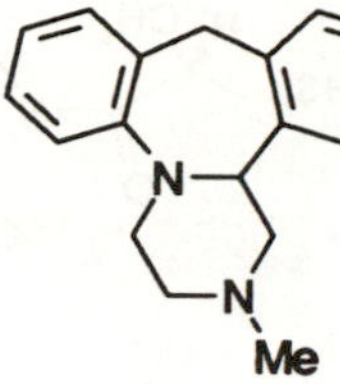

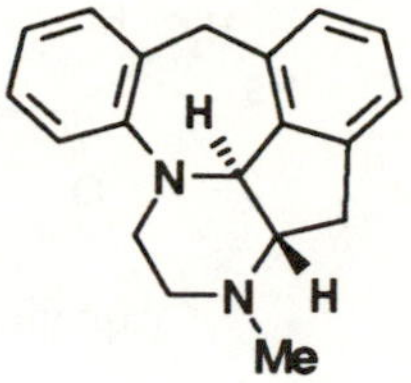

(±) BRL 34849

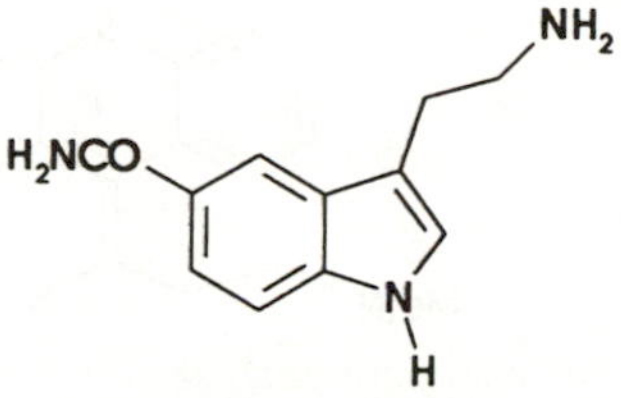

5-CT: 5-HT$_{1A}$ > 5-HT$_{1D}$

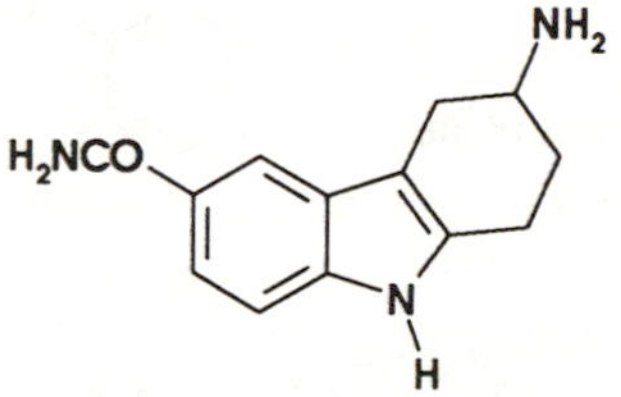

BRL 56905: 5-HT$_{1D}$ > 5-HT$_{1A}$

tional restriction of the basic side chain, BRL 34849 was obtained which retained the 5-HT$_2$ and α_1 antagonist activity but was devoid of H$_1$ activity.[3]

Similar selectivity can be achieved with agonists. For example, chemists at Glaxo found that replacement of the 5-OH group of 5-HT with a 5-carboxamido group gave 5-carboxamidotryptamine (5-CT) which is selective for 5-HT$_{1A}$ and 5-HT$_{1D}$ receptors, but more potent at 1A. Subsequently we found that conformational restriction to give the 3-amino-6-carboxamidotetrahydrocarbazole (BRL 56905) very much reduced the 5-HT$_{1A}$ receptor binding affinity, but retained the 5-HT$_{1D}$ affinity and the functional agonism.[4]

Increase in Receptor/Enzyme Affinity

Using a conformational restriction approach one might expect to increase affinity at the receptor or enzyme for two possible reasons:

1. a reduced adverse entropy effect
2. stabilisation of a high energy 'active' conformation.

When a flexible molecule binds to a receptor, the molecule is constrained resulting in a reduction in the number of degrees of freedom and a marked adverse change in entropy, which reduces the beneficial free energy change on binding. This effect is probably more marked for compounds which bind with a high entropy term, for example lipophilic antagonists, rather than those which bind mainly by enthalpic interactions, for example small agonists. As conformational restriction retains the same binding functionalities, the change in enthalpy is likely to be small. In contrast conformational restriction can inherently reduce the number of degrees of freedom, in spite of the additional bonds; hence the adverse entropy change on binding can be reduced, resulting in a greater free energy change.

A simpler concept is where the molecule is not binding to the receptor in its lowest energy state. For example, if a *gauche* orientation needs to be invoked, an

relative potency = 1

captopril
relative potency = 10

relative potency = 0.1

chlorprothixene

energy penalty must be paid to orientate the functionalities for binding to the enzyme or receptor. However if that high energy state can be mimicked by, for example, a lower-energy state of a 1,2-disubstituted carbocycle, the molecule may now be able to bind in a low energy conformation without an energy penalty.

There are numerous examples where simple conformational restriction has had a significant effect upon activity, and by way of example two cases are given here. In the first, the simple addition of an α-methyl group to give the angiotensin-converting enzyme (ACE) inhibitor captopril increased potency by 10-fold over the des-methyl compound.[5]

The effect of the introduction of the methyl group could be due simply to an interaction with a 'lipophilic pocket', but it could also be due to a restriction in the rotational freedom and to differences in the low energy conformations. It is interesting that there is also a 100-fold difference between the enantiomers, so that the effect is highly stereospecific. This is often the case as the interacting proteins are also chiral. A second example is the introduction of unsaturation which defines the relative orientation of the functionalities. In this case it is orientation of the dimethylamino and chloro substituents for which the Z-isomer, chlorprothixene, is a more potent anti-psychotic than the E isomer.[6]

Definition of the 'Pharmacophore'

The pharmacophore can be defined as the spatial arrangement of the functionalities of a molecule which interact with the receptor, and can also take into account sterically allowed and excluded volumes. At present the refinement of the G-protein receptor models is not sufficiently accurate that useful pharmacophores can be generated by *ab initio* methods. For enzymes, many have had their tertiary structures identified, with and without substrates or inhibitors, and therefore useful pharmacophores can be generated. However, many enzymes have not had the structure of their active site resolved and hence the medicinal chemist has to fall back on other techniques. To try to rationalise the SAR for interaction with these structurally unknown proteins, the medicinal chemist has to rely on structural overlaps of active molecules to build up a picture of the common

sumatriptan $t_{1/2}$ MAN ca. 2h   GR 85548 $t_{1/2}$ MAN ca. 5h

interacting functionalities, allowed areas of space, and their relative positions, *i.e.* the pharmacophore. From this information, 3-D databases can be searched to identify novel leads, or the structures can be inserted into the protein models for further refinement. Great difficulties are encountered when overlapping a number of very flexible molecules, and often a number of different possible pharmacophores can be found. It is possible to test each of these possibilities by synthesis of conformationally restricted analogues which rigidly define the binding functionalities in the possible 'active' orientation. Whereas a positive result can define the pharmacophore, a negative result does not necessarily rule out that conformation, as other factors such as steric hindrance may have come into play.

Metabolic Stabilisation

Metabolic instability of amide bonds of peptides is a major problem which, in general, prevents their use as oral drugs. Cyclisation of a peptide can be used as part of an overall strategy of peptide stabilisation. This is presumably based on the conformational restriction preventing optimum alignment of the peptide at the active site of the peptidase enzyme whilst retaining the desired pharmacological activity.

Other functional groups can be rapidly metabolised and stabilisation can similarly be achieved by cyclisation. A recent example of this is the prevention of the rapid oxidative metabolism of the aminoethyl side chain of the anti-migraine drug sumatriptan (blood half-life of 2 h) to the inactive indole acetic acid. A cyclic piperidine analogue, GR 85548, retains the anti-migraine activity, but has a much longer duration (blood half-life about 5 h), the half-life now being limited by metabolism of the 5-substituent.[7]

Reduced Intrinsic Activity of Agonists

There are far fewer examples of successful drugs which are receptor agonists than antagonists. One reason for this is that potent, long acting agonists can over stimulate the receptor, leading to desensitisation. One possible approach to overcome this is to design partial agonists which have a lower maximum stimulatory effect. It may also be possible to gain regional selectivity with an agonist by exploiting environmental differences between the same receptor located in different tissues. In a particular tissue the receptor may be well coupled to its secondary messenger system with a large receptor reserve, whilst in other tissues it may be less well coupled, with a low receptor reserve. In the latter case a higher receptor occupancy would be required, *i.e.* a higher concentration of drug, to elicit the same response. These differences could be amplified with a partial agonist. Within a series of conformationally restricted agonists, small differences in the relative orientations of the functionalities may not adversely affect binding, but may affect the efficiency of activating the receptor.

Table 3: *Muscarinic agonists*

R =

STRUCTURE	INTRINSIC ACTIVITY*	STRUCTURE	INTRINSIC ACTIVITY*
	130		360
	84		5

* Intrinsic activity = IC_{50} Antagonist/IC_{50} Agonist: >100 = Agonist; 1><100 = partial agonist

A series of acetylcholine mimetics from our muscarinic agonist group based on oxadiazole-substituted azabicycles exemplifies the possibilities (Table 3). For their study the intrinsic activity of the agonist was defined by the ratio of binding displacement affinity of radiolabelled antagonist and agonist. A ratio of >100 correlated with full agonist efficacy whereas a ratio of between 100 and 10 was indicative of partial agonism. By subtle alteration of the relative position of the basic nitrogen, agonists of varying 'partial' nature were identified down to an almost silent antagonist profile.[8]

Peptides: Mimicry of the Tertiary Structure of Proteins

Large proteins and peptides normally have a defined tertiary structure which is essential for their biological activity. Often the biological activity resides with two or three amino acid residues, and nature has used size and conformational restriction in the form of stabilised turns, sheets, and S–S bonds to orientate these key residues. It is a major challenge to medicinal chemists to identify small molecules which retain the biological activity of these macromolecules and one approach is to identify small peptides, up to six amino acid residues, which contain all the biologically active functionality of the large protein. Unfortunately, small peptides do not normally form definite tertiary structures and therefore it is necessary to build in conformational restriction to orientate the side

β-TURN MIMICKED BY: **γ-TURN MIMICKED BY:**

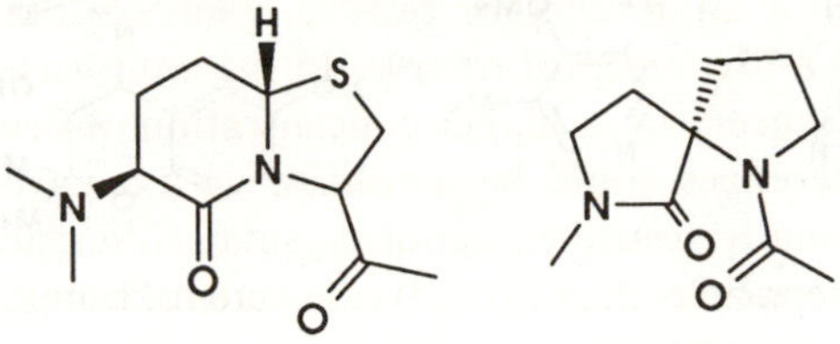

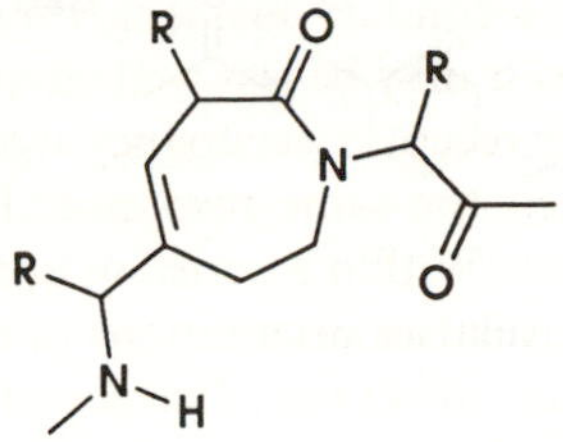

chain functionalities correctly. This can be achieved by using β- or γ-turn mimetics to induce appropriate turns in the peptide, and also improve stability with the removal of some of the amide bonds. Numerous examples have appeared in the literature, an example of which from our own US laboratories is a γ-turn mimetic incorporated into active HIV protease inhibitors.[9]

Novel Structural Types

Often the starting leads for the medicinal chemists are known compounds in the literature and a key task is to identify novel structural types with a good pharmacological profile based on these lead structures. Conformational restriction inevitably leads to chemical entities distinct from these lead structures and hence having a high probability of originality. Because there are no fixed rules for the success of this approach, each lead compound and each biological target has to be assessed individually. At the outset, the desired conformational restriction is normally unknown, though computational graphics techniques are becoming increasingly helpful as more models of enzymes and receptors are created. However, even with computational modelling techniques, the total effect of particular conformational restrictions on biological activity is unknown and still unpredictable. Thus when entering a conformational restriction approach, one is immediately entering uncharted territory for which no relevant *prior art* normally exists.

In conclusion, for a number of reasons, conformational restriction is a very powerful approach to the optimisation of lead compounds. The final section of this chapter will be devoted to a Case History to further illustrate the principles and opportunities for success.

4 PRO-DRUGS

The two previous sections have addressed the problem of optimising the potency and selectivity of a lead compound. However, often good *in vitro* potency is achieved but when the compounds are tested *in vivo*, only poor activity is observed. This could be due to a number of factors, including poor absorption, rapid metabolism, and/or clearance or poor penetration to the site of action. Other factors, such as toxicity, may be an issue and often these problems are resolved by returning to the *in vitro* selection to identify compounds which do not have these problems. Occasionally, however, these problems are endemic to the

nabumetone   omeprazole   cromakalim

series of compounds and cannot be readily avoided. This is where a pro-drug approach may be appropriate.

A **pro-drug** is defined as an **inactive compound**, which when absorbed is converted into an **active** form which then produces the desired pharmacological response. This should not be confused with a **soft drug**, which is **active**, but is **inactivated** in a controlled fashion. Clearly, a pro-drug cannot be identified from *in vitro* screening unless some activation mechanism is included. There are many early examples of pro-drugs which were identified using *in vivo* disease models, an approach to testing which nowadays is generally out of fashion. Two such examples are nabumetone, in which the ketone side chain is metabolised to the biologically much more active arylacetic acid and omeprazole, which is activated in the acidic environment of the acid-secreting parietal cell to inhibit irreversibly the H^+/K^+ ATPase responsible for secretion of acid into the stomach. For both of these are examples where there is a definite advantage to progress the inactive form. Nabumetone does not cause the same degree of gastric damage as other arylacetic acid anti-inflammatories, and omeprazole achieves a unique enzyme selectivity. However, other cases exist where it has been preferred to develop the active form. For example the K-channel activator cromakalim originally came from a series of amines which were only active because of metabolism to the amide. In this case the activated form had the better properties.

With a major concentration of lead optimisation based on *in vitro* screening, a more rational approach to pro-drug design is needed. This is an extremely complex subject beyond the scope of this book, but there have been numerous reviews to which the reader can refer for further guidance.[10-12] Briefly a pro-drug strategy can offer:

• improved solubility and/or formulation
• improved absorption and distribution
• site specificity and reduced toxicity
• stability and/or prolonged release
• better patient acceptability

Pro-drugs can be classified as *carrier-linked pro-drugs*, in which the active drug is linked to an easily removed carrier, and *bioprecursors*, in which the molecular modification produces the active principle. Omeprazole is an example of a bioprecursor. Carrier-linked pro-drugs, on the other hand, usually have some labile group, similar to a protecting group used in organic synthesis, which is cleaved off to release the active drug. These can be further subdivided into *bipartate* which is the combination of one carrier and the drug, and *tripartate* in which the carrier is connected *via* a linker to the drug. Commonly the groups masked are highly polar functionalities, such as alcohols, amines, sulphonamides, or acids which have poor pharmacokinetics. Many of the 'protecting groups' are very similar to those used in organic synthesis, such as esters, amides, carbamates, and imines, but the aim is to design groups which are relatively chemically stable, but cleaved enzymatically at a desired rate. This desired rate is often difficult to achieve. The group must be stable to gastric acid and enzymes to ensure bioavailability, but sufficiently labile to ensure cleavage once absorption has occurred. A summary of some of those carrier groups frequently investigated is included in Table 4.

However, the pro-drug approach is not without problems, though many spectacular successes have been achieved. There are often large inter-species variations between the rate of enzymatic cleavage; thus a compound which looks good in animal models may not be so good in man. This problem can be overcome to a certain extent by investigating the *in vitro* stability to human enzymes. Another problem is that the cleavage produces by-products which, in some cases, have been found to be toxic, for example formaldehyde and some aliphatic acids. Great care is therefore necessary in the choice of carrier and linker, especially where intended chronic therapy requires long-term, high-dose toxicology.

Table 4: *Examples of carriers for pro-drugs*

Drug-OH →Drug-OX

X = -(C=O)R -(C=O)CH_2NR_2 -(C=O)CH_2CH_2COOR -(C=O)Ph -PO_3^{2-}

  -(C=O)-CH_2SO_3H -(C=O)$CH_2CH_2NR_2$

Drug-NH →Drug-NX

X= -(C=O)R -(C=O)$CHRNH_2$ -(C=O)OPh -CH_2NH(C=O)Ar =CHAr

  =NAr -CHR-O(C=O)R   -CH_2—$\overset{+}{N}$⟨ ⟩ -(C=O)CH_2NR_2 -CH_2NR_2

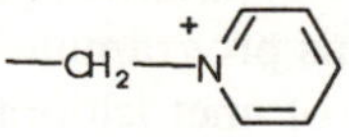

Drug>C=O → Drug>C(X)Y

>C(X)Y = >C=NR >C=NOR >C(OR)$_2$

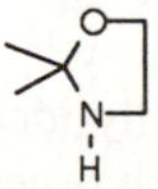

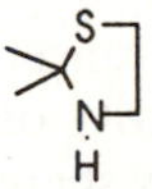

Drug-CO_2H → Drug-CO_2X

X = -R -CHR-O(C=O)R -CHR-O(C=O)NR_2 -CH_2(C=O)NR_2

  -CHR-O(C=O)OR   -CH_2CH_2OH

5 CASE HISTORY: FROM METOCLOPRAMIDE TO SELECTIVE DOPAMINE, 5-HT$_3$ AND 5-HT$_4$ RECEPTOR ANTAGONISTS AND 5-HT$_4$ RECEPTOR AGONISTS

Metoclopramide is a member of the class of compounds called 'orthopramides' derived from the *ortho*-methoxybenzamide structure.[13]

Metoclopramide has been used as an anti-emetic and gastric motility stimulant for over 20 years. It is a weak dopamine and 5-HT$_3$ receptor antagonist and 5-HT$_4$ receptor agonist. We started a chemical programme based on metoclopramide in 1975 with the initial aim of identifying a gastric motility stimulant which was free from the extrapyramidal side effects common to centrally acting dopamine receptor antagonists. At that time only its dopamine receptor antagonist properties had been identified and it was unclear as to whether all of its biological activity was mediated through dopamine antagonism, possibly involving unknown receptor subtypes, or whether other unknown mechanisms were involved. The gastric motility enhancing properties had been identified in the clinic, and it was believed that this property of metoclopramide was unique amongst known dopamine receptor antagonists.

As the mechanism of gastric stimulation was unclear, our primary screen was based on an *in vivo* model in the rat which involved the continuous measurement of changes in intra-duodenal pressure. Metoclopramide causes a dose-dependent increase in mean basal intra-duodenal pressure up to a maximum, then has reduced activity at higher doses – a 'bell-shaped' dose–response curve. The advantage of this test was that there was no bias towards a particular activity, such as if the pressure had been artificially reduced by application of an exogenous agent, such as dopamine. In later investigations we used a Heidenhain pouch dog model of intra-gastric pressure which proved to be more sensitive and more specific for 5-HT$_4$ receptor mediated effects. For a measure of central dopamine D$_2$ receptor antagonist activity, we used the inhibition of climbing behaviour in mice induced by the dopamine agonist, apomorphine.

Shortly after embarking on this programme, John Fozard identified the 5-HT$_3$ receptor antagonist properties of metoclopramide.[14] Some time later Gareth Sanger, in our laboratories, linked this activity to the ability of high-dose metoclopramide to inhibit both the chemical and radiation-induced emesis encountered in cancer therapy.[15] This anti-emetic activity was different from the anti-emetic activity originally identified with conventional doses of metoclopramide, an activity shared with other dopamine receptor antagonists. In response to this finding, a new target became the identification of potent and selective 5-HT$_3$

metoclopramide   5-HT   dopamine receptor antagonists for use in conjunction with highly emetogenic anti-cancer treatments. For this activity we used as the primary screen the inhibition of the Bezold–Jarisch reflex in the rat. A bolus *i.v.* injection of 5-HT causes a reflex bradycardia which is mediated by 5-HT$_3$ receptors located in the heart and is dose-dependently inhibited by 5-HT$_3$ receptor antagonists. It is these three activities, intragastric pressure (rat, dog), inhibition of apomorphine-induced climbing (mouse), and inhibition of Bezold–Jarisch reflex (rat) which will be referred to throughout the chapter for comparing potencies.

The key structural features of metoclopramide are the flexible basic side chain, which is regarded as the 'primary binding site' (probably to an aspartate of the receptor), a possible intramolecular H-bond between the NH and the *ortho*-OMe, and the aromatic substitution pattern. The aromatic amine is a very weak base and not normally protonated. The spatial orientations are such that one can imagine the basic aliphatic amino group interacting at the same site as the amino of dopamine and 5-HT, with the amide possibly mimicking the binding of the hydroxyl groups. These three key structural features are areas of conformational freedom which have potential for investigation by conformational restriction and I shall discuss the results both we, and others, have obtained from conformational restriction of each of these in turn.

Conformational Restriction of the Side Chain

Early work by the group at Almirall concentrated on replacement of the aminoethyl side chain with a 4-piperidine ring.[16] From this work, clebopride was identified which incorporated a more lipophilic benzyl group. Clebopride was more potent than metoclopramide as a dopamine receptor antagonist and roughly equivalent as a gastric motility stimulant. From this work we believed that there could be a large degree of variation allowable on the side chain and our first investigations were further to conformationally restrict the side chain in the form of the fused azabicycles, the 6,6-quinolizidines, and the 6,5-indolizidines.

We investigated all isomers round the rings and the only convincing motility stimulant activity was found with the '4' isomers corresponding to the 4-substitution in clebopride. The equatorial isomer retained both dopamine receptor antagonism and weak motility stimulant activity. However, the axial isomers retained only the desired motility stimulant activity. Thus both the axial quinolizidine and axial indolizidine were more potent than metoclopramide as gastric motility stimulants and 5-HT$_3$ antagonists, these two activities appearing to run roughly in parallel.[17]

From this series we selected BRL 20627 for development as the first gastric motility stimulant effectively devoid of dopamine receptor antagonist activity. Before this compound, it was believed that the gastric motility stimulant properties of metoclopramide were *via* dopamine receptor antagonism. BRL 20627 reached early clinical trials and was found to be an effective gastric motility stimulant in man but eventually failed on toxicology grounds.

In order to retain dopamine receptor antagonist activity we incorporated a phenyl group as in clebopride. Activity was retained only with the indolizidines in

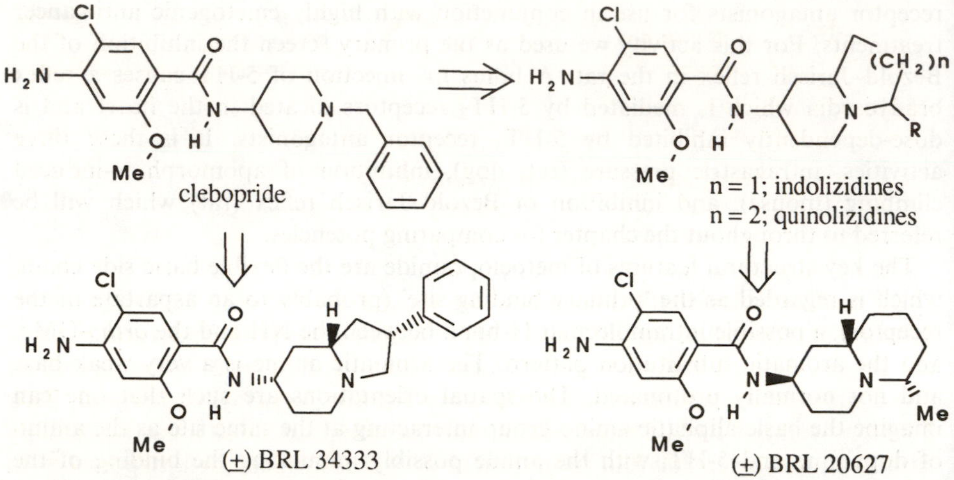

clebopride

n = 1; indolizidines
n = 2; quinolizidines

(±) BRL 34333

(±) BRL 20627

which the phenyl group was at the β position to the basic nitrogen. Interestingly, the pharmacological profile was different depending upon the orientation of the phenyl group. With the phenyl group 'up', BRL 34333, a potent and selective dopamine antagonist, was obtained. However with the phenyl group 'down', 5-HT$_4$ agonist activity, as evident from gastric motility assessment, was retained with much reduced dopamine antagonist activity.[18] Thus the properties of clebopride had been separated. In both cases the axial isomers were much less active.

In the meantime we also investigated further the effects of conformational restriction, focusing especially on those ring systems which contained a piperidine moiety, but which differentiated between axial and equatorial isomers. One such ring system was the tropane. As with the indolizidines, the equatorial tropanes retained dopamine receptor antagonism and BRL 25594, which incorporated the *N*-benzyl group, was found to be some 500 times more potent than metoclopramide.[19] Thus simply bridging across the piperidine ring of clebopride had increased dopamine antagonist potency by about 30-fold.

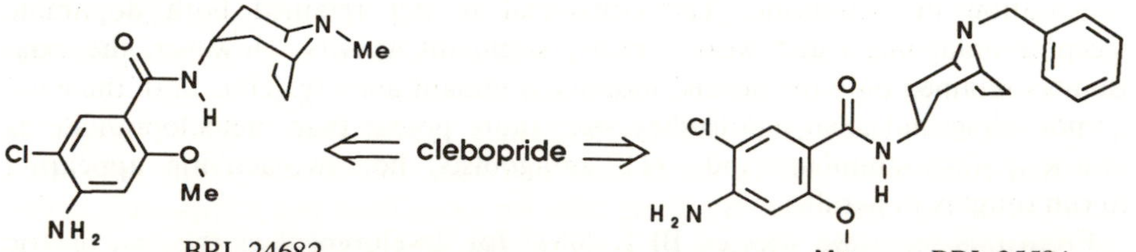

BRL 24682   ⇐ clebopride ⇒   BRL 25594

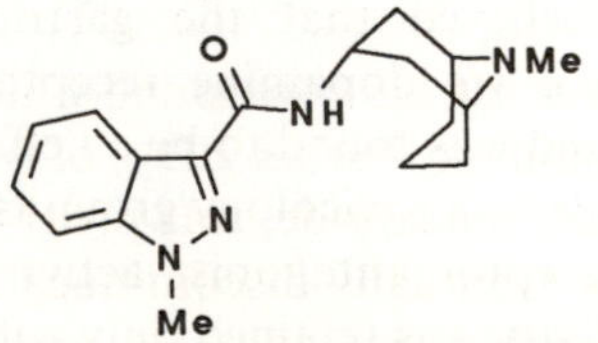

granisetron

N inversion $\Longleftrightarrow$ boat - chair $\Longleftrightarrow$

N inversion $\Longleftrightarrow$

By analogy with the indolizidines, we looked at tropanes with smaller N-substituents for gastric motility and 5-HT$_3$ antagonist activity, and again most of the activity resided with the axial isomers. None of these axial compounds had any significant dopamine antagonist activity and the *N*-methyl compound, BRL 24682, was about 10-fold more potent than metoclopramide as a gastric motility stimulant, and over 300-fold more potent as a 5-HT$_3$ receptor antagonist.[20] In contrast, the *N*-ethyl compound was relatively inactive at the 5-HT$_3$ receptor. The related granatane, with a propylene bridge, also had a low potency as a motility stimulant but was even more potent than the tropane as a 5-HT$_3$ receptor antagonist. In part it was this finding that helped us to identify granisetron as a highly potent and selective 5-HT$_3$ receptor antagonist now marketed in many countries as an anti-emetic.[21]

To summarise, dopamine receptor antagonist activity resides in the equatorial isomer, with lipophilic substitution such as benzyl preferred, and the tropane is about as potent as the granatane. In contrast, for gastric motility stimulant (5-HT$_4$ receptor agonist) activity, the axial isomer is preferred, with methyl being more potent than benzyl and tropane more active than granatane. For 5-HT$_3$ receptor antagonism, again axial isomers are potent, and again methyl is optimal, but now granatane is roughly equivalent to tropane. Thus from this series, we identified selective dopamine and 5-HT$_3$ receptor antagonists but failed to achieve a 5-HT$_4$ agonist free from 5-HT$_3$ antagonist activity.

In an attempt to achieve this, we looked at alternative conformational restriction of the piperidine ring in the form of 'tied back' azabicycles. We rationalised this investigation in considering the relative potencies of the quinolizidines and indolizidines. The indolizidines were more potent, and they also have a lower energy barrier to nitrogen inversion.

We therefore looked at azabicycles which mimic these higher energy, N-inverted conformations. To do this we tied back the N-substituent onto the β position of the piperidine. By doing this, we again identified compounds devoid of dopamine receptor antagonist activity, but which retained high potency as gastric motility stimulants (5-HT$_4$ receptor agonists) and also 5-HT$_3$ receptor antagonists.

The most selective compound was the 6,5 compound which had a lowest active dose of 5 μg kg^{-1} as a gastric stimulant, but an ED$_{50}$ of only 30 μg kg^{-1} at the 5-HT$_3$ receptor. The 6,6 compound, renzapride, was progressed to the clinic as a gastric motility stimulant but was eventually discontinued as it was found to be teratogenic at high doses. Renzapride was resolved and we found that both

X	n	IGP[#]	B-J[$]
CH_2	0	0.005	30
*CH_2	1	0.01	3.3
O	1	0.01	19
S	1	0.01	-

[#]Intragastric pressure in dog, lowest active dose mg/kg sc
[$]Inhibition of Bezold-Jarisch reflex ID_{50} µg/kg iv
* BRL 24924 (renzapride)

enantiomers showed virtually identical activity.[22] We also investigated the introduction of oxygen and sulphur into the side chain of renzapride, in order to investigate the effects of altering basicity. In this series the oxa-analogue retained 5-HT$_4$ receptor agonist potency but showed a small reduction in 5-HT$_3$ receptor antagonism. This result contrasts with our findings for granatanes where oxygen insertion into the propylene bridge actually improved 5-HT$_3$ antagonist potency.

n	IGP[#]	B-J[$]
1	0.01	-
2	0.01	3.4 ± 1.3
(+) renzapride	0.01	4.2 ± 1.7
(-) renzapride	0.01	3.9 ± 1.7

[#]Intragastric pressure in dog, lowest active dose mg/kg sc
[$]Inhibition of Bezold-Jarisch reflex ID_{50} µg/kg iv

The equivalence of the enantiomers of renzapride prompted us to investigate the aza-tricyclic combining the carbon framework of each enantiomer. As expected, a similar profile of activity to renzapride was obtained confirming a lack of steric differentiation at the receptor. Finally we investigated the 4-quinuclidine which very rigidly held the amide and nitrogen in a fixed position. This compound retained the 5-HT$_4$ receptor agonist activity with the best selectivity over both 5-HT$_3$ and dopamine.

In conclusion, conformational restriction of the side chain of metoclopramide led us to identify compounds selective for dopamine receptor antagonism, with a 500-fold potency increase, selective for 5-HT$_4$ receptor agonism with a potency increase of between 10- and 50-fold, and selective for 5-HT$_3$ receptor antagonism with potency increases in the order of 200–300-fold.

Conformational Restriction of the Amide

In combination with some of these highly potent side chains, we investigated conformational restriction of other parts of the molecule. For both the dopamine antagonist and selective 5-HT$_4$ agonist side chains, we investigated cyclisation of the amide NH and the *ortho*-methoxy group with little success. However, in the 5-HT$_3$ area more success was achieved. For the benzamides, the 4-amino-5-chloro substituents were found to be optimal for 5-HT$_3$ antagonist activity. By mimicking the H-bond by forming the benzotriazinones, we obtained a series of highly potent compounds which qualitatively showed a similar SAR with respect to substituents as the benzamides.[20]

From this we concluded that the active conformation of the benzamides at the 5-HT$_3$ receptor is with the carbonyl group in plane, held by the intramolecular H-bond.

B-J*	R	B-J*
12	H	14
0.17	NH$_2$	0.7

* Inhibition of Bezold-Jarisch reflex ID$_{50}$ µg/kg iv

ondansetron: 4-fold more potent

The results from this cyclisation were similar to that found by Glaxo in their ondansetron series, where cyclisation of the ketone back onto the indole gave a four-fold increase in potency.[23]

It is worth noting that the lack of success with similar conformational restriction of the amide when applied to the other areas of dopamine and 5-HT$_4$ raises question marks over the orientation of the amide at these receptors.

Cyclisation of the *ortho*-Alkoxy Group

We had previously investigated cyclisation of the *ortho*-alkoxy group back onto the free 3-position of the aromatic ring with only moderate success in the dopamine antagonist area, and with no success in the 5-HT$_4$ agonist area. However, in the mid 1980s, a number of groups simultaneously applied this approach to the 5-HT$_3$ antagonist area, which resulted in a number of highly potent antagonists being identified. Two are given here by way of example, zatosetron from Lilly[24] and Y-25130 from Yamanouchi.[25] In all these series, the chloro substituent was vital for high potency.

Despite our earlier failures with this approach to 5-HT$_4$ receptor agonists, we have applied this methodology more recently to the identification of selective 5-HT$_4$ receptor antagonists. Metoclopramide is a weak partial agonist at the 5-HT$_4$

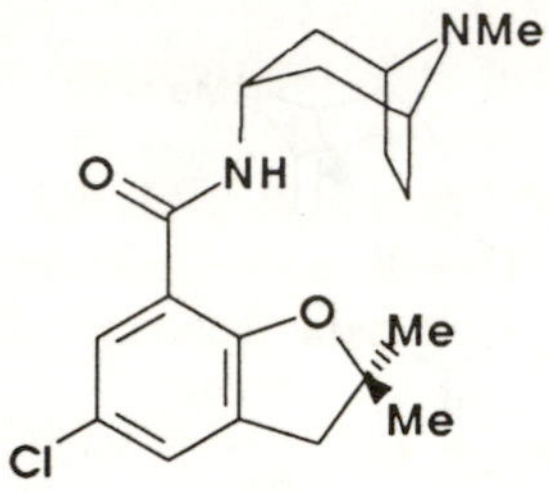

zatosetron

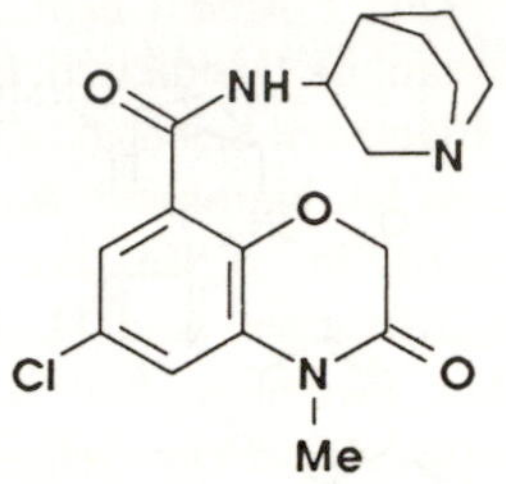

Y-25130

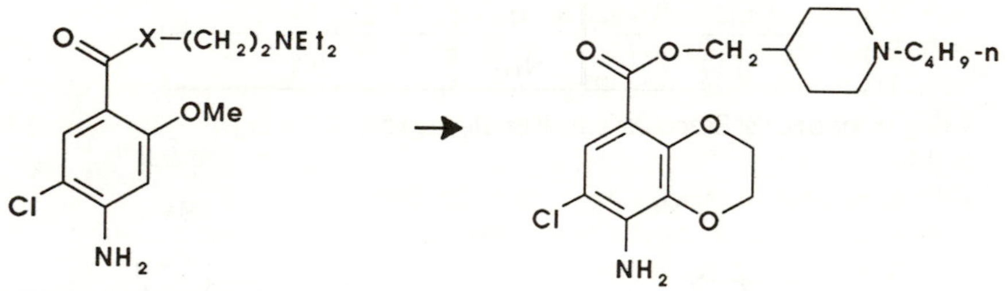

X = NH; Metoclopramide
X = O   SDZ 205557

SB 204070

receptor. However, workers at Sandoz identified the ester, SDZ 205557, as a weak, but selective, antagonist.[26] We had previously identified the *N*-butyl-4-piperidinylmethylbenzamide as a more potent partial agonist than metoclopramide. Applying the amide to ester interchange still gave us a very low-efficacy partial agonist with increased potency. This potency was further dramatically increased on cyclisation of the methoxy group to give a benzodioxan, SB 204070, which is a selective 5-HT$_4$ receptor antagonist approximately 1000-fold more potent than SDZ 205557.

In conclusion we, and a number of other companies, have used metoclopramide as a lead and, by using the conformational restriction approach, have identified a number of highly potent and selective agents acting at both dopamine and 5-HT receptors.

6 REFERENCES

1. C.W. Thornber, *Chem. Soc. Rev.*, 1979, **8**, 563.
2. C.A. Lipinski, *Annu. Rep. Med. Chem.*, 1986, **21**, 283.
3. Blaney and Orlek (personal communication).
4. F.D. King *et.al.*, *J. Med. Chem.* 1993, **36**, 1918.
5. M.J. Wyvratt and A.A. Patchett, *Med. Res. Rev.*, 1985, **5**, 483.
6. 'Burgers Medicinal Chemistry', 4th Edn., Part 3, Chap. 56.
7. R.D. Kempsford *et al.* Presented at the British Pharmacological Society Meeting in Aberdeen, 14th–16th April 1993.
8. B.S. Orlek *et al.*, *J. Med. Chem.*, 1991, **34**, 2726.
9. W.F. Huffman in 'Medicinal Chemistry for the 21st Century', ed., C.G. Wermuth, Blackwell Scientific Publications, 1992, p. 247.
10. N. Bodor and J.J. Kaminski, *Ann. Rep. Med. Chem.*, 1987, **22**, 303.
11. H. Bundgaard, in 'A Textbook of Drug Design and Development', ed. P. Krogsgaard-Larsen and H. Bundgaard, Harwood Academic Publishers GmbH, Chur, Switzerland, 1991.
12. H. Bundgaard, *Adv. Drug Delivery Rev.*, 1989, **3**, 39.
13. G.J. Sanger and F.D. King, *Drug Design and Delivery*, 1988, **3**, 273.
14. J.R. Fozard and M. Host, *Br. J. Pharmacol.*, 1982, **77**, 520P.
15. W.D. Miner and G.J. Sanger, *Br. J. Pharmacol.*, 1986, **88**, 497.
16. D.J. Roberts, *Curr. Ther. Res.*, 1982, 51.
17. M.S. Hadley, *et al.*, *BioMed. Chem. Lett.*, 1992, **2**, 1147.
18. F.D. King, *et al.*, *J. Med. Chem.*, 1988, **31**, 1708.
19. M.S. Hadley, in 'Chemical Regulation of Biological Mechanisms', ed. A.M. Creighton, and S. Turner, The Royal Society of Chemistry, London, 1982, p. 140.
20. F.D. King *et al.*, *J. Med. Chem.*, 1990, **33**, 2942.
21. J. Bermudez *et al.*, *J. Med. Chem.*, 1990, **33**, 1924.
22. F.D. King *et al.*, *J. Med. Chem.*, 1993, **36**, 683.
23. A.W. Oxford *et al.*, in 'Progress in Medicinal Chemistry', ed. G.P. Ellis and D.K. Luscombe, Elsevier, Amsterdam, 1992, **29**, 239.
24. D. W. Robertson *et al.*, *J. Med. Chem.*, 1992, **35**, 310.
25. T. Kawakita *et al.*, *Chem. Pharm. Bull.*, 1992, **40**, 624.
26. K. H. Bucheit *et al.*, *N.S. Arch. Pharmacol.*, 1992, **345**, 387.
27. L. M. Gaster *et al.*, *J. Med. Chem.*, 1993, **36**, 4121.

CHAPTER 15

The Design and Synthesis of Selective Protein Kinase C Inhibitors

CHRISTOPHER H. HILL

1 INTRODUCTION

It has been estimated that approximately one third of the plethora of proteins which are expressed in a typical mammalian cell are covalently bonded to phosphate.[1] The regulation of the phosphorylation state of these intracellular proteins is controlled by a large number of protein kinases and phosphatases. Genomic sequencing suggests that about 2–3% of all eukaryotic genes may code for protein kinases, of which perhaps 200 have been identified.

Protein kinase C (PKC) is a family of serine/threonine-specific protein kinases, consisting of at least ten isoenzyme species, which is believed to play a central role in cellular signal transduction processes. Activation of PKC following receptor occupation leads to the catalytic transfer of the γ-phosphate of adenosine triphosphate to serine or threonine residues in acceptor proteins. The consequent alteration in the properties of these substrate proteins propagates the signal. PKC is therefore able to modulate mechanisms of cell proliferation and gene expression and is implicated in the pathogenesis of a number of diseases.

The PKC isoenzymes are single polypeptide chains[2] which consist of two major functional domains.[3] The catalytic carboxyl terminal halves of the molecules contain the binding sites for the nucleotide and protein substrates. The ATP binding sites are highly conserved between isoenzymes and resemble those of other protein kinases. The regulatory domains differ between isoenzymes but, in the 'conventional' isoenzyme family, contain binding sites for Ca^{2+} and anionic phospholipids such as phosphatidylserine. Diacylglycerols are required for optimal activity of PKC by increasing its affinity for Ca^{2+} and phospholipid. A tandem repeat of a cysteine-rich sequence found in the regulatory domain of PKC has been suggested to be the probable binding site for diacylglycerol, and also for phorbol esters which are believed to be potent and highly selective activators of PKC.[4] All PKC isoenzymes contain a pseudosubstrate sequence[5] in their regulatory domain. This sequence resembles the substrate phosphorylation site and is proposed to interact with the enzyme active site, thereby preventing binding of substrate. It is believed that binding of cofactors induces a conformational change which uncouples this interaction resulting in enzyme activation.

Receptor occupation by a variety of cytokines, hormones, neurotransmitters, and growth factors, either *via* a G-protein or *via* tyrosine-specific protein kinase activity, results in activation of phospholipase C. This enzyme, when activated, catalyses the hydrolysis of inositol phospholipids in the inner leaflet of the plasma membrane to generate inositol triphosphate, which promotes release of Ca^{2+} from intracellular stores, and diacylglycerol (DAG) which is the physiological activator of PKC.[6] DAG may also result from hydrolysis of phosphatidylcholine by phospholipase D to yield phosphatidic acid which is converted to DAG by removal of its phosphate.[7] Physiological activation of PKC appears to involve its translocation from the cytosol to the membrane and binding to the membrane results in activation of a Ca^{2+}-dependent neutral proteinase which then catalyses limited proteolysis of the kinase to produce a form that is Ca^{2+}-independent.[8]

Isolated PKC has a broad substrate specificity and it is clear from studies with phorbol esters, which are used as DAG mimetics, that PKC can phosphorylate a large number of different proteins in cells. Despite this, relatively few proteins have been identified as physiological substrates for PKC. Phorbol esters can induce a wide range of cellular responses and it is tempting to speculate that physiological agonists which induce the same responses will also utilise PKC-dependent pathways. The degree of redundancy involved in these processes, however, is not properly understood. Moreover, recent results with selective PKC inhibitors suggest that these agents will block phorbol ester, but not C5a-induced adhesion of neutrophils to endothelial cells. It would seem, therefore, that PKC is not involved or is not a rate-limiting step in C5a-induced adhesion.[9] Results such as these imply that PKC inhibitors will have a selective action that is not immediately apparent from the wide range of cellular processes in which this enzyme has been implicated.

2 IN PATHOLOGICAL PROCESSES

Inappropriate PKC activation may occur in a number of disease states. Proliferation of particular T cell populations in response to antigen is believed to underlie autoimmune diseases such as rheumatoid arthritis and multiple sclerosis, and several lines of circumstantial evidence support the hypothesis that PKC is involved in antigen-driven T cell proliferation.[10] It has been shown that common proteins are phosphorylated in T cells in response to both phorbol esters and to stimulation by antigen. Also, down-regulation of PKC activity in T cells by chronic stimulation with phorbol esters renders the cells unresponsive to activation. Finally, selective PKC inhibitors will block proliferation of T cell clones following exposure to antigen-pulsed autologous cells.[11] PKC may also be involved in diseases of the central nervous system such as Alzheimer's disease, malignant transformation, and in viral entry into cells (*e.g.* HIV entry into $CD4^+$ T cells). Additionally, changes in cellular PKC activity have also been associated with several cardiovascular conditions (hypertension, cardiac hypertrophy, ischaemia).[12]

This evidence would suggest that a very wide range of potential therapeutic applications exist for PKC inhibitors. Much of the evidence for PKC involvement in the diseases mentioned above, however, contains serious flaws. It relies on the use of phorbol esters to stimulate a physiological process but this, of course, does not preclude alternative pathways which might be used by physiological agonists. The increased concentrations of PKC, translocation of PKC and/or altered phosphorylation patterns in cells derived from diseased tissues may actually represent an attempt to redress some imbalance caused by the initial lesion. Studies with inhibitors such as H7, staurosporine, and K252a are inconclusive since these agents lack the required selectivity for PKC over closely-related protein kinases.[12] The therapeutic potential for PKC inhibitors in these areas therefore needs to be explored using highly selective inhibitors.

3 INHIBITOR DESIGN

The microbial metabolite staurosporine has been widely used to investigate the role of PKC in signal transduction processes following the initial report describing it as a potent inhibitor of this Ca^{2+}/phospholipid-dependent protein kinase.[13] It rapidly became apparent, however, that this indolocarbazole was also a potent inhibitor of a variety of other kinases.[14] Nonetheless it does represent an attractive lead for the design of selective PKC inhibitors.

Initially, we set out to synthesize the aglycone of staurosporine to see whether this would retain any of the inhibitory activity of the parent system.

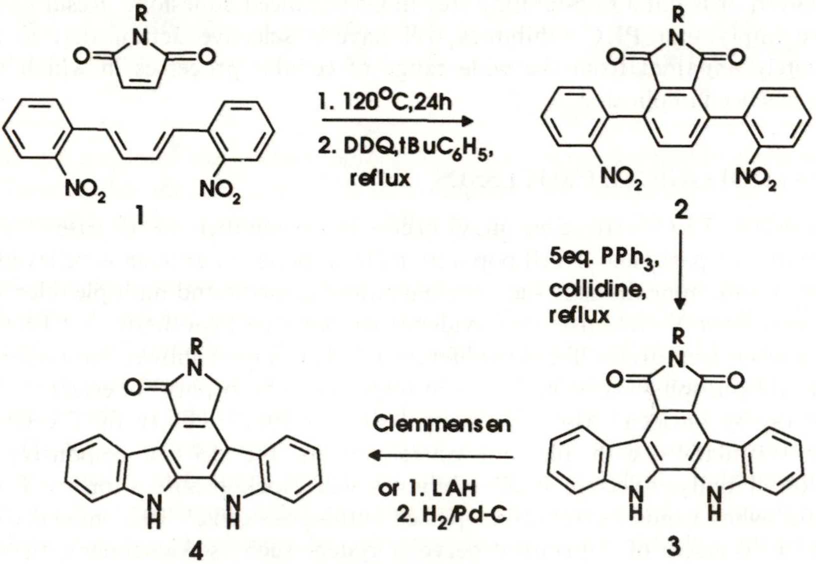

Scheme 1

The approach that we adopted involved a modification of Raphael's route[15] to such indolocarbazoles and required a Diels–Alder reaction of diene 1 with maleimide, followed by aromatisation of the initial adduct with DDQ to afford phthalimide 2 in good yield (Scheme 1). Access to the indolocarbazole was then achieved *via* a double nitrene insertion into the central phthalimide ring using an

Table 1: *Selectivity profile of staurosporine and related analogues*

	IC$_{50}$ (nM)		
	PKC	**PKA**	**PhK**
5 Staurosporine	9	120	0.5
6 K252a	500	100	1.7
4 Aglycone	1400	2800	4

excess of triphenylphosphine in refluxing collidine. The desired lactam **4** was then obtained by a two-step process; reduction of the imide **3** to the corresponding hydroxylactam with lithium aluminium hydride followed by catalytic hydrogenolysis.

The aglycone was considerably less active than staurosporine itself and, like other indolocarbazoles such as K252a, it had little selectivity for PKC over other related kinases (Table 1). The difference in potency between staurosporine and the other two indolocarbazoles was intriguing and we reasoned that this was likely to be due to the presence of the methylamino substituent on the pyranose ring of staurosporine. A number of analogues of the aglycone were prepared and it was found that alkylation of the lactam nitrogen resulted in a total loss of inhibitory activity. In contrast the corresponding imide appeared to retain the potency of the aglycone, although determination of a precise IC$_{50}$ was hampered by the physical properties of this compound.

Although the aglycone appeared to be an interesting lead, none of these early compounds exhibited any significant selectivity for protein kinase C over related kinases and we wished to investigate other systems which did not contain flat polyaromatic ring systems with the potential for DNA intercalation. Indeed it was known that such a compound containing an indolocarbazole, rebeccamycin, is able to induce single-strand breaks in DNA,[16] possibly through intercalation. We therefore wished to investigate the activity of non-planar analogues of the

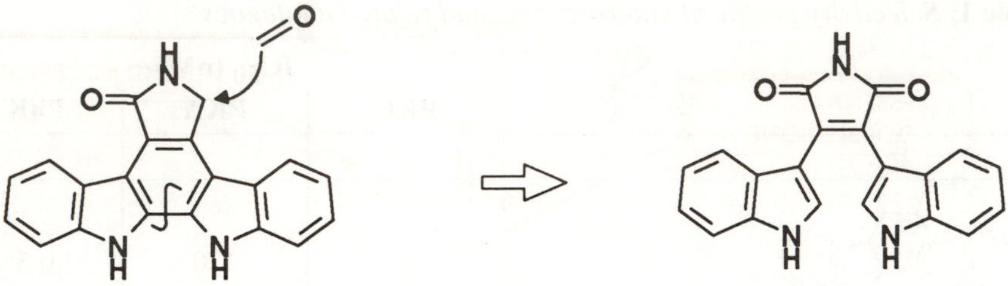

Figure 1

aglycone. One approach involved formal removal of the 12a–12b bond in the aglycone coupled with the introduction of a second carbonyl into the lactam ring (Figure 1).

Molecular mechanics calculations (within MOLOC[17]) on the resulting bisindolylmaleimides suggested that there is a significant barrier for either indole ring to achieve coplanarity with the maleimide. It was pleasing to find that this compound was a slightly more potent PKC inhibitor than the aglycone, but the crucial discovery was that it also demonstrated a forty-fold selectivity for PKC over PKA (Table 2).

Clearly, this compound represented an exciting new lead for the design of selective PKC inhibitors and it was systematically modified to identify the structural features required for inhibitory activity (Figure 2).[18] The imide NH is absolutely essential for activity, presumably as a hydrogen bond donor; both alkylated imides and the corresponding maleic anhydrides are totally inactive. The imide double bond appears to be essential since both *cis-* and *trans-*succinimides lose all inhibitory activity. Both carbonyls also appear to be required for optimal activity, as indicated by the twenty-fold drop in potency for the corresponding lactam.

Replacement of the indole ring with a variety of aryl and heteroaryl ring systems all resulted in reduced activity. The more active compounds appeared to be those with an aryl ring which more closely resembles that of indole, *e.g.* 3-benzothiophene, 1-naphthalene, whereas substituents which would occupy significantly different spatial volumes exhibited much reduced activity.

Substitution around the indole rings was also investigated with a variety of substituents possessing different electronic, steric, and lipophilic properties, but these were generally less active than the parent system. The only position in the

Table 2: *Bisindolylmaleimides are selective inhibitors of PKC*

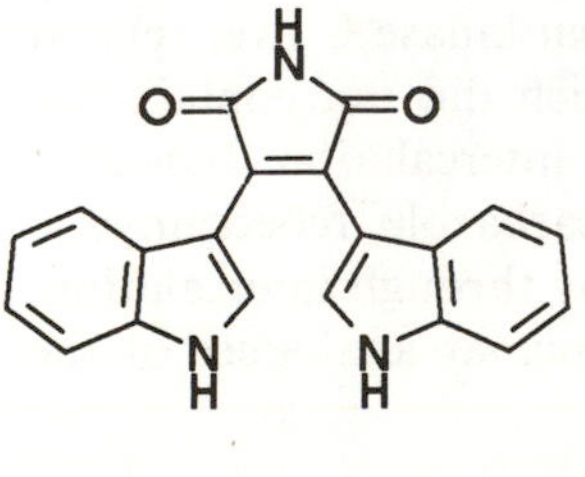

	IC_{50} (nM)
PKC	600
PKA	26000
PhK	1700

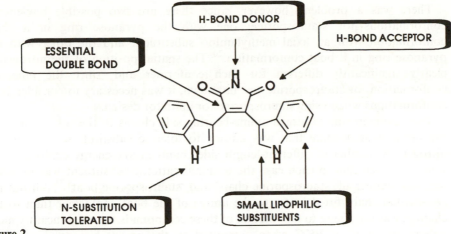

Figure 2

molecule which would tolerate any significant substitution (*e.g.* n-propyl) was the indole nitrogen which fortunately was a convenient point for further elaboration of these systems. Small lipophilic substituents were also tolerated at the 2-, 4-, 5-, and 7- positions.

An examination of the SAR of staurosporine analogues points to a significant role for the 4'-methylamino substituent and the three orders of magnitude loss of activity reported for the compound resulting from replacement of the methylamino substituent with hydroxyl[19] gives credence to the hypothesis that there is a potential cationic binding site for these inhibitors. Since we now wished to improve the potency of our relatively selective PKC inhibitors we wanted to take advantage of this putative amine binding site. We therefore proposed a common mode of binding for our inhibitors and staurosporine based upon some common structure–activity relationships. In both series of compounds imides are active, but alkylation of the imide or lactam rings is not tolerated and it was thought that this was likely to be a common region for interaction with the enzyme. The imide ring of the bisindolylmaleimides could therefore be matched onto the lactam of staurosporine and the indoles were brought as close as possible to the plane of the indolocarbazole ring system without paying any significant energy penalty. This was therefore a low-energy conformation of the bisindolylmaleimide.

Table 3: *Improved potency of aminoalkyl substituted bisindolylmaleimides*

Compound	n	IC$_{50}$ (nM)
8	2	64
9	3	70
10	4	44
11	5	76

There was a problem, however, since there are two possible low-energy conformations for staurosporine; one with the pyranose ring in a chair conformation with an axial methylamino substituent and the other with the pyranose ring in a boat conformation.[20] The spatial position of the nitrogen is clearly significantly different for each conformer and, since the bioactive conformation for staurosporine was unknown, it was necessary to consider both conformations when using staurosporine for inhibitor design.

The next step was to attach amine-bearing side chains to the sole position in the bisindolylmaleimide that was known to tolerate substitution – the indole nitrogen. A number of different-length side chains in low-energy conformations were evaluated and in each case the terminal cationic substituent was matched onto the amines of 'staurosporine chair' and 'staurosporine boat'.[21] All but the two-carbon chain fitted better to the amine of the boat conformer than to the chair. It was gratifying to find that all of these compounds were significantly more potent inhibitors of PKC when compared to the parent bisindolylmaleimide (Table 3), suggesting that the amine substituents were interacting favourably with the enzyme. It is likely that this is an electrostatic interaction, since a quaternary amine retained activity but alcohols were less active.

Replacement of the amino group with a variety of alternative cationic species identified amidines, guanidines, and isothioureas as more potent analogues in which the potency was dependent on chain length (Table 4). This was in contrast to the amine series and is consistent with a carboxylate–bifurcated cation interaction which one would expect to be more geometry dependent than a carboxylate–ammonium interaction. At this stage a number of compounds were evaluated on oral dosing to rats and compounds such as the isothiourea **13** gave very little PKC inhibitory activity in plasma. The amine **9**, however, appeared to have a considerably better pharmacokinetic profile and significantly higher levels of PKC inhibitory activity were observed, despite its lower *in vitro* potency.

This amine was still significantly less active than staurosporine and an improvement in the potency of amine **9** was therefore sought. One way to achieve this could be to conformationally restrict the amine side chain. Potentially this could be accomplished by cyclising around from the indole nitrogen to the

Table 4: *Bifurcated cationic side chains confer greater potency*

Compound	n	X	IC_{50} (nM)
12	2	SC(NH)NH$_2$	45
13	3	SC(NH)NH$_2$	10
14	4	SC(NH)NH$_2$	34
15	3	C(NH)NH$_2$	54
16	4	C(NH)NH$_2$	30
17	5	C(NH)NH$_2$	130
18	3	NHC(NH)NH$_2$	23

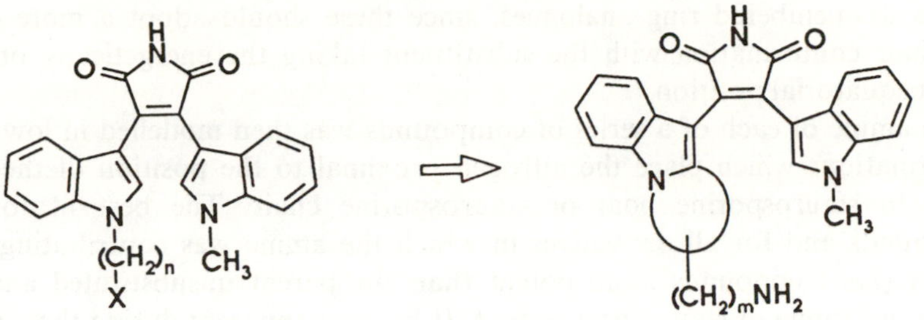

Figure 3

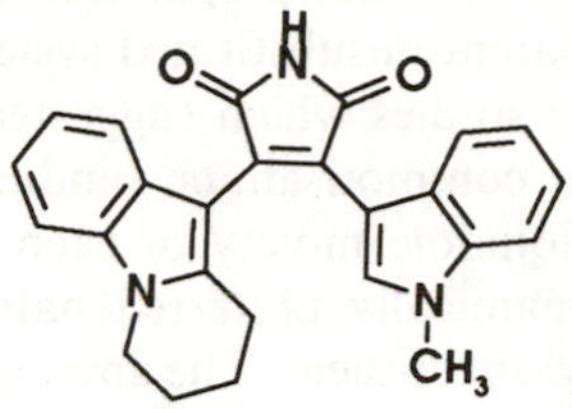

Figure 4

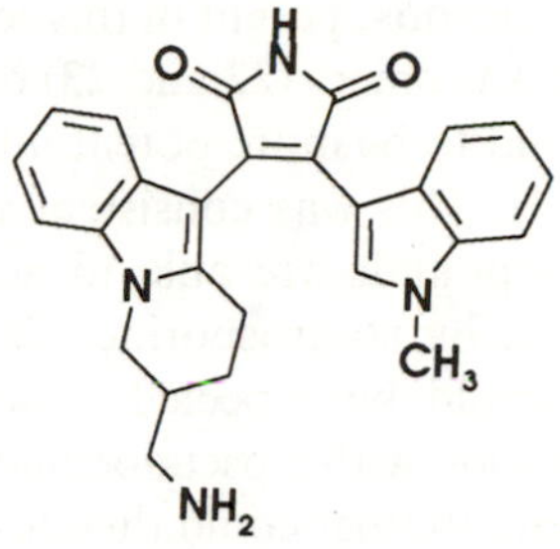

2-position (Figure 3), since it was known from our earlier work that small, lipophilic substituents were tolerated here.

Modelling studies suggested that the formation of such a ring would result in an ideal template for appending desired substituents which could favourably interact with the putative cationic binding site. The parent tetrahydropyrido[1,2-*a*]indole system (**19**, Figure 4) was initially constructed in order to test whether this extra ring could be accommodated by the enzyme. The activities of this compound (**19**, IC$_{50}$ 155 nM) and the five and seven ring analogues clearly indicated that such a template would be useful for the design of more potent inhibitors.[22] Compounds were then designed which had an amine-containing group attached to the template ring. The focus of attention initially was centred

Table 5: *Conformationally restricted amines*

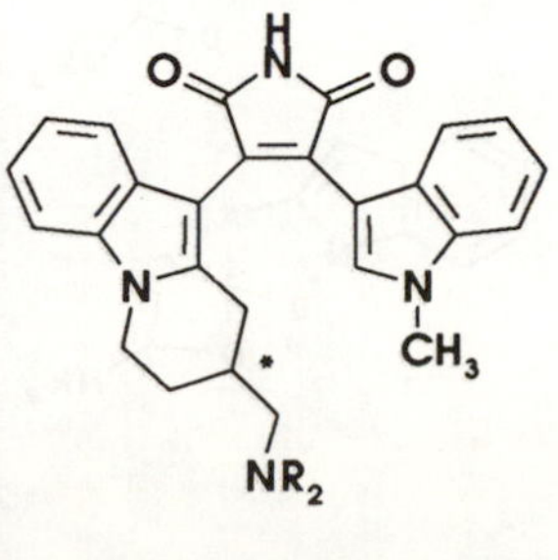

Compound		R	*	IC$_{50}$ (nM)
21	Ro 31-8425	H	R,S	7.6
22	Ro 31-9875	H	S	4.1
23	Ro 31-9877	H	R	10
24	Ro 31-8830	Me	R,S	42
25	Ro 32-0432	Me	S	19

on the six-membered ring analogues, since these should adopt a more defined half-chair conformation with the substituent taking the energetically preferred pseudoequatorial position.

The amine of each of a series of compounds was then modelled in low energy conformations which place the nitrogen proximal to the position of the amino group in staurosporine boat or staurosporine chair. The best fit for most compounds and for all derivatives in which the amine was contributing to the activity (*i.e.* compounds more potent than the parent unsubstituted analogue) was to the amine of staurosporine boat. It became apparent during the course of these studies that, as expected, the spatial position of the amine of staurosporine boat was not optimal for our inhibitors. The compound which fits the model best is the 7-aminomethyl derivative (**20**) but the 8-aminomethyl analogue (**21**) was found to be most potent in this series (Table 5).

The enantiomers (**22** and **23**) of primary amine **21** were also prepared and both were found to be more potent inhibitors than the parent unsubstituted system, **19** (Figure 4). This was consistent with the modelling studies which suggested that both compounds are able to access the proposed common amine binding site recognised by staurosporine. The tetrahydropyridoindole moiety of each enantiomer would be expected to adopt a thermodynamically preferred half-chair conformation with a pseudoequatorial aminomethyl substituent. The amine group of each enantiomer could therefore occupy a similar spatial position, although any effects due to steric differences between the two compounds would not be predicted.

On dosing the primary amine **21** orally to rats it was found that very poor plasma levels of PKC inhibitory activity were attained. In contrast significant plasma concentrations of PKC inhibitory activity were achieved with the corresponding tertiary amine **24** despite a loss of *in vitro* potency for this compound. The relative selectivity for Ro 31-8830 over other related kinases was retained; however it was now desirable to increase further the potency of such a tertiary amine. We therefore needed to define an amino pharmacophore model based upon our most potent compounds in order to guide the design of the next generation of bisindolylmaleimide inhibitors.

A large number of potential further conformationally restricted targets could be envisaged (Figure 5) and in order to select those compounds most likely to

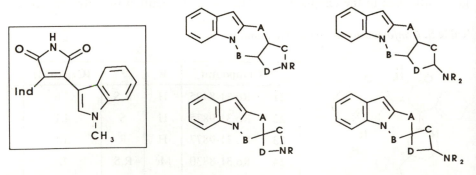

Figure 5

have the best activity, a model was established which should allow the identification of the more promising synthetic targets.

Three of the most potent compounds from the previous series were thus modelled in low-energy conformations with the amine nitrogens proximal to the amine of staurosporine boat and the spatial positions of these nitrogens were used to identify an amine pharmacophore model. The candidate further conformationally restricted compounds were then modelled to bring their respective amine nitrogens proximal to the centroid of the triangle representing the amine binding site. Using this approach many possible candidates were eliminated since the spatial positions of the nitrogens would clearly be relatively remote to the preferred site. A small number of compounds were thus selected for synthesis and one of the most promising targets is shown (Figure 6). This tertiary amine is significantly more potent (IC_{50} 4 nM) than those from the earlier series.

A number of bisindolylmaleimides have recently been evaluated against five PKC isoenzymes (PKC-α, βI, βII, γ, and ε), all of which showed a slight selectivity for PKC-α over the other isoforms tested.[23] The most selective compound reported to date (Ro 32-0432) exhibits a ten-fold selectivity for PKC-α and a four-fold selectivity for PKC-βI over PKC-ε.

4 CELLULAR AND *IN VIVO* STUDIES

Having achieved the initial goal of designing selective PKC inhibitors, it was important to establish whether or not these compounds could access and block the enzyme in an intracellular environment. This can be directly measured by

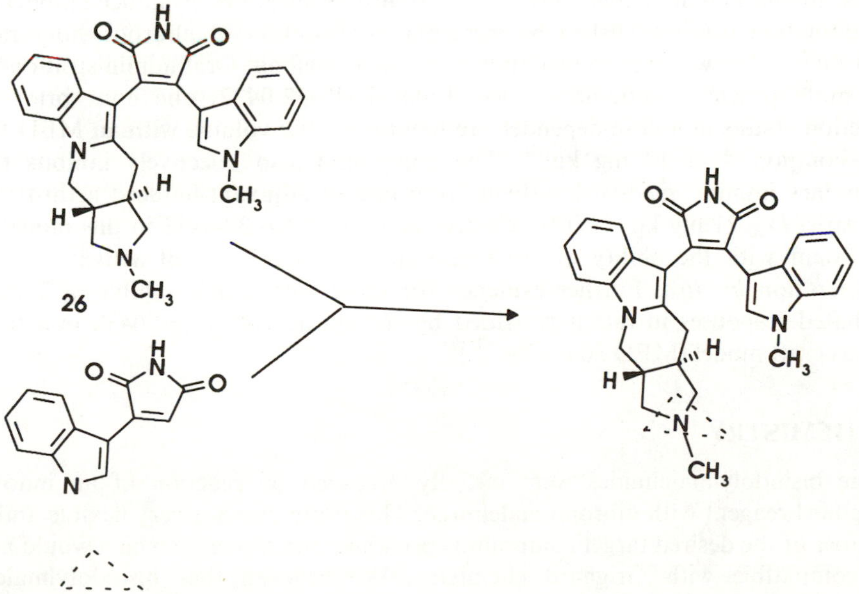

Figure 6

prelabelling human platelets with [^{32}P]orthophosphate and following the phosphorylation of specific proteins after treatment with phorbol ester. These bisindolylmaleimides are all able to antagonise, in a dose-dependent fashion, PKC mediated phosphorylation of a 47 kDa protein in platelets[24] and therefore represent powerful tools for the elucidation of the function of PKC in cells. The compounds do appear to be less potent in an intracellular environment, but this is probably explained by the fact that these inhibitors are competitive with ATP and whilst the concentration of ATP in the isolated enzyme assay is 10 μM; in cells it is in the millimolar range.

We next wished to study *in vitro* models of antigen induced T cell proliferation and initially the compounds were evaluated in an allogeneic mixed lymphocyte reaction. The inhibitors exhibited a dose-dependent inhibition in this system and also antagonised the antigen-driven proliferation of a T cell clone.[25] The compounds also inhibit PHA-induced IL-2 receptor expression and IL-2 secretion in human peripheral blood T cells. They do not, however, appear to antagonise IL-2 induced proliferation of peripheral blood T cells. The resulting effect of inhibiting PKC in T cells therefore appears to be much the same as for cyclosporin, although clearly the mechanism of action is totally different. Cyclosporin interferes with the activation of the calcium-dependent type 2B serine/threonine-specific phosphatase, calcineurin,[26] and has no effect on the PKC pathway whilst PKC inhibitors have no effect on calcium driven responses. Both PKC inhibitors and cyclosporin seem to cause arrest in the G0-G1 transition stage of the cell cycle but do not have an effect on post IL-2 receptor mediated signal transduction (G1-S cell cycle transition).

The PKC inhibitors were next evaluated *in vivo* to ascertain if they could gain access to and inhibit endogenous PKC. Initially a phorbol ester-induced model of inflammation was established by intra-plantar injection of phorbol dibutyrate into the hind paws of mice resulting in a rapid swelling. Oral administration of the more potent enantiomer of Ro 31-8830 (Ro32-0432) one hour prior to injection results in a dose-dependent reduction in paw volume with an MED for this compound of 10 mg kg^{-1}. The compound also selectively inhibits the secondary immune-mediated systemic response of adjuvant-induced arthritis in the rat (ED$_{50}$ 11 mg kg^{-1}). The selective activity of Ro 32-0432 in this model is consistent with the ability of the compound to inhibit T cell activation and proliferation *in vitro*. Further evidence for these compounds inhibiting T cell-mediated responses in rats is provided by the efficacy of Ro 32-0432 in a host versus graft model (MED 50 mg kg^{-1}).

5 CHEMISTRY

Some bisindolylmaleimides were initially prepared by reaction of an indolyl Grignard reagent with dibromomaleimide. This route was not very flexible and a number of the desired target compounds possessed functionality which would not be compatible with Grignard chemistry. We believed that bisindolylmaleic anhydrides could be useful intermediates for the synthesis of the required imide, but literature preparations of diaryl anhydrides would not work or were otherwise unsuitable for our purposes and a new method for preparing these anhydrides was developed. Suitably protected indoles **27** are reacted with oxalyl chloride to afford the corresponding indolylglyoxylyl chlorides **28**. These can react with indolylacetic acids **29** in the presence of an excess of a suitable base, such as triethylamine, to give the desired bisindolylmaleic anhydrides **31** directly (Scheme 2).[27] Presumably the reaction proceeds *via* the mixed anhydride **30** which

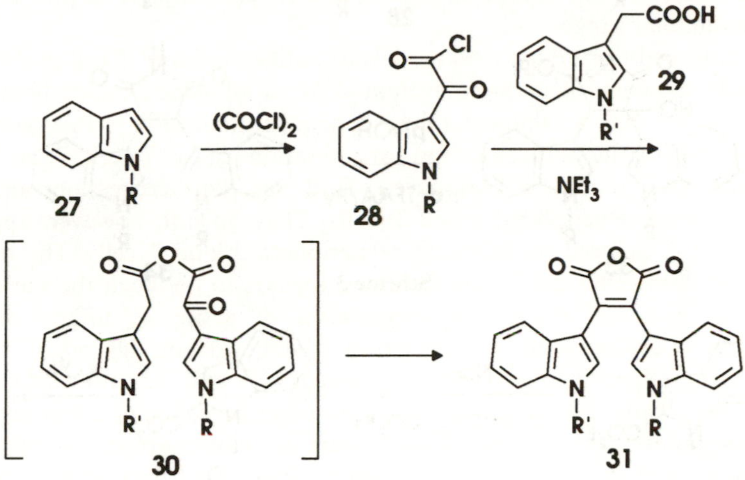

Scheme 2

can undergo an intramolecular Perkin reaction. Typically these bisindolylmaleic anhydrides are conveniently elaborated to the corresponding maleimides by heating to 140 °C in a bomb with 880 ammonia. Concomitant deprotection of the acetate in the side chain is also achieved under these conditions, allowing conversion of the resulting alcohol into the desired amines *via* the corresponding triflates.

This convenient and flexible coupling method has proved extremely useful for the preparation of a large number of analogues; however the yields were modest, typically around 30%. We therefore required a more efficient method for the construction of the bisindolylmaleimide system and decided to examine the possibility of directly accessing the maleimide from imidate **32**. This approach has proved very fruitful and reaction of isopropyl 3-indolylacetimidate **32** with an indolylglyoxylyl chloride **28** affords the hydroxypyrroline **33**, which in the presence of *p*-toluenesulphonic acid undergoes dehydration and hydrolysis to give the desired product **34** in good yield[28] (Scheme 3). An alternative way of promoting the dehydration/hydrolysis for compounds with acid-sensitive substituents using trifluoroacetic anhydride in pyridine was also developed.

The more complex substituted fused [1,2-*a*]indoles required for these coupling reactions have generally been made by a Dieckman and ring expansion approach,[29] an example of which is shown in Scheme 4.

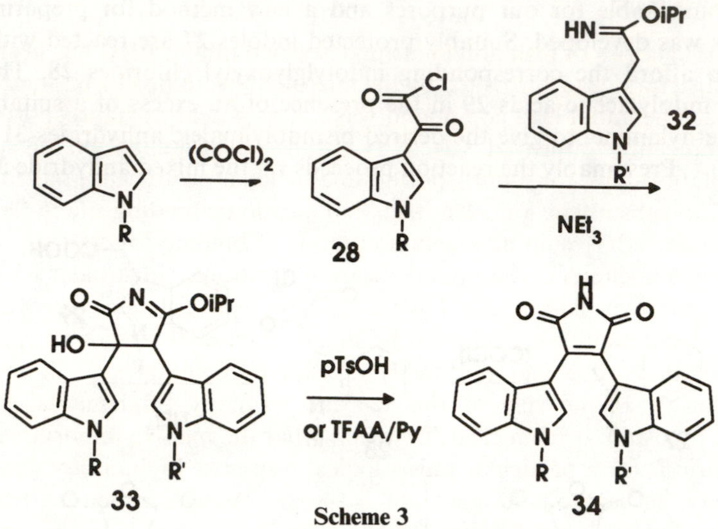

Scheme 3

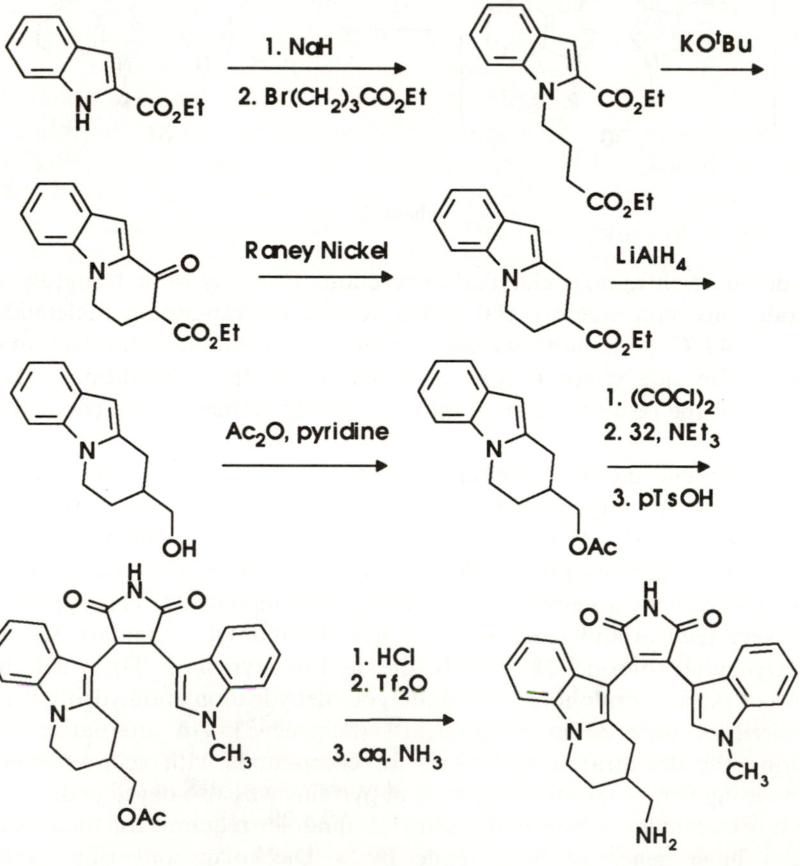

Scheme 4

6 CONCLUSION

In summary, a series of bisindolylmaleimides which inhibit PKC has been derived from the structural leads provided by the microbial broth products, staurosporine and K252a. The initial lead compound was not as potent as staurosporine, but it had a significantly improved selectivity profile. By examination of structure–activity relationships for staurosporine analogues a significant role for the 4'-methylamino substituent was identified, and a cationic binding site in the enzyme active site inferred. Assuming a common mode of binding for staurosporine and the bisindolylmaleimides, compounds bearing a cationic substituent which could access the putative binding site have been designed. Further improvements in potency and selectivity were achieved by a conformational restriction approach.

The availability of potent and highly selective PKC inhibitors will now permit the elucidation of the role of this enzyme in many fundamental biological processes. It is still far from clear, however, what the relative importance of each PKC isoform is for a particular physiological response. Preliminary data suggest that it may be possible to generate isozyme selective inhibitors from these bisindolylmaleimides, but for significant progress to be made in this area X-ray crystal structure information would be desirable. To date only two protein kinases have proved amenable to crystallographic analysis,[30,31] but it can only be a matter of time before other examples, including PKC, are reported.

The results we have obtained with an orally available, selective protein kinase C inhibitor demonstrate the crucial role for this enzyme in T cell activation and T cell driven chronic inflammatory responses *in vivo*. Inhibition of PKC clearly represents an important mechanistic approach to prevent T cell activation and compounds of this type could prove to be of valuable therapeutic benefit in the treatment of autoimmune diseases such as rheumatoid arthritis. The enormous potential for new, useful therapies for a variety of poorly treated diseases will ensure that PKC inhibitors will retain a high profile for many years to come.

7 REFERENCES

1. M.J. Hubbard and P. Cohen, *TiBS*, 1993, **18**, 172.
2. M. Inoue, A. Kishimoto, Y. Takai, and Y. Nishizuka, *J. Biol. Chem.*, 1977, **252**, 7610.
3. P.J. Parker *et al.*, *Science*, 1986, **233**, 853.
4. M. Castagna *et al.*, *J. Biol. Chem.*, 1982, **257**, 7847.
5. C. House and B.E. Kemp, *Science*, 1987, **238**, 1726.
6. Y. Nishizuka, *Nature*, 1984, **308**, 693.
7. J.H. Exton, *J. Biol. Chem.*, 1990, **265**, 1.
8. E. Melloni *et al.*, *Proc. Natl. Acad. Sci.*, 1985, **82**, 6435.
9. J.A. Sullivan, J.E. Merritt, and T.J. Hallam, *Br. J. Pharmacol.*, in press.
10. N. Berry and Y. Nishizuka, *Eur. J. Biochem.*, 1990, **189**, 205.
11. J.S. Nixon *et al.*, *Biochem. Soc. Trans.*, 1992, **20**, 419.
12. D. Bradshaw *et al.*, *Agents Actions*, 1993, **38**, 135.
13. T. Tamaoki *et al.*, *Biochem. Biophys. Res. Comm.*, 1986, **135**, 397.

14. L.H. Elliott *et al.*, *Biochem. Biophys. Res. Comm.*, 1990, **171**, 148.
15. I. Hughes, W.P. Nolan, and R.A. Raphael, *J. Chem. Soc., Perkin Trans. 1*, 1990, 2475.
16. J.A. Bush *et al.*, *J. Antibiot.*, 1987, **40**, 668.
17. P.R. Gerber, K. Gubernator, and K. Mueller, *Helv. Chim. Acta*, 1988, **71**, 1429.
18. P.D. Davis *et al.*, *J. Med. Chem.*, 1992, **35**, 177.
19. H. Osada *et al.*, *J. Antibiot.*, 1990, **43**, 163.
20. P.D. Davis *et al.*, *J. Chem. Soc., Chem. Commun.*, 1991, 182.
21. P.D. Davis *et al.*, *J. Med. Chem.*, 1992, **35**, 994.
22. R.A. Bit *et al.*, *J. Med. Chem.*, 1993, **36**, 21.
23. S.E. Wilkinson, P.J. Parker, and J.S. Nixon, *Biochem. J.*, 1993, **294**, 335.
24. P.D. Davis *et al.*, *FEBS Lett.*, 1989, **259**, 61.
25. A.M. Birchall *et al.*, *J. Pharm. Exp. Ther.*, in press.
26. A.L. DeFranco, *Nature*, 1991, **352**, 754.
27. P.D. Davis, R.A. Bit, and S.A. Hurst, *Tetrahedron Lett.*, 1990, **31**, 2353.
28. R.A. Bit, P.H. Crackett, W.Harris, and C.H. Hill, *Tetrahedron Lett.*, 1993, **34**, 5623.
29. R.A. Bit, P.D. Davis, C.H. Hill, E. Keech, and D.R. Vesey, *Tetrahedron*, 1991, **47**, 4645.
30. J. Zheng *et al.*, *Biochemistry*, 1993, **32**, 2154.
31. H.L. De Bondt *et al.*, *Nature*, 1993, **363**, 595.

CHAPTER 16

Discovery of 1069C – A Novel Synthetic Antitumour Agent with Low Cross-Resistance Potential

SIMON T. HODGSON

1 INTRODUCTION

Cancer today is still an important clinical problem with the prognosis for the majority of tumours remaining relatively poor. Surgery, radiotherapy, and chemotherapy all have an important role to play in the treatment of cancer, either alone or when combined with each other to form a more effective strategy. Advances in chemotherapy have often been made with compounds which work through new mechanisms. A good example in recent years is Etoposide, which is useful in small-cell lung and testicular carcinomas, and works *via* inhibition in the enzyme topoisomerase II.

The disruption of microtubule function is another important biological target in cancer chemotherapy. The natural product *Vinca* alkaloids, Vincristine and Vinblastine[1] (Figure 1), have been successfully used in the clinic for some 30 years. They disrupt microtubule (MT) assembly by interaction with α- and β-tubulin protein dimers, which leads to inhibition of cell division. Although the precise mechanism of how MT assembly is blocked is not clear, it is apparent that specific high- and low-affinity tubulin binding sites[2,3,4] exist for the *Vinca* alkaloids. Currently there is great interest in another series of naturally derived MT inhibitors, Taxol[5] and the semi-synthetic derivative, Taxotere[6] (Figure 1).

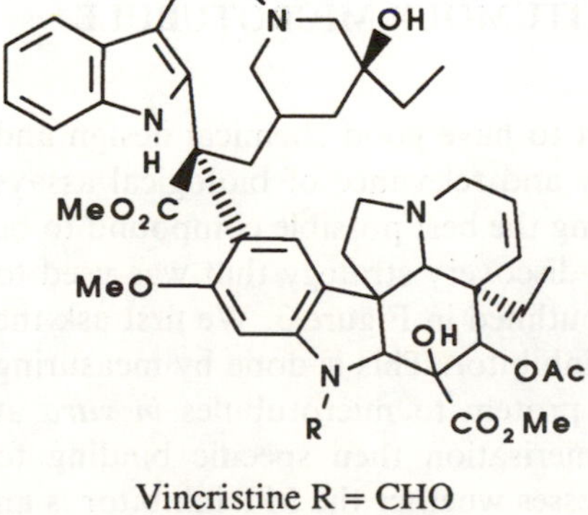

Vincristine R = CHO
Vinblastine R = Me

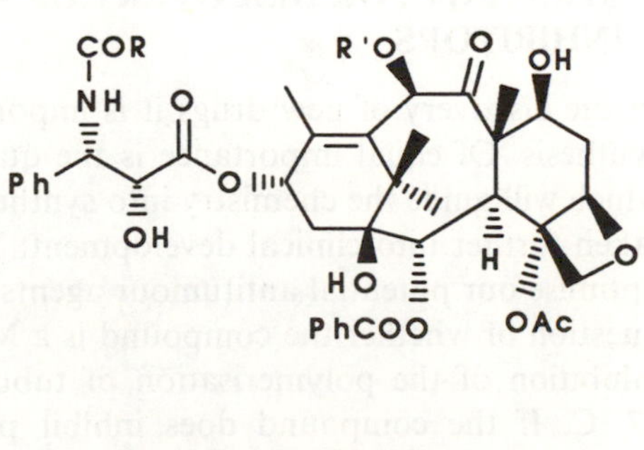

Taxol R = Ph, R' = Ac
Taxotere R = t-BuCO, R' = H

Figure 1: *Natural product microtubule inhibitors*

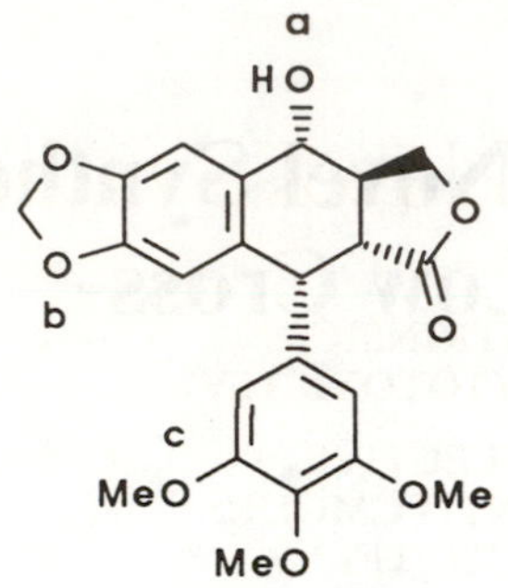

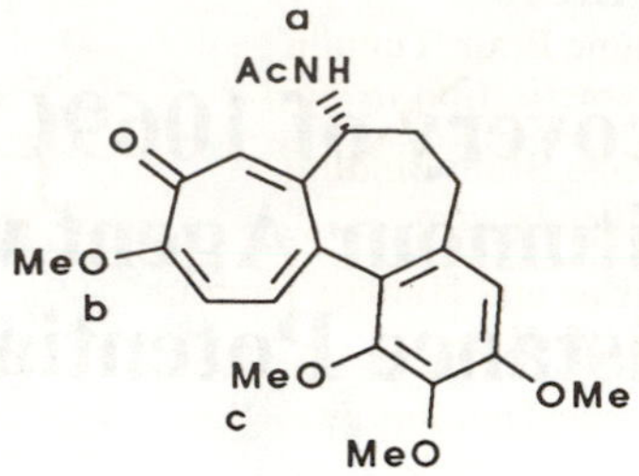

Podophyllotoxin   Colchicine

Figure 2: *Natural products binding at the colchicine site on tubulin*

In contrast to the *Vinca* alkaloids which inhibit tubulin polymerisation, Taxol[7,8] disrupts MT function through the promotion of tubulin polymerisation and stabilisation of MTs. Taxol has shown activity against a number of cancer types in clinical trials, such as ovarian carcinoma, malignant melanoma, and breast cancer. The drawback to Taxol's use has been the limited supply from the bark of the Pacific yew tree. Extensive resources are being channelled into alternative methods of production of Taxol and Taxotere, which may involve semi-synthetic chemistry.

Several years ago we were attracted to MTs as a therapeutic target for cancer because of the success of the *Vinca* alkaloids and the possibility of interfering with MTs through different mechanisms. On tubulin proteins there exists a site, distinct from the *Vinca* site(s), which binds the natural products Colchicine and Podophyllotoxin (Figure 2) with high affinity. It seemed to us that producing antagonists at the 'Colchicine binding site' was an attractive approach to new antitumour agents since this had not been exploited fully, and an antitumour agent working *via* a new mechanism might lead to novel therapeutic effects in the clinic.

2 STRATEGY FOR DISCOVERY OF ANTITUMOUR MICROTUBULE INHIBITORS

In the discovery of new drugs it is important to have good chemical design and synthesis. Of equal importance is the quality and relevance of biological assays which will guide the chemistry into synthesising the best possible compound to be taken further into clinical development. The discovery strategy that was used to optimise our potential antitumour agents is outlined in Figure 3. We first ask the question of whether the compound is a MT inhibitor. This is done by measuring inhibition of the polymerisation of tubulin protein to microtubules *in vitro* at 37 °C. If the compound does inhibit polymerisation then specific binding to tubulin can be measured. The next phase assesses whether the MT inhibitor is an anti-proliferative agent, *i.e.* it can penetrate tumour cells and stop growth *in vitro*. This assesses intrinsic cytotoxicity against growing tumour cells. The next and

1. Design and Chemical Synthesis

2. Equine Brain Tubulin
   Polymerisation *In vitro*

3. Equine Brain Binding   } → MT EFFECTS
   Studies *In vitro*

4. Murine and Human Tumour   → INTRINSIC
   Cells *In Vitro*   CYTOTOXICITY?

5. Murine Tumours *In vivo*   → SELECTIVE
                                ANTITUMOUR
                                ACTIVITY?

↓

OPTIMUM COMPOUNDS   → SAFE?
                              BIOAVAILABLE?
                              FORMULATION?

Figure 3: *Strategy for discovery of new antitumour microtubule inhibitors*

most important phase is to show whether the compound is able to kill selectively the tumour cells *in vivo* without too much damage to normal healthy cells. Clearly each result through different phases is fed back into the chemistry, with the ultimate goal of optimising the antitumour activity *in vivo*. Once a sufficiently effective compound has been identified then it will undergo various pre-clinical development activities, such as formulation, chemical synthesis scale-up, and safety evaluation. It is only during the clinical phase, when a new compound will be tested against a range of tumour types, that the true antitumour potential will be realised.

3 DISCOVERY OF THE LEAD COMPOUND

All the antitumour microtubule inhibitors used clinically are natural compounds or semi-synthetic derivatives. Our decision was to find synthetic molecules because these would be more accessible (*cf.* the problems with Taxol) and more amenable to optimisation through analogue synthesis. Furthermore, it is reasonable to expect that synthetic antitumour agents are less likely to suffer resistance problems than natural compounds (*vide infra*).

A number of benzimidazole carbamates are known to be microtubule inhibitors and are marketed products, such as benomyl[9] (a plant antifungal agent) and oxfendazole[10] (an anthelmintic agent). In addition, the benzimidazole carbamate, nocodazole,[11] has several properties (antifungal, anthelmintic, and antitumour) in experimental models.

Our lead compounds at Wellcome came from certain imidazo[1,2-*b*]pyridazine carbamates which had very potent anthelmintic activity against the nematode *N. Brasiliensis* (Table 1). We suspected that these early imidazopyridazine carbamates were probably selective inhibitors of the nematode tubulin polymerisation. They were singularly inactive against mammalian tubulin polymerisation and P388 leukaemia cell proliferation (Table 1).

Table 1: *Anthelmintic Imidazopyridazine carbamates*

	IC$_{50}$ (μM) Tubulin Polymerisation	IC$_{50}$ (nM) P388 Leukaemia Cell Poliferation	IC$_{50}$ (μM) *N. Brasiliensis*
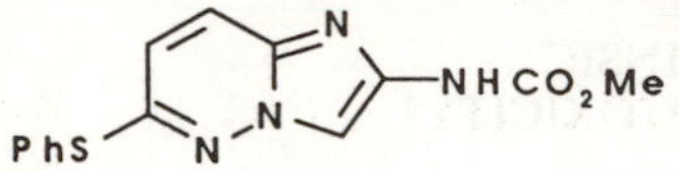 PhS—[imidazopyridazine]—NHCO$_2$Me	28.6	>10,000	0.011
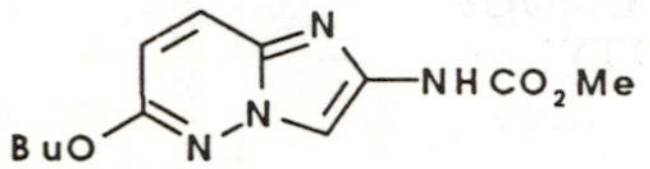 BuO—[imidazopyridazine]—NHCO$_2$Me	10.6	>1000	0.064

The key challenge we were faced with was how to design in the effects against mammalian tubulin in the imidazopyridazine carbamate series. Clearly the imidazopyridazine carbamate structures are very different from the natural products Colchicine and Podophyllotoxin, both of which bind to the same 'Colchicine Site' on tubulin. Margulis[12] had suggested from *X*-ray structures of Colchicine and Podophyllotoxin that certain atoms were common and over-lapped well (marked as a, b, c in Figure 2). However, the 'a' site cannot be critical since 4-deoxy-podophyllotoxin retains the same activity as Podophyllotoxin itself.

Based on a hunch that it is the trimethoxyphenyl rings in Colchicine and Podophyllotoxin that are important for tubulin binding, we modified the 6-position in the imidazopyridazines and incorporated a trimethoxybenzyl group. This led to 1069C (Figure 4) which, remarkably, is a very potent inhibitor of mammalian tubulin polymerisation and potent inhibitor of P388 leukaemia cell proliferation. In contrast, 1069C is not active against the nematode *N. Brasiliensis*.

The 6-trimethoxybenzyl substituent has therefore reversed the selectivity between antitumour and anthelmintic effects by approximately 1000-fold. When compared against other MT inhibitors (Table 2) 1069C is a very potent inhibitor

1069C   [structure: MeO, MeO, MeO trimethoxybenzyl-O-imidazopyridazine-NHCO$_2$Me]

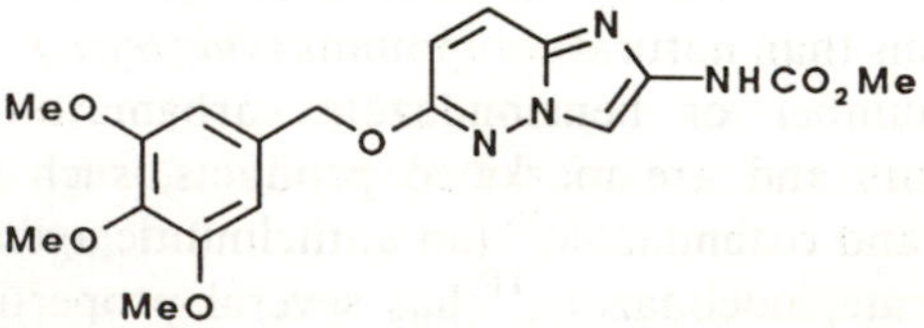

IC$_{50}$ (μM) Tubulin Polymerisation	IC$_{50}$ (nM) P388 Leukaemia Cell Proliferation	IC$_{50}$ (μM) *N. Brasiliensis*
0.31	8.9	>10

Figure 4: *1069C - an imidazopyridazine carbamate with selectivity for mammalian tubulin*

Table 2: *Comparative microtubule inhibitory and cytotoxic effects of 1069C and natural products*

	IC_{50} (µM) ETP	EC_{50} (nM) P388 CMSD	IC_{50} (nM) P388 P	IC_{50} (nM) P388 CF
1069C	0.31	6–9	8.9	13
Colchicine	1.5	–	0.6	71
Vincristine	0.22	20–40	4.7	190
Vinblastine	–	–	1.7	8.2

ETP = Equine Tubulin Polymerisation; CMSD = Cell Mitotic Spindle Disruption; P = Proliferation; CF = Colony Formation.

of tubulin polymerisation. Furthermore, 1069C disrupts mitotic spindles in intact P388 leukaemia cells at similar concentrations required to block cell proliferation, providing support for the mode of the action of 1069C as a MT inhibitor in tumour cells. Either as a MT inhibitor or a cytotoxic agent, 1069C appears to be one of the most potent known compounds.

4 COMPUTER MODELLING OF 1069C AND NATURAL PRODUCT LIGANDS AT THE COLCHICINE SITE

In tubulin binding studies 1069C was a competitive inhibitor of [^{3}H]-Colchicine binding but had no effect on [^{3}H]-Vinblastine binding. Thus, having shown that 1069C binds to the Colchicine site it was of great interest to understand how the very different structures of 1069C and Colchicine could be related by computer modelling. Conformational minimisation of 1069C using Sybil showed a number of low energy states. One such example is a folded conformation (Figure 5) where the trimethoxybenzyloxy side chain is bent around and almost underneath the heterocyclic ring system. A very interesting picture emerged when this structure was overlaid with Colchicine (Figure 6): with the two trimethoxyphenyl rings coincident, the tropolone methoxy O-atom of Colchicine and the N-atom at position-3 of the imidazopyridazine system in 1069C fitted each other. Both atoms would be capable of acting as hydrogen bond acceptors. Oxygen would be expected to be a stronger H-bond acceptor, but CNDO calculations showed that there is a larger negative charge on the nitrogen of 1069C [$q(O) = -186$ for Colchicine and -212 for Podophyllotoxin; $q(N) = -296$ for 1069C]. Interestingly, the carbamate group contributes greatly to this high negative nitrogen charge in 1069C.

When 1069C, Colchicine, and Podophyllotoxin were fitted together and their electrostatic potential surfaces were examined (Figure 7) we discovered a striking similarity between these molecules. We therefore discovered that the Colchicine binding receptor seems to recognise molecules with a particular shape and charge distribution, and showed for the first time how the synthetic carbamates can mimic the natural product ligands, Colchicine and Podophyllotoxin.

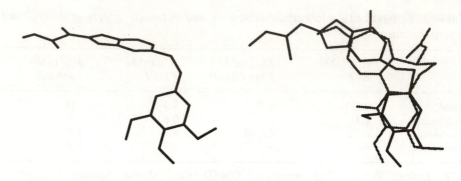

Figure 5: *The folded conformation of 1069C*   **Figure 6:** *Overlay of 1069C and colchicine*

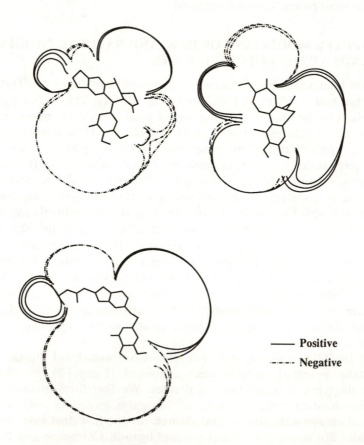

—— Positive

----- Negative

Figure 7: *Electrostatic potential maps of podophyllotoxin, colchicine and 1069C*

5 SAR STUDIES *(IN VITRO)*

1069C was one of the earliest examples in the imidazopyridazine series to show potent antitumour effects. A range of analogues were synthesised in order to investigate the series more fully.

Side-chain Aromatic Group

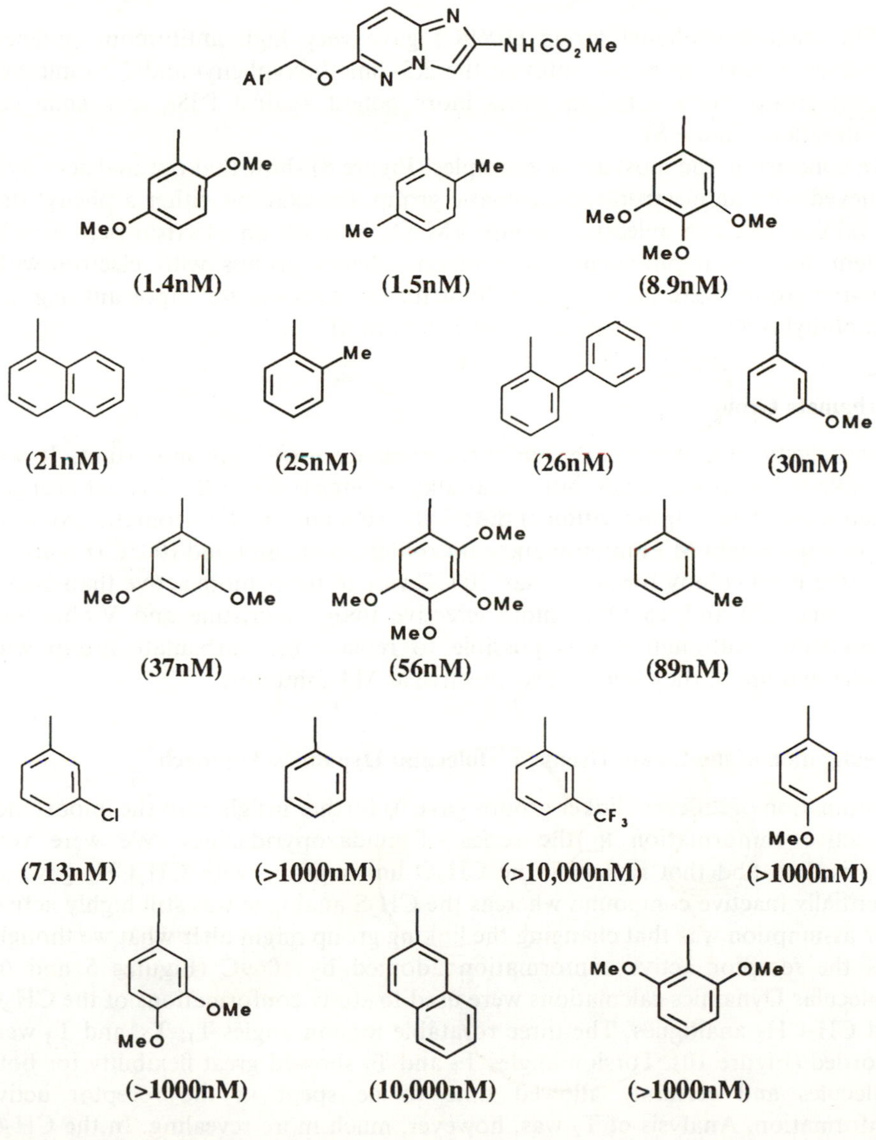

Figure 8: *SAR of aromatic groups (vs P388 in vitro)*

1005C

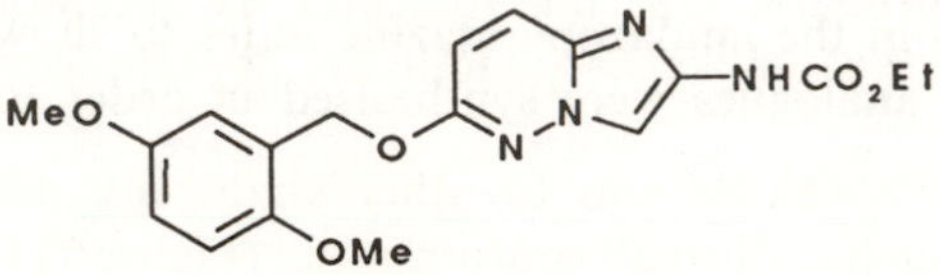

Tubulin Polymerisation IC_{50} 0.14 μM

P388 Proliferation IC_{50} 0.43 nM

Figure 9: *An exceptionally potent imidazopyridazine carbamate*

The trimethoxyphenyl group (1069C) gave very high antitumour potency. However, this group is not optimal: the 2,5-dimethoxyphenyl and 2,5-dimethyl-phenyl groups were some six times more potent against P388 leukaemia cell proliferation (Figure 8).

In conclusion, the most active examples (Figure 8) show that optimal activity is achieved with an electron-rich aromatic group, for example either a phenyl ring containing electron releasing groups (MeO, Me) or an electron-rich bicyclic system such as naphthalene. In contrast, phenyl groups with electron-with-drawing groups were poorly active. Substitution patterns are important (*e.g.* the 2-naphthyl is 500 times less active than 1-naphthyl).

Carbamate Group

Lipophilicity and steric effects in the carbamate group are important. It was possible to increase potency with linear alkyl groups (n-Pr, n-Bu, Et) but decrease potency with t-Bu. Optimisation of the alkyl carbamate and the aromatic group led to our most potent MT inhibitor and antiproliferative compound 1005C (Figure 9).

In the P388 colony forming assay 1005C was 26 times more active than 1069C and some 380 and 16 times more effective than Vincristine and Vinblastine, respectively. Although it was possible to replace the carbamate group with amides and ureas, they were not so effective as MT inhibitors.

Investigation of the Linker Group: a Molecular Dynamics Approach

Examination of different linker groups gave us further insight into the importance of active conformation in the series of imidazopyridazines. We were very surprised to find that replacing the CH_2O linker group with CH_2CH_2 gave an essentially inactive compound whereas the CH_2S analogue was still highly active. Our assumption was that changing the linking group might alter what we thought was the receptor active conformation adopted by 1069C (Figures 5 and 6). Molecular Dynamics calculations were used to study conformations of the CH_2O and CH_2CH_2 analogues. The three rotatable torsion angles T_1, T_2, and T_3 were recorded (Figure 10). Torsion angles T_1 and T_3 showed great flexibility for both molecules and certainly allowed time to be spent in the receptor active conformation. Analysis of T_2 was, however, much more revealing. In the CH_2O analogue (1069C) torsion T_2 showed values 70°, 180° and 290° (*i.e.* two *gauche* and one *trans* conformations) whereas the CH_2CH_2 analogue remained exclusively in the *trans* $T_2 = 180°$ conformation (the line indicates the receptor active conformation in Figure 10) and thus unlikely to adopt the hypothesised folded conformation (Figure 5, p. 246).

We extended the Molecular Dynamics calculations to other analogues and calculated the time spent in the receptor active ('fitted') conformation (Figure 11).

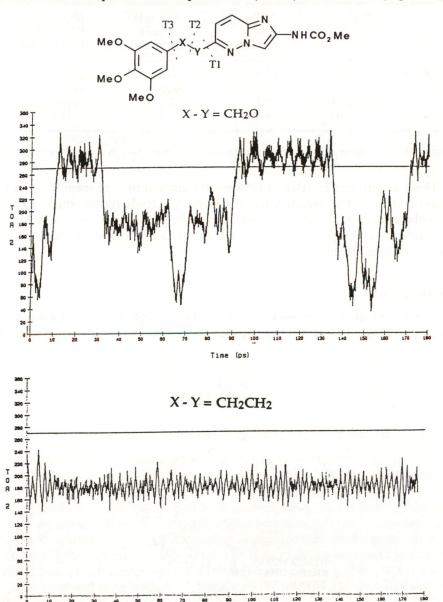

Figure 10: *Molecular dynamics study of torsion T_2 in CH_2O and CH_2CH_2 linker analogues*

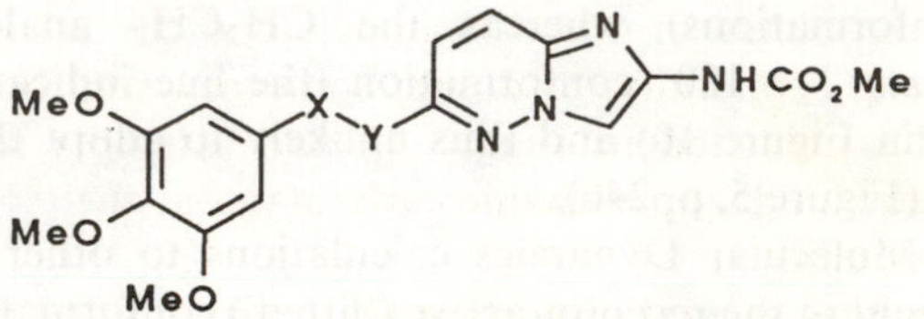

	X-Y	% Time in Fitted Conformation	IC$_{50}$ (μM) Tubulin Polymerisation	IC$_{50}$ (nM) P388 Cell Proliferation
1069C	CH$_2$O	12.5	0.42	8.9
	CH$_2$S	1.6	0.55	95
	CH$_2$CH$_2$	0.3	10	1000
	CH$_2$S(O)	0.0	> 20	> 10,000

Figure 11: *Correlation between biological potency and time spent in fitted (receptor active) conformation*

There is a striking correlation between the amount of time spent in the active conformation and biological activity. Clearly this lends further support to our hypothesis that the flexible carbamate type MT inhibitors need to achieve a particular conformation for optimal activity at the Colchicine binding receptor on mammalian tubulin.

Working Model

Usually, Medicinal Chemists have to work without three-dimensional structures of biological targets. Thus chemists will often evolve a conceptual model

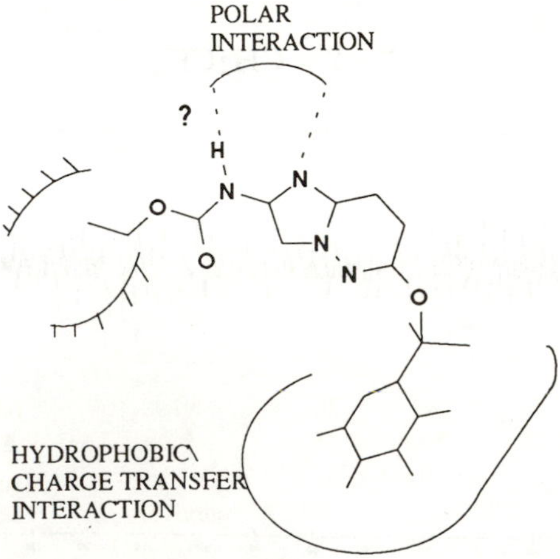

Figure 12: *Working model for interaction of imidazopyridazine carbamates at the colchicine binding receptor*

within a series of compounds in order to understand the activity of molecules already synthesised and, hopefully, to design some new and better compounds. Our working model is depicted in Figure 12 and attempts to rationalise the activity of the synthetic imidazopyridazine carbamates at the Colchicine receptor site on mammalian tubulin.

The model encapsulates several important features: a folded conformation, an electron rich system, presumably binding with the receptor *via* an hydrophobic or charge transfer interaction; an H-bond accepting N-atom; an H-bonding donating NH group; and steric constraints in the carbamate group.

6 *IN VIVO* ANTITUMOUR ACTIVITY

Thus far we have focused very much on biochemical activity of MT inhibitors and how this translates into cytotoxicity to tumour cells growing in culture. The key property of any new antitumour agent is an ability to kill tumour cells actively proliferating in an animal system without causing undue damage to the animal itself. Of the many animal model systems used over the years the P388 mouse model was well established and used by the American National Cancer Institute. The principle of the assay (Figure 13) is that mouse P388 cells are injected (i.p.) on day 0 and after a certain period, usually about 10 days, the mice will have died due to tumour (P388 leukaemia) overload. For a new compound to show antitumour efficacy, an increase in life-span (ILS) must be achieved. Exceptionally effective compounds will produce 60 day survivors, which are regarded as true cures because surviving mice at this stage rarely die subsequently of tumour. For 60 day survivors to be achieved every last tumour cell must have been eradicated by the antitumour agent after dosing on days 1, 5, and 9.

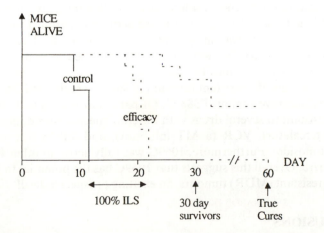

Figure 13: *Mouse P388 survival assay (NCI) – [10^6 P388 cells implanted IP; drug given IP on days 1, 5, and 9]*

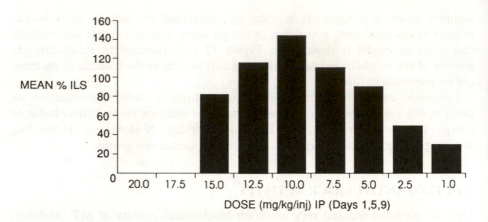

Figure 14: *Dose–response antitumour effect of 1069C against P388 in vivo*

From our *in vitro* structure–activity studies in the imidazopyridazine carbamates we produced a number of exceptionally potent MT inhibitors with exceptional activity against proliferating tumour cells (*e.g.* 1005C, 1069C). After we evaluated a number of compounds in the mouse P388 model, 1069C stood out from the rest as having the best combination of potency and antitumour efficacy, *i.e.* 1069C gave the highest %ILS values for the lowest dose. In addition, 60 day survivors (cures) were often noted at certain doses. A dose–response relationship was seen (Figure 14) where antitumour efficacy increases from the 1 mg kg^{-1} dose to an optimum at 10 mg kg^{-1}. At higher doses antitumour efficacy starts to decrease as the drug begins to produce toxicity. This feature is common to all so-called cytotoxic antitumour drugs. The largest number of 60 day survivors was seen at doses of 10–15 mg kg^{-1} of 1069C.

As mentioned earlier, treatment of cancers by chemotherapy has been successful only for certain tumour types. Failure of chemotherapy may be due to intrinsic resistance of the tumour to a given drug or acquired resistance of the tumour in response to the drug. It was important to evaluate the lead compound 1069C against resistant tumours. We were pleasantly surprised to find in P388 tumours made resistant to several clinically used drugs (Figure 15), that 1069C appeared to be as effective against the resistant tumours, P388/Vincristine or P388/Adriamycin, as the normal sensitive tumour P388/O. Of particular note is that the P388/ADR tumour is resistant to several drugs with differing mechanisms of action, *i.e.* ADR (a DNA intercalator), VCR (a MT inhibitor), and VP-16 (the topoisomerase inhibitor, etoposide). Furthermore, 1069C was fully active in other P388-resistant tumours *in vivo*. Overall this suggests that 1069C has the potential to be effective in multi-drug-resistant (MDR) tumours, an exciting prospect indeed!

7 CONCLUSIONS

In summary we have manipulated a series of imidazopyridazine carbamates to be effective at the Colchicine receptor site on mammalian tubulin. As in much work

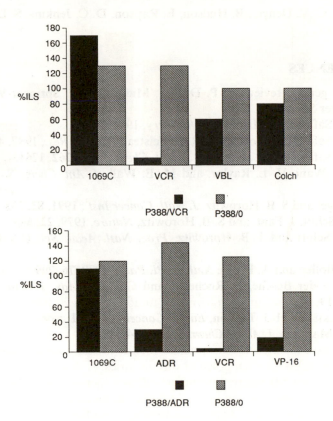

Figure 15: *Antitumour efficacy of 1069C against P388-resistant tumours in vivo – a comparison with other drugs (VCR = Vincristine, VBL = Vinblastine, Colch = Colchicine, ADR = Adriamycin, VP-16 = etoposide)*

in medicinal chemistry we do not have a 3D picture of our target receptor. However, we have used computer modelling techniques to develop a receptor active conformation and can now suggest, for the first time, how synthetic carbamate MT inhibitors relate to the natural product ligands at the Colchicine binding receptor on mammalian tubulin. The optimal compound 1069C has a very interesting profile: it is a very potent inhibitor of microtubule function in P388 tumour cells and demonstrates potent antitumour efficacy *in vivo*. Furthermore, 1069C has a remarkable activity against murine tumours which are resistant to a wide range of clinically used antitumour drugs. If this property translates into the clinic then 1069C would become an important drug in cancer chemotherapy.

8 ACKNOWLEDGEMENTS:

There is a large number of people who have contributed to this work. In particular, I should mention A. W. Randall, J. Wilkinson, D. J. Davies,

M. Reddy, C .V. Denyer, B. Hudson, E. Rapson, D. C. Jenkins, S. D. M. Watts, and V. Knick.

9 REFERENCES

1. For a general review see P. Dustin, 'Microtubules', Springer-Verlag, 1984, Chapter 5.
2. A. R. Safa and E. Hamel, *Biochemistry*, 1987, **26**, 97.
3. A. R. Safa, C. J. Glover, and R. L. Felstead, *Cancer Res.*, 1987, **47**, 5149.
4. A. R. Safa and R. L. Felstead, *J. Biol. Chem.*, 1987, **262**, 1261.
5. M. C. Wani, H. L. Raylor, and M. E. Wall, *J. Am. Chem. Soc.*, 1971, **93**, 2325.
6. I. Ringel and S. B. Horowitz, *J. Natl. Cancer Inst.*, 1991, **83**, 288.
7. P. B. Schift, J. Fant, and S. B. Horowitz, *Nature*, 1979, **22**, 665.
8. P. B. Schift and J. B. Horowitz, *Proc. Natl. Acad. Sci. U.S.A.*, 1980, **77**, 1561.
9. G. J. Bollen and A. Fuchs, *Neth. J. Pl. Path.*, 1970, **76**, 299.
10. H. Van der Bosche, F. Rochette, and C Horig, *Adv. Pharm. Chemother.*, 1982, **19**, 67.
11. C. Atassi and H. J. Tagnon, *Eur. J. Cancer*, 1975, **11**, 599.
12. T. N. Margulis, *J. Amer. Chem. Soc.*, 1974, **96**, 899.

The Design and Biological Properties of 'Dipeptoid' Antagonists

DAVID C. HORWELL

1 INTRODUCTION

Peptides are widely distributed in mammalian tissue. More than 100 mammalian peptides have been cited as acting as neurotransmitters, neuromodulators, and trophic factors (growth hormones). Some of the more well characterised peptides and their most common fragments that occur in mammalian central nervous system tissue are shown in Table 1.

A goal of research and drug discovery in the pharmaceutical industry is to produce drugs that may have therapeutic application by their ability to regulate the action of neuropeptides in disease states. Such drugs we call 'peptoids' and they are defined in Figure 1.

Our approach to design small molecule non-peptide analogues 'peptoids' of the neuropeptide cholecystokinin CCK26-33[1-3] (Figure 2, **1**) has led to the discovery of CCK-A and CCK-B antagonist 'dipeptoids' of general formula **2**. CCK receptors exist in at least two forms termed CCK-A and CCK-B/gastrin. CCK-A receptors are found in abundance in the pancreas and in smaller amounts in other tissue including the central nervous system. Activation of this receptor in the pancreas by CCK26-33 (sulphated) leads to release of amylase and this effect is blocked by the selective CCK-A antagonist Devazepide. CCK-B receptors

Table 1: *Neuropeptides in mammalian central nervous system and their most abundant forms.*

Neuropeptide	No. of amino acids in most abundant form	Neuropeptide	No. of amino acids in most abundant form
ACTH	39	GHRH	44
Angiotensin	8	LHRH (GnRH)	10
Bombesin	14	α-MSH	13
Bradykinin	9	Neuromedin B	32
Calcitonin	32	Neuropeptide K	36
Cholecystokinin	8	Neuropeptide Y	36
Dynorphin A	17	Oxytocin	9
β-Endorphin	31	TRH	3
Leu-enkephalin	5	VIP	28
Met-enkaphalin	5	Vasopressin	9
Glucagon	29	Substance P	11

PEPTOID:
A credible drug candidate that mimics or blocks the action(s) of an endogenous peptide
CREDIBLE DRUG CANDIDATE:
1. Demonstrable efficacy as an agonist or antagonist of the peptide receptor
2. Oral bioavailability
3. Pharmaceutically useful half-life (hours)
4. Manufacturable on a plant scale

Figure 1: *Definition of 'peptoid'.*

occur in the brain and appear to be the same as gastrin receptors in the gut. Both are activated by the CCK/gastrin selective agonist pentagastrin and the effects are blocked by CCK-B antagonists such as L365260 and CI-988.

The dipeptoid CI-988 (PD134308) **3** has high affinity $(K_i = 1.7$ nM) and selectivity for the CCK-B receptor (CCK-A/B ratio is 2500:1), and shows anxiolytic properties in several anxiogenic models by both s.c. and *oral* routes of administration over a wide dose range. The rational design of this compound is described in this article.

Asp-Tyr(OSO3H)-Met-Gly-Trp-Met-Asp-Phe-NH2
26 27   28   29   30   31   32   33
(1)

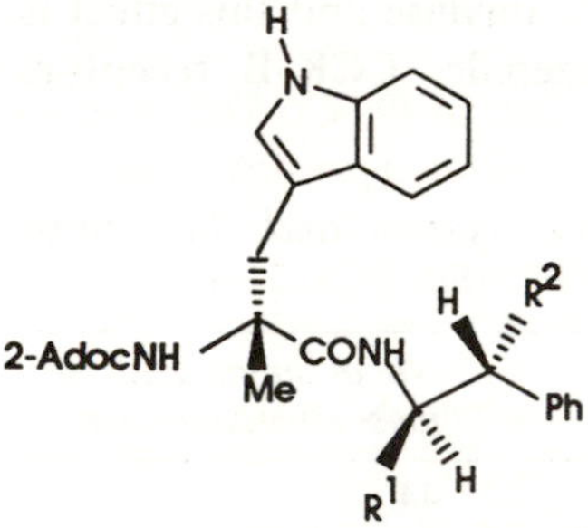

(2)

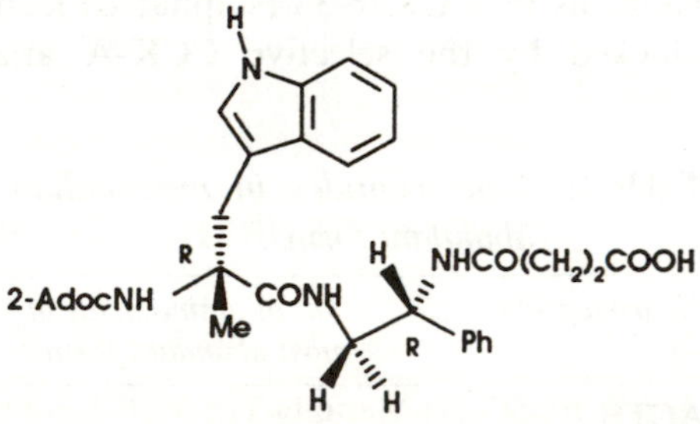

(3) CI-988 (PD134308)

Boc ———————— Trp ———————— Phe-NH2
(4)

Boc = t-butyloxycarbonyl-; 2-Adoc = 2-adamantyloxycarbonyl-

Figure 2: *Structures for compounds 1–4*

2 IDENTIFICATION OF THE DIPEPTIDE CHEMICAL LEAD

The design of these 'dipeptoids' **2** from CCK26-33, using the mouse cerebral cortex CCK-B binding assay with displacement of tritiated pentagastrin as the radioligand, involved identification of the *non-contiguous* dipeptide fragment of CCK, Boc-Trp-Phe-NH$_2$ **4** with low micromolar affinity (Tables 2 and 3).

Table 2 shows the binding affinities of fragments of CCK26-33 in the mouse cerebral cortex assay. Removal of the Asp-26 residue has no effect on binding whereas removal of the Phe-33 residue leads to loss of affinity. This shows that the phenylalanine residue is essential for receptor binding. The *C*-terminal tetrapeptide CCK30-33 retains full nanomolar binding affinity, but the two tripeptides CCK31-33 and CCK30-32 lose activity. It is therefore concluded that the Trp- and Phe-residues *together* are essential for high binding to CCK-B receptors. The tetrapeptide CCK30-33 retains comparable nanomolar affinity with the full octapeptide 26-33.

Table 3i shows that the nanomolar affinity of CCK30-33 can be increased ten-fold by replacing the *N*-terminal with simple peptide blocking groups such as Boc and Amoc. Table 3ii shows that the nature of the spacer group between the Boc-Trp-Phe-derivatives is important. Nanomolar affinity is seen only with CCK30-33. The simple dipeptide Boc-Trp-Phe-NH$_2$ has low micromolar affinity comparable with glycine-modified full tetrapeptides a–c.

The dipeptide Boc-Trp-Phe-NH$_2$ may be considered to act as a contiguous message equivalent to the non-contiguous message of the full tetrapeptide CCK30-33 (Figure 3). It is proposed that the receptor 'reads' the ligands comprising of the side chains of Trp- and Phe- in the dipeptide in the same way as the folded, possibly α-helical tetrapeptide.[4] These two lipophilic ligands would be expected to contribute binding energy equivalent to the observed low micromolar affinity. Chemical stabilization of the *single* peptide bond in this molecule

Table 2: *Structure–affinity relationships of CCK fragments at the CCK-B receptor from mouse cerebral cortex by displacement of tritiated pentagastrin*

FRAGMENTS OF THE *C*-TERMINAL OCTAPEPTIDE CCK 26-33

26	27		28	29	30	31	32	33	affinity K$_i$ (nM)
					*CCK-B receptor*				

Sequence	affinity K$_i$ (nM)
Asp-Tyr(OSO$_3$H)-Met-Gly-Trp-Met-Asp-Phe-NH$_2$	2.5
Tyr(OSO$_3$H)-Met-Gly-Trp-Met-Asp-Phe-NH$_2$	2.4
Tyr(OSO$_3$H)-Met-Gly-Trp-Met-Asp-NH$_2$	Inactive 10^{-4}M
Trp-Met-Asp-Phe-NH$_2$	3.1
Met-Asp-Phe-NH$_2$	10^5
Trp-Met-Asp-NH$_2$	Inactive 10^{-3}M

Conclusion:
a. Trp-Met-Asp-Phe-NH$_2$ fragment retains nanomolar affinity
b. Trp and Phe residues *together* are essential for high binding affinity to central CCK-B receptors

Table 3: *Binding affinities of modified CCK fragments*

X-Trp-Y-Phe-NH$_2$
i. The affect of altering the N-tryptophan protecting group
    X with Y = Met-Asp as in CCK 30-33

X	Structure	CCK receptor affinity (K_i)
H	H-Trp-Met-Asp-Phe-NH$_2$	3.1×10^{-9}M
Amoc	Amoc-Trp-Met-Asp-Phe-NH$_2$	2.7×10^{-10}M
Boc	Boc-Trp-Met-Asp-Phe-NH$_2$	3.0×10^{-10}M

Conclusion:
Asp-Tyr(SO$_3$H)-Met-Gly- of CCK-26-33 can be replaced by simple groups like Boc and retain nanomolar affinity

ii. The effect of altering the spacer group Y
1. Replacing the amino acid spacers with glycine

Y	Structure	CCK receptor affinity (K_i)
a. Gly-Gly	Boc-Trp-Gly-Gly-Phe-NH$_2$	5.0×10^{-3}M
b. Gly-Asp	Boc-Trp-Gly-Asp-Phe-NH$_2$	2.0×10^{-6}M
c. Met-Gly	Boc-Trp-Met-Gly-Phe-NH$_2$	2.7×10^{-5}M
d. Met-Asp	Boc-Trp-Met-Asp-Phe-NH$_2$	3.0×10^{-10}M

2. Altering spacer by methylene groups

Y	Structure	CCK receptor affinity (K_i)
–	Boc-Trp———Phe-NH$_2$	7.0×10^{-5}M
–CH$_2$–	Boc-Trp-Gly——Phe-NH$_2$	10^{-4}M
–(CH$_2$)$_2$–	Boc-Trp-Bala—Phe-NH$_2$	2.5×10^{-5}M
–(CH$_2$)$_3$–	Boc-Trp-Gaba–Phe-NH$_2$	5.0×10^{-3}M
–(CH$_2$)$_4$	Boc-Trp-Dava–Phe-NH$_2$	10^{-3}M

Conclusion:
The simple dipepetide Boc-Trp-Phe-NH$_2$ has affinity comparable with full modified tetrapeptides a–c rather than sub-nanamolar with Boc-CCK-30-33 (d).

together with identification of a third auxiliary ligand perhaps corresponding to the Met- or Asp- side chains of CCK30-33 (Figure 3) should then produce a low molecular weight, metabolically stable, and nanomolar affinity 'peptoid'.[5]

3 ENHANCEMENT OF THE BOC-TRP-PHE-NH$_2$ DIPEPTIDE CHEMICAL LEAD

A key modification of the dipeptide **4** involved replacement of the natural L-tryptophan by the non-genetically coded D-α-methyltryptophan moiety. The binding affinities of the α-methyltryptophan derivatives are shown in Table 4. The D-α-methyltryptophan residue enhances affinity 10-fold over the corresponding

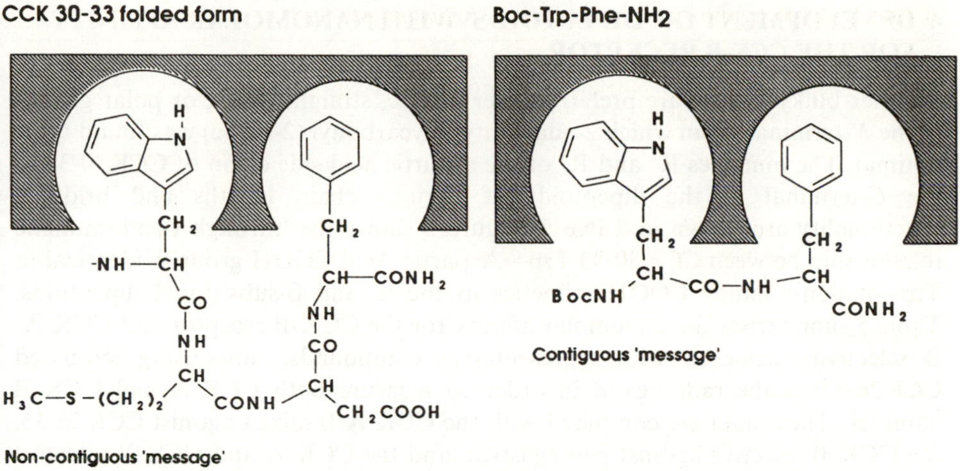

CCK 30-33 folded form

Boc-Trp-Phe-NH₂

Non-contiguous 'message'

Contiguous 'message'

Figure 3: *Cartoon comparison of folded form of CCK 30-33*

L-α-methyltryptophan diastereomer as well as the unsubstituted dipeptide **4**. This compound, PD122263 (Figure 4), on further chemical modification gave racemic PD125325 with the same receptor affinity. This showed that the *C*-terminal amide is not necessary for binding, the phenyl group can be replaced by simple heterocyclic groups such as pyridine, and the *N*-terminal Boc-group may be replaced by the much more sterically bulky, lipophilic, yet more acid and alkali stable TcBoc-group. Hence this compound would likely be more metabolically stable than PD122263 (TcBoc = CCl₃CMe₂OCO-).

Table 4: *Binding affinities of α-methyl-Trp-Phe derivatives compared with the simple dipeptide*

Compound	CCK receptor affinity (K_I)
[L] [L] Boc-Trp-Phe-NH₂	7.0×10^{-5}M
[DL] [L] Boc-(α-Me)-Trp-Phe-NH₂	1.6×10^{-5}M
[L] [L] Boc-(α-Me)-trp-Phe-NH₂	6.7×10^{-5}M
[D] [L] Boc-(α-Me)-Trp-Phe-NH₂	6.0×10^{-6}M

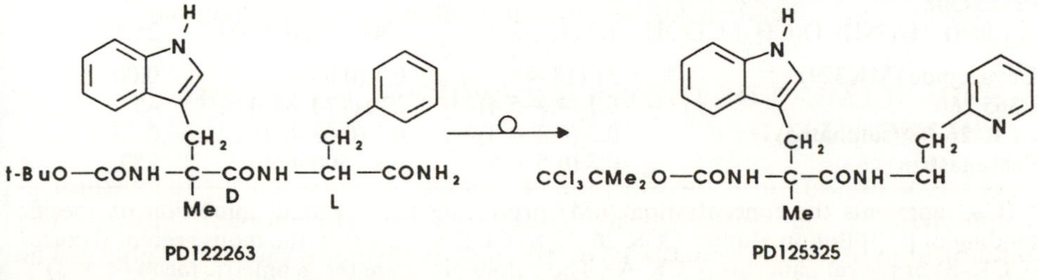

PD122263

PD125325

Figure 4: *Development of PD125325 from PD122263*

4 DEVELOPMENT OF 'DIPEPTOIDS' WITH NANOMOLAR AFFINITY FOR THE CCK-B RECEPTOR

Other bulky groups are preferred over TcBoc, straight chain, or polar groups at the *N*-terminal, from which 2-adamantyloxycarbonyl (2-Adoc) was found to be optimal. The mimetics R^1 and R^2 of the aspartic acid side chain of CCK30-33 at the *C*-terminal of the dipeptoids of various chain lengths and bridging functionality are shown in Table 5. Figure 5 shows the 'through bond' mimetic relationship between CCK30-33 Trp→Aspartic Acid COOH group is identical to Trp→malonic amide COOH mimetics in the α- and β-substituted dipeptoids. Table 5 summarises the nanomolar affinity for the CCK-B receptor and CCK A/B selectivity achieved with representative compounds, now using iodinated CCK26-33 as the radioligand in order to measure both CCK-A and CCK-B affinities. These data are compared with the CCK A/B mixed agonist CCK26-33, the CCK-B selective agonist pentagastrin, and the CCK-A and CCK-B selective antagonists Devazepide and L365,260 respectively.

Table 5: *Binding affinities of 'dipeptoid' ligands[a] to CCK-A and CCK-B receptors*

		IC_{50} (nM)		
R^1	R^2	CCK-B	CCK-A	A/B ratio
CH$_2$NHCOCH$_2$COOH	H	2.6 (1.8–3.5)	500 (390–600)	190
CH$_2$NHCO(CH$_2$)$_2$COOH	H	4.2 (2.9–6.3)	950 (740–1100)	230
CH$_2$NHCO(CH$_2$)$_3$COOH	H	4.6 (4.0–6.0)	1100 (1000–1400)	250
H	NHCOCH$_2$COOH	0.8 (0.5–1.0)	870 (620–1500)	1100
PD134308 (CI-988) H	NHCO(CH$_2$)$_2$COOH	1.7 (1.3–2.7)	4300 (1200–8500)	2500
Devazepide (MK329)		31 (18–43)	0.1 (0.03–0.2)	0.0032
L365,260		5.1 (4.6–5.4)	230 (170–380)	45
CCK 26–33 (sulphated)		0.3 (0.2–0.3)	0.1 (0.08–0.2)	0.33
Pentagastrin		0.8 (0.5–0.9)	600 (500–660)	750

[a] IC_{50} represents the concentration (nM) producing half-maximal inhibition of specific binding of [^{125}I] Bolton Hunter CCK 26–33 to CCK receptors in the mouse cerebral cortex (CCK-B) or the rat pancreas (CCK-A). The values given are the geometric mean ($n = 3$).
[b] 2 Adoc: 2-adamantyloxycarbonyl

CCK 30-33

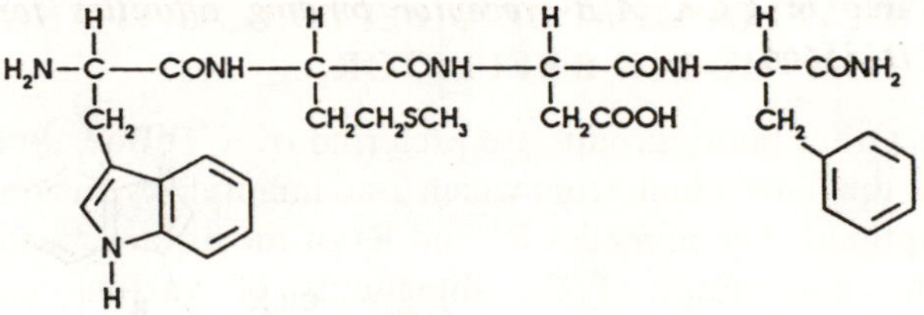

Asp - side chain mimetic on the α-phenylethylamide carbon atom

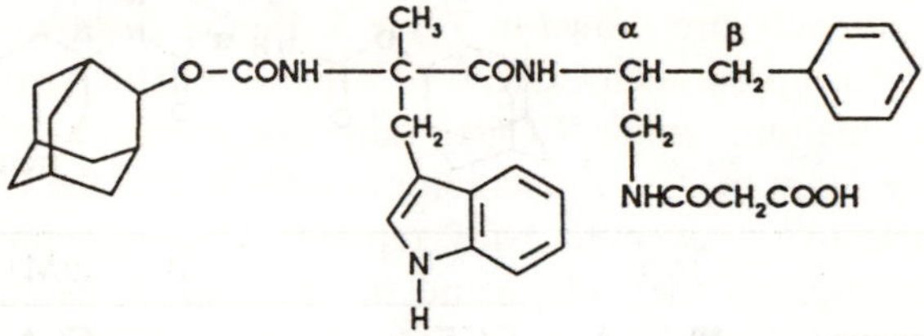

Asp - side chain mimetic on the β-phenylethylamide carbon atom

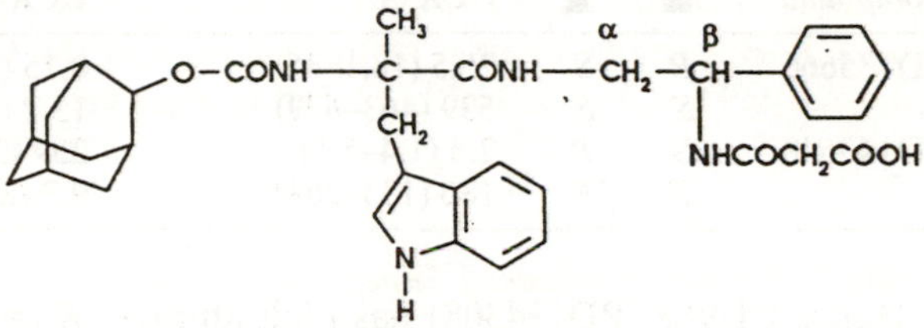

Figure 5: *Through bond mimetic of Trp → Asp carboxylic acid side chain*

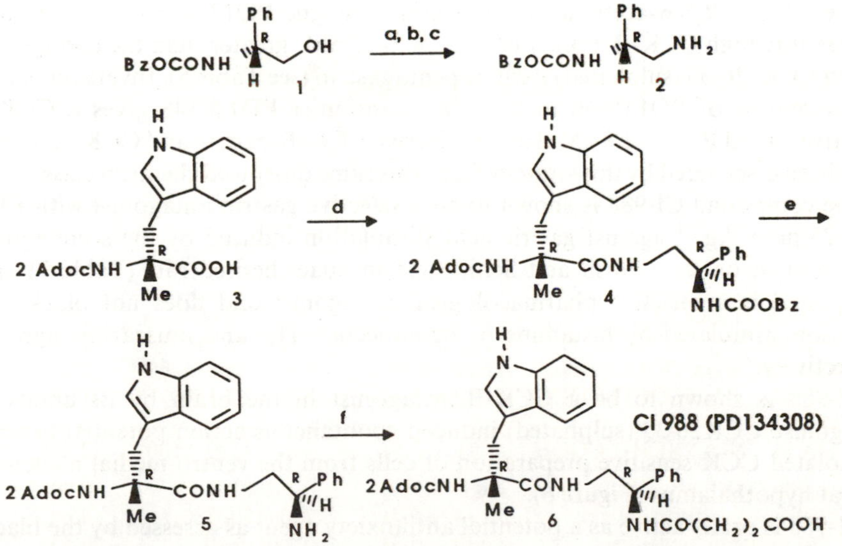

Scheme 1: *Synthesis of CI 988 (PD134308)*

CI 988 (PD134308)

Reagents: a) pTsCl, Et₃N, CH₂Cl₂, 81%; b) NaN₃, DMF, Δ, 88%; c) H₂, Lindlar, EtOAc, ~100%; d) DCC, HOBt, (2), EtOAc, 96%; e) Pearlman's Catalyst, H₂, EtOH, ~100%; f) succinic anhydride, EtOAc, 60%

Table 6: *CCK A/B- receptor binding affinities for all four stereoisomers of PD135666*

| Compound | ■ | ▲ | IC50 (nM) | | A/B ratio |
			CCK-A	CCK-B	
PD135666	R	S	25.5 (18.1–35.8)	0.15 (0.09–0.21)	170
	S	S	539 (463–629)	13.2 (10.4–16.9)	41
PD140548	S	R	2.8 (1.4–5.1)	259 (208–292)	0.01
	R	R	186 (133–268)	9.3 (8.4–10.5)	20

Hence CI-988 (PD134308) has high affinity (K_i = 1.7 nM) and selectivity for the CCK-B receptor with an A/B ratio of 2500:1. This novel 'dipeptoid' mimics the Trp-30, Phe-33, and Asp-32 side chain message found in CCK26-33 and represents a new chemical class of CCK-B receptor antagonists.[6] The synthesis of CI-988 is given in Scheme 1.

The related *R,S* α-acetic acid side chain analogue PD135666 (Table 6) has a remarkably high CCK-B affinity of IC_{50} = 0.15 nM, greater than the endogenous ligand CCK-26-33 (sulphated) itself or pentagastrin (see Table 5). Inversion of *both* stereo centres of PD135666 to the *S,R* enantiomer PD140548 gives a CCK-A selective ligand IC_{50} = 2.8 nM. Hence selective CCK-B/gastrin and CCK-A ligands have been discovered by this strategy from this same dipeptoid chemical class.

The compound CI-988 is shown to be a selective gastrin antagonist with ED_{50} = 0.25 μmol kg^{-1} against gastric acid stimulation induced by the secretagogue pentagastrin on the Ghosh and Schild test in anaesthetised rats (Table 7). The compound is a selective pharmacological antagonist and does not block acid secretion stimulated by histamine or bethanechol, H_2- and muscarinic agonists respectively.[7]

CI-988 is shown to be a CCK-B antagonist in the brain by its ability to antagonise CCK26-33 (sulphated) induced spontaneous action potential firing in an isolated CCK-sensitive preparation of cells from the ventro-medial nucleus of the rat hypothalamus (Figure 6).

CI-988 is orally active as a potential antianxiety agent as assessed by the black–white test box in mice over a wide dose range. This is compared with control where the mice spend more time in the black (darkened) compartment, whereas after oral administration of CI-988 the mice spend more time in the white (light) compartment (Figure 7).[6,8] This effect is also seen with clinically effective anxiolytics such as Diazepam and Alprazolam.

Table 7: *Potency[a] of selected agents on inhibition of gastric acid secretion in Gosh and Schild test*

Compound	Pentagastrin	Histamine	Bethanechol
CI-988 (PD134308)	0.25 (0.06–1.05)	> 25	> 25
L-365,260	1.61 (0.61–4.21)	> 160	> 160
Devazepide (MK329)	> 300	> 300	> 300
Ranitidine	0.19 (0.11–0.36)	0.20 (0.08–0.49)	0.25 (0.03–2.30)
Atropine	> 0.2	> 0.2	0.002 (0.0003–0.012)
Omeprazole	0.47 (0.17–1.33)	0.23 (0.03–1.96)	0.19 (0.09–0.40)

[a] ED_{50} in μmol kg^{-1}, 95% confidence limits

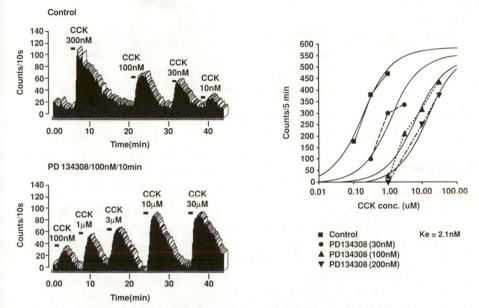

Figure 6: *Antagonism of CCK-induced spontaneous action potential firing by CI-988 (PD134308).*

5 CONCLUSION

To our knowledge these are the first examples of neuropeptide receptor antagonists that have been designed starting *solely* with the chemical structure of the target endogenous mammalian neuropeptide.

Small molecule ligands for other neuropeptide receptors may also be designed using a similar strategy.

6 ACKNOWLEDGEMENTS

I thank Dr E. Roberts and Dr M. Pritchard for their valuable synthetic work, Dr J. Hughes for valuable discussions and Professor B. Costall for anxiolytic data on these compounds.

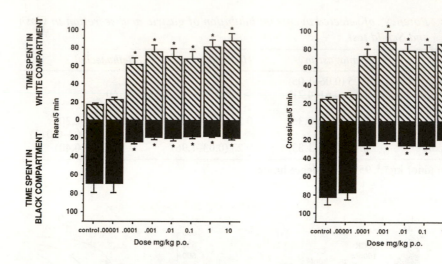

n = 5. *P < 0.001 (anxiolytic action). Pretreatment time 40 min

Figure 7: *Anxiolytic activity of CI-988 (PD134308) by oral administration (mouse black:white test box)*

7 REFERENCES

1   D.C. Horwell *et al.*, *J. Med. Chem.*, 1987, **30**, 729.
2   D.C. Horwell 'Peptoids' from CCK-8, in 'Topics in Medicinal Chemistry', 4th SCI–RSC Medicinal Chemistry Symposium, ed. P.R. Leeming, Special Publication No. 65, The Royal Society of Chemistry, London, 1988, p. 62.
3   B. Birchmore *et al.*, *Euro. J. Med. Chem.*, 1990, **25**, 53.
4   M.R. Pincus *et al.*, *Peptides*, 1988, **9**, 145.
5   P.S. Farmer and E.J. Ariëns, *TiPS*, 1982, 362.
6   D.C. Horwell *et al.*, *J. Med. Chem.*, 1991, **34**, 404.
7   N.J. Hayward *et al.*, *Br. J. Pharmacol.*, 1991, **104**, 973.
8   J. Hughes *et al.*, *Proc. Natl. Acad. Sci. USA*, 1990, **87**, 6728.

CHAPTER 18

Migraine Therapy – from Serotonin to Sumatriptan

PETER C. NORTH*

1 THE SYMPTOMS AND PREVALENCE OF MIGRAINE

Migraine headache is a common disorder which affects approximately one in ten of the adult population. The headache is often one-sided, throbbing in nature, and can be associated with nausea, vomiting, and acute sensitivity to light and sound. In addition to these core-symptoms, approximately 15% of sufferers experience an 'aura' usually within one hour before the incidence of the headache. The nature of this 'aura' is variable but can include visual disturbances such as flashing lights or tunnel vision, sensory disturbances such as tingling, or motor dysfunction such as partial paralysis of the limbs.[1] Approximately one third of all sufferers experience two or more severe attacks each month and, with some attacks lasting up to three days, the quality of life of many migraine sufferers is poor.[2] In addition to the profound effects it can have on the lifestyle of individuals, migraine is also a significant cause of lost productivity through sickness or inefficiency in the workplace.[3]

Although little is known about the mechanisms that cause migraine, some sufferers are aware of trigger factors which will precipitate an attack. These trigger factors can be dietary (*e.g.* red wine, cheese), environmental (*e.g.* excessive noise, extremes of temperature), or hormonal (*e.g.* at certain times during the menstrual cycle) and vary considerably between individuals. The majority of migraine sufferers are, however, unaware of specific trigger factors and find it difficult or impossible to avoid an attack.

2 ACUTE THERAPY

Historically, many migraine sufferers have resorted to self medication using 'over the counter' analgesics based mainly on aspirin or paracetamol, sometimes in combination with caffeine or codeine. Although readily available without prescription, these remedies are often ineffective and may cause gastro-intestinal damage on chronic use. Those sufferers seeking professional medical advice were often prescribed drugs based on ergotamine for the treatment of acute attacks.

This alkaloid, originally isolated from a parasitic fungus found on rye plants, is a potent vasoconstrictor and has been in clinical use for over sixty years.[4] Its use

* Co-authors: A.W. Oxford, W. Fenuik, P.P.A. Humphrey, and H.E. Connor

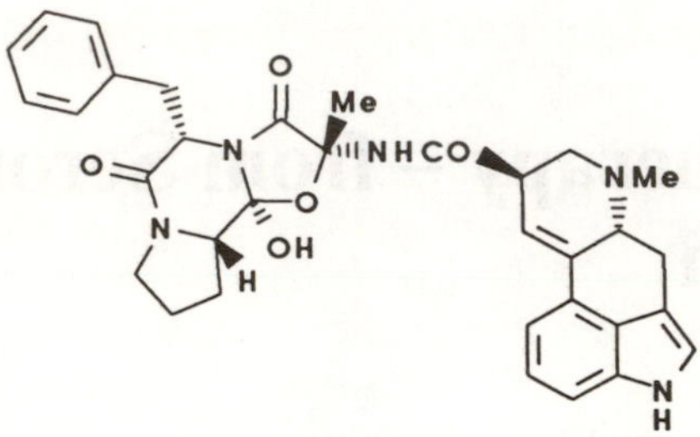

Ergotamine

in the treatment of acute migraine is, however, limited by variable efficacy and a variety of well-documented adverse reactions including nausea, vomiting, and constriction of peripheral blood vessels (peripheral vasoconstriction), the severity of which requires careful monitoring of both dose and frequency of administration.[5] Ergotamine is a non-selective drug and has been shown to interact with 5-hydroxytryptamine, dopamine, and noradrenalin receptor sub-types with varying degrees of efficacy.[6]

3 THE ROLE OF 5-HYDROXYTRYPTAMINE IN MIGRAINE

5-Hydroxytryptamine (5-HT, serotonin), a ubiquitous biogenic amine biosynthesised from dietary tryptophan, is an important neurotransmitter found mainly in the gut, brain, and blood platelets. Although the cause of migraine is still not fully understood, there is considerable circumstantial evidence to implicate 5-HT

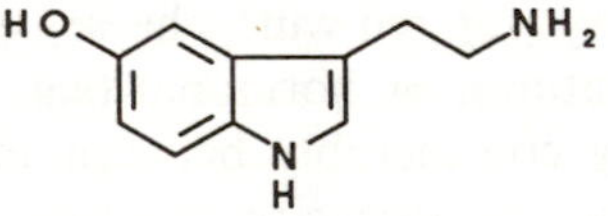

5-HT

in the disease. It has been found, for example, that blood platelet 5-HT levels fall by up to 40% at the onset of migraine[7] and that the urinary excretion of the 5-HT metabolite, 5-hydroxyindoleacetic acid, is increased during an attack.[8] It has also been reported that reserpine, an amine-depleting drug, can induce a migraine-like headache in migraine sufferers but not in non-sufferers.[9] In addition, it is interesting to note that many of the drugs that have been used clinically to treat migraine interact, albeit non-selectively, with 5-HT receptors.[10] Perhaps the most intriguing evidence implicating 5-HT in migraine, however, is the observation that 5-HT will itself abort an established migraine when given intravenously.[11] Notwithstanding the latter observation, the fact that 5-HT is intrinsically non-selective at 5-HT receptor sub-types and has relatively poor pharmacokinetics[12] renders it unsuitable as a drug for the treatment of migraine.

4 SELECTIVE 5-HT AGONISTS – A NOVEL MECHANISM TO TREAT MIGRAINE?

We first became interested in the treatment of migraine in the mid 1970s. We recognised that migraine was a very widespread disease which was inadequately treated by old and relatively ineffective drugs. Our initial research proposal was based on the idea that the pain of migraine might stem from the vasodilatation of certain pain-sensitive blood vessels in the head.[13] This view was supported by the knowledge that non-specific vasoconstrictors, such as ergotamine and 5-HT, will abort a migraine attack[4,11] and on the observation that ergotamine treatment of migraine is associated with a concomitant reduction in the amplitude of pulsations of the temporal artery.[4]

We therefore began to consider how we might achieve a *selective* vasoconstriction of the pain-sensitive blood vessels in the head *via* a novel mechanism. The achievability of this goal was supported by three important clues that were in the literature at the time. Firstly, it had been shown by Saxena[14] that the migraine prophylactic drug methysergide, known as a 5-HT antagonist, had a selective and dose-dependent vasoconstrictor effect on the blood vessels in the head supplied

Methysergide

by the carotid artery (carotid arterial bed) when administered intravenously to the anaesthetised dog, while having little effect on blood pressure or heart rate. Secondly, Saxena had also shown[18] that 5-HT was able to elicit the same vasoconstrictor effect in the carotid arterial bed and that the response was not blocked by the 5-HT receptor antagonists available at the time. Finally, a comparative clinical trial of several drugs used to prevent migraine attacks (prophylactic drugs) showed methysergide to be the most effective treatment even though it was no more potent as a 5-HT antagonist *in vitro* than the other drugs under evaluation.[19] Taken together these observations suggested that the 5-HT antagonist methysergide could be acting as an *agonist* or *partial agonist* at a novel 5-HT receptor sub-type mediating selective vasoconstriction of the carotid arterial bed in the head. Encouraged by this possibility, we set about characterising this putative carotid vascular 5-HT receptor focusing initially on the pharmacology of our only lead, methysergide.

5 THE PHARMACOLOGY OF METHYSERGIDE

Although it was apparent that several types of 5-HT receptor existed, only two sub-types had been defined in the mid 1970s: the 'D-receptor' mediating generalised vasoconstriction and contraction of smooth muscle and the 'M-receptor' mediating the depolarisation of cholinergic nerves. These receptor sub-types, so called because they were known to be blocked by the drugs dibenzyline (an anti-hypertensive) and morphine (an analgesic) respectively, were later to be extensively characterised using more selective antagonist tools and are now known as the 5-HT$_2$ and 5-HT$_3$ receptor sub-types respectively.[17] The fact that the vasoconstrictor activity of methysergide and 5-HT in the carotid bed of the dog was not blocked by 5-HT$_2$ antagonists clearly excluded the involvement of this receptor sub-type, which is very widespread in most other blood vessels. Similarly, although we had shown that methysergide could constrict the rabbit isolated perfused ear artery *via* an agonist effect at α-adrenoceptors,[18] its vasoconstrictor activity in the carotid circulation in the dog was not blocked by phentolamine (an α-adrenoceptor blocker), thereby excluding an effect *via* α-adrenoceptors.

Encouraged by these observations we set out to explore the effect of methysergide and 5-HT on other isolated blood vessels from the dog *in vitro*. Although we quickly established that the large arteries from the carotid bed of the dog contained only the widespread 5-HT$_2$ receptor, our search was rewarded when we examined the dog saphenous vein (DSV), a peripheral blood vessel found in the hind leg. In this tissue, both 5-HT and methysergide caused a dose-dependent contraction and neither could be antagonised by 5-HT$_2$ receptor antagonists.[19] Further studies with this tissue, however, revealed that the contractile effect of both agents could be antagonised by the non-selective biogenic amine blocker, methiothepin, with a similar degree of antagonism. This observation strongly suggested that both 5-HT and methysergide were acting at a common and, as yet, uncharacterised 5-HT receptor.[20]

Although further encouraged by these findings, we were still puzzled and frustrated by our inability to identify this novel receptor on isolated blood vessels from the carotid circulation in the head, the existence of which was pivotal to our goal of exploiting a novel mechanism to treat of migraine. We therefore postulated that if the novel receptor identified on the dog saphenous vein was indeed present in the carotid circulation, then it must be predominantly located on the small resistance blood vessels which, for technical reasons, were much more difficult to study *in vitro* than the larger arteries. In order to test this hypothesis we returned to studying the detailed effects of methysergide *in vivo* in the anaesthetised dog. By injecting methysergide directly into the carotid artery of the anaesthetised dog, and by measuring increases in vascular resistance (seen as a decrease in flow) using an electromagnetic flow probe,[14] we were able to obtain consistent and reproducible dose–response curves. Furthermore, by using this model, we were able to establish that the vasoconstrictor effect of methysergide *in vivo* was not antagonised by doses of the 5-HT antagonist cyproheptadine sufficient to cause 5-HT$_2$ antagonism but was specifically antagonised by methiothepin.

This experimental evidence *in vivo* was sufficient to convince us that the carotid circulation of the dog did indeed contain a novel 5-HT receptor sub-type, identical to that found on the dog saphenous vein *in vitro*, and that a selective agonist at this novel receptor would selectively constrict the carotid circulation in the dog. This novel receptor, like the 'D' and 'M' receptors, was subsequently well characterised and called the 5-HT$_1$-like receptor[17] because it is pharmacologically similar, but not identical, to certain 5-HT$_1$ radioligand binding sites found in brain tissue.

6 PROJECT OBJECTIVES AND MEDICINAL CHEMICAL STRATEGY

Having identified and characterised the new 5-HT$_1$-like receptor, our chemical objective was to identify a selective agonist for the receptor, suitable for administration to man, in order to determine whether or not such a compound would have clinical efficacy for the acute treatment of migraine. Although, at first sight, methysergide would seem to be an obvious starting point for a chemical programme we were keen to avoid the intrinsic lack of selectivity associated with ergot-like derivatives. We were aware, for example, that methysergide had activity not only at different 5-HT receptor sub-types, but also at α-adrenoceptors and histamine receptors.[21] Additionally, methysergide is known to be metabolised *in vivo* by *N*-demethylation of the indole nitrogen to give methylergometrine which interacts with a variety of receptors including dopamine D$_2$ receptors.[22] We had also shown that methysergide was only a partial agonist in the dog saphenous vein preparation and, because methysergide is only clinically effective as a prophylactic migraine therapy, we reasoned that a full agonist would be more efficacious in treating *acute* migraine.

In view of these considerations we decided to initiate a chemical programme based on the systematic modification of 5-HT using a strategy that would allow us to determine which structural features of 5-HT were important for activity at the 5-HT$_1$-like receptor and then to apply this knowledge to design novel, selective, and full agonists. In this respect our discovery that the 5-HT$_1$-like receptor is fortuitously present on the dog saphenous vein was particularly useful as it provided us with a robust functional assay *in vitro* with which to assess new compounds for both efficacy (*i.e.* full agonist, partial agonist, or antagonist) and relative potency compared to 5-HT. Other functional assays used to determine the receptor specificity of new compounds included contraction of the isolated rabbit aorta to detect 5-HT$_2$ receptor efficacy and depolarisation of the rat vagus nerve to detect 5-HT$_3$ receptor efficacy.

7 EARLY MILESTONES

The chemistry programme initially embarked on the systematic modification of the 5-hydroxyl group of 5-HT in order to ascertain which properties of this group, if any, were important for activity and selectivity at the 5-HT$_1$-like receptor. This exercise afforded some very useful structure–activity relationships (SAR) a selection of which are shown in Table 1. Thus, replacement of the hydroxyl group of 5-HT with a hydrogen atom (1) and a selection of functional groups (2–7) afforded compounds which were both weaker than 5-HT at the 5-HT$_1$-like receptor and non-selective with respect to the 5-HT$_2$ receptor.

Table 1: *In vitro activity of selected 5-substituted tryptamines*

No	R	5-HT$_1$-like (DSV) EPMR (5-HT=1)	5-HT$_2$ (RA) EPMR (5-HT=1)
(1)	H	171	48
(2)	MeO	10	2
(3)	Me	14	8
(4)	Cl	58	33
(5)	NH$_2$	9	14
(6)	HOCH$_2$	39	14
(7)	MeCO	5	7
(8) 5-CT	**H$_2$NCO**	**0.4**	**26**

The functional *in vitro* activity of compounds at the 5-HT$_1$-like receptor on the dog saphenous vein (DSV) and 5-HT$_2$ receptor on the rabbit aorta (RA) is expressed as an equipotent molar ratio (EPMR) with 5-HT = 1. Thus, compounds with a higher or lower agonist potency relative to 5-HT have an EPMR of less than or greater than one respectively.

We also established that, in most instances, modification to the hydroxyl group greatly reduced agonist activity at the 5-HT$_3$ receptor thus rendering the routine screening for 5-HT$_3$ agonist activity on the rat vagus nerve unnecessary for the majority of new compounds. A significant early milestone from this work was the 5-carboxamido derivative of 5-HT, 5-carboxamidotryptamine (8). 5-Carboxami-dotryptamine (5-CT) was found to be *ca.* two-fold more potent as a 5-HT$_1$-like agonist and *ca.* 25 times less potent as a 5-HT$_2$ agonist compared to 5-HT *in vitro*. With this degree of potency and selectivity at the 5-HT$_1$-like receptor we felt that 5-CT was a good prototype to examine *in vivo* in the anaesthetised dog in order to established whether it would have the predicted vasoconstrictor activity on the carotid circulation. To our surprise, and initial disappointment, we found that 5-CT actually caused a *vasodilatation* of the carotid circulation in the dog, and led to a profound fall in blood pressure (hypotension) in conscious dogs, cats, and rats.[23] In order to explain this unexpected activity *in vivo* we further examined the action of 5-CT on a series of isolated blood vessels *in vitro* and discovered that it was a very potent agonist at a poorly characterised 5-HT receptor mediating vascular relaxation.[24]

This new receptor, shown to be present in the cat saphenous vein (CSV) and porcine vena cava, is pharmacologically similar to the 5-HT$_1$-like receptor in the dog saphenous vein in that both receptors are activated by 5-CT, both are antagonised by methiothepin, and neither is blocked by 5-HT$_2$ or 5-HT$_3$ antagonists.[25] Despite their similarities, however, it was clear to us that the two receptors were pharmacologically distinct[26] and that it was necessary to design compounds that were selective for the DSV 5-HT$_1$-like receptor not only with

Table 2: In vitro *activity of selected analogues of 5-CT*

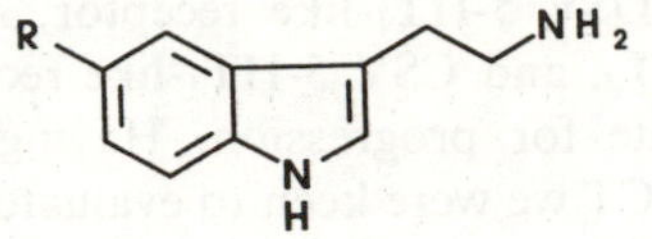

No.	R	*5-HT₁-like (DSV) EPMR (5-HT=1)*	*5-HT₁-like (CSV) EPMR (5-HT=1)*	*5-HT₂ (RA) EPMR (5-HT=1)*
(8)	H_2NCO	0.4	0.02	26
(9)	MeNHCO	3	0.3	352
(10)	Me_2NCO	4	8	100
(11)	^iPrNHCO	3	16	43
(12)	H_2NSO_2	36	85	261
(13)	$MeSO_2$	8	60	49
(14)	MeSO	16	27	22
(15)	H_2NCOCH_2	9	201	>1696
(16)	$H_2NSO_2CH_2$	16	>79	>94
(17)*	**$MeNHCOCH_2$**	**4**	**>100**	**>1000**

*** AH25086**

The functional *in vitro* activity of compounds at the 5-HT₁-like receptor on the dog saphenous vein (DSV), the 5-HT₁-like receptor on the cat saphenous vein (CSV), and 5-HT₂ receptor on the rabbit aorta (RA) is expressed as an equipotent molar ratio (EPMR) with 5-HT = 1.

respect to 5-HT₂ and 5-HT₃ receptors, but also with respect to the vascular 5-HT₁-like receptor mediating vascular relaxation. Our finding that the latter mediated relaxation of the cat saphenous vein (CSV) provided us with an additional functional assay with which to test new compounds for activity and selectivity.

Using 5-CT as a lead, we further modified the 5-carboxamido substituent in an attempt to retain activity at the DSV 5-HT₁-like receptor but reduce or eliminate activity at the other subtypes. We had, by now, established that 5-CT was *ca.* 50-fold more potent than 5-HT at the CSV 5-HT₁-like receptor and was *ca.* 20-fold more selective for this receptor over the DSV 5-HT₁-like receptor (Table 2). Alkylation of the primary amido function of 5-CT with two methyl groups (10) or an isopropyl group (11) afforded compounds which were marginally selective for the DSV 5-HT₁-like receptor over the CSV receptor albeit at the expense of potency at both sub-types. Similarly, replacing the carboxamide group with sulphonamide, sulphone, and sulphoxide groups (12–14) afforded compounds which again were marginally selective for the DSV receptor but lacked sufficient potency and selectivity to warrant serious consideration for progression.

A very significant advance was made, however, when we introduced a methylene group between the indole ring and the carboxamido function to give the 5-CT homologue (15). This modification gave a compound that was essentially inactive at the 5-HT₂ receptor and *ca.* 20-fold more selective for the DSV over the CSV 5-HT₁-like receptor. Although a similar pattern emerged when the homologated sulphonamide (16) was prepared, the homologated *N*-

methylcarboxamide, (17) [AH25086], was the compound which emerged as having by far the best *in vitro* profile at the time. Thus, although four-fold less potent than 5-HT at the DSV 5-HT$_1$-like receptor, AH25086 was essentially inactive at the 5-HT$_2$, 5-HT$_3$, and CSV 5-HT$_1$-like receptors[27] and accordingly became a leading candidate for progression. Having now identified a more selective compound than 5-CT we were keen to evaluate its properties in the dog. As originally predicted, AH25086 produced a pronounced vasoconstrictor action in the carotid arterial bed of the anaesthetised dog when given intravenously and had little effect on blood pressure, heart rate, or total peripheral resistance.[28] Unlike the non-selective agonist, 5-CT, AH25086 did not cause vasodilatation or hypotension.

Having identified a compound with the required profile *in vitro* and *in vivo*, we were keen to test our initial hypothesis that a selective 5-HT$_1$-like agonist would be clinically effective in the treatment of acute migraine. We were aware that a beneficial clinical effect in man was crucial, not only to support our initial hypotheses, but also to the future of the project. The acceptable tolerability of AH25086 in human volunteers led to its clinical evaluation which unequivocally established, for the first time, that a selective 5-HT$_1$-like agonist was indeed very effective in alleviating all the symptoms of an acute migraine attack when given intravenously.[29,30]

8 THE DISCOVERY OF SUMATRIPTAN

AH25086 was not suitable for progression into full development and our chemistry therefore focused on identifying an alternative compound that would be suitable for both oral and parenteral administration. Encouraged by the finding that the homologated sulphonamide (16), like the amides (15) and (17), also gave good selectivity for the DSV 5-HT$_1$-like receptor we focused on modifying this group further and, at the same time, began to examine alternatives to the primary amino group in an attempt to inhibit or hinder its metabolism *via* oxidative de-amination, which was known to be a major metabolic pathway of 5-HT in man.

Modification of the homologated sulphonamide (16) proved to be a fruitful exercise and established that good potency and selectivity could be obtained with the *N*-methylsulphonamide (18) (Table 3). Larger, more lipophilic groups, as exemplified by (19)–(23), afforded compounds which lacked sufficient agonist potency at the DSV 5-HT1-like receptor to warrant further progression. Of particular interest was the finding that substitution of a methyl group in either the 1-, 2-, or β-position, (24–26), completely abolished agonist activity at the DSV 5-HT$_1$-like receptor, indicating an intolerance of steric hindrance at these positions.

In order to investigate the effect of changes to the basic amino group we chose to systematically modify the *N*-methylsulphonamidomethyltryptamine (18) because this compound had one of the best potency/selectivity profiles and as such was a good basis on which to develop further SAR. An example of some chemistry that can be used to prepare such compounds is shown in Scheme 1. Thus, although the desired agonist potency was lost with the isopropylamino

Table 3: In vitro *activity of selected 5-sulphonamidomethyl tryptamines*

No.	R	5-HT$_1$-like (DSV) EPMR (5-HT=1)	5-HT$_1$-like (CSV) EPMR (5-HT=1)	5-HT$_2$ (RA) EPMR (5-HT=1)
(16)	H$_2$N	16	> 79	> 94
(18)	**MeNH**	**9**	**1470**	**> 294**
(19)	EtNH	19	NT	973
(20)	Pr^{i}NH	48	NT	645
(21)		57	NT	> 419
(22)		15	NT	300
(23)	PhNH	78	NT	> 316
(24)	H$_2$N (2-methyl)	> 2000	NT	> 436
(25)	MeNH (1-methyl)	984	NT	> 655
(26)	MeNH (β-methyl)	> 811	NT	> 381

The functional *in vitro* activity of compounds at the 5-HT$_1$-like receptor on the dog saphenous vein (DSV), the 5-HT$_1$-like receptor on the cat saphenous vein (CSV), and 5-HT$_2$ receptor on the rabbit aorta (RA) is expressed as an equipotent molar ratio (EPMR) with 5-HT = 1. NT = Not Tested.

(29), pyrrolidinyl (30), and anilino (31) compounds we actually saw a potency enhancement with the both the methylamino (27) and dimethylamino (28) compounds (Table 4).

More importantly, the dimethylamino analogue, (28) [GR43175], first prepared in 1984, was shown to cause selective carotid vasoconstriction in the anaesthetised dog *via* both the intravenous route (50% of maximum vasoconstriction occurring with 35–40 µg kg^{-1} i.v) and the intraduodenal route of administration suggesting that the compound had potential for good oral activity.

Further experiments *in vitro* established that GR43175 had remarkable receptor selectivity for the DSV 5-HT$_1$-like receptor subtype being devoid of activity at 5-HT$_2$, 5-HT$_3$, adrenergic, dopaminergic, muscarinic and benzodiazepine receptors. In addition, more detailed haemodynamic measurements in dogs and cats established that the vasoconstrictor activity of GR43175 was selective within the carotid vascular bed and had no vasoconstrictor activity which might compromise the blood supply to important major organs such as the brain, heart, liver, and kidney. GR43175, subsequently named sumatriptan, quickly became

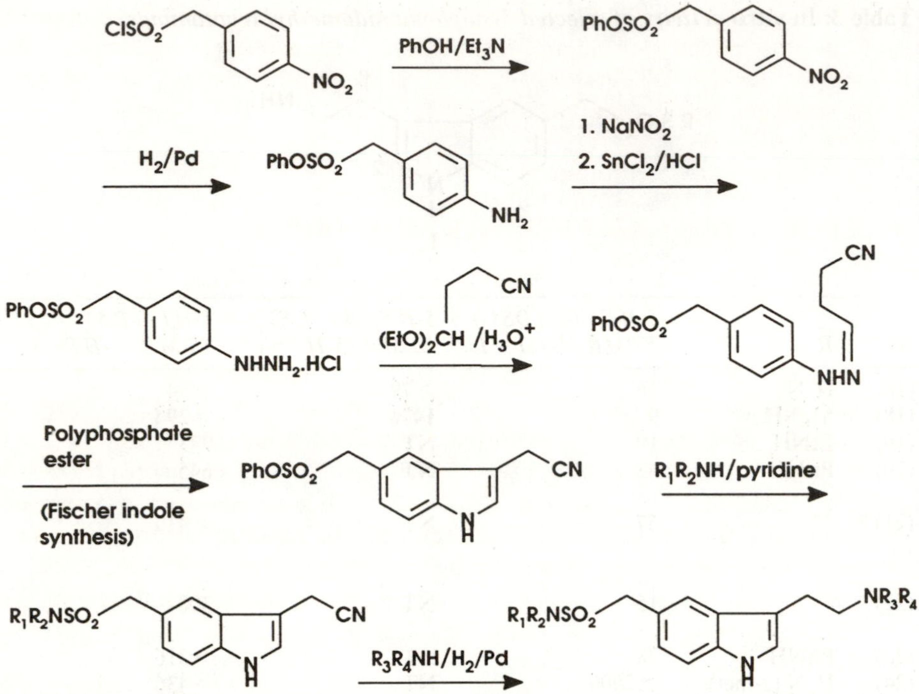

Scheme 1: *General synthesis of sulphonamido-tryptamine derivatives*

Table 4: In vitro *activity of selected amino derivatives*

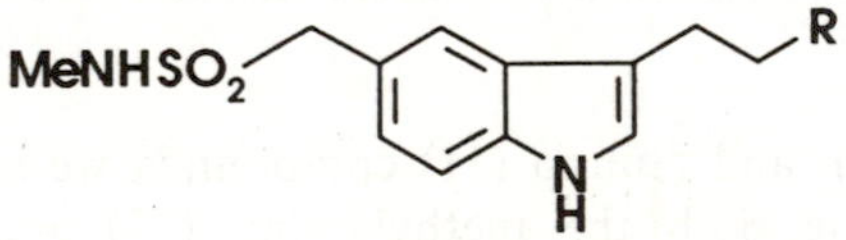

No.	R	5-HT$_1$-like (DSV) EPMR (5-HT=1)	5-HT$_1$-like (CSV) EPMR (5-HT=1)	5-HT$_2$ (RA) EPMR (5-HT=1)
(18)	NH$_2$	9	1470	> 294
(27)	NHMe	5.3	NT	> 342
(28)*	**NMe$_2$**	**4.6**	**> 100**	**> 1000**
(29)	NH^{i}Pr	633	NT	> 132
(30)		100	NT	> 87
(31)	NHPh	> 92	NT	> 128

* GR43175

The functional *in vitro* activity of compounds at the 5-HT$_1$-like receptor on the dog saphenous vein (DSV), the 5-HT$_1$-like receptor on the cat saphenous vein (CSV), and 5-HT$_2$ receptor on the rabbit aorta (RA) is expressed as an equipotent molar ratio (EPMR) with 5-HT = 1. NT = Not Tested.

our leading compound and was later shown to be well tolerated in volunteers[31] and clinically effective in migraine patients.[32,33] As a result the compound was progressed through full development and first launched as a novel therapy for the acute treatment of migraine[34] in June 1991.

9 CLINICAL TRIAL RESULTS WITH SUMATRIPTAN

Sumatriptan has undergone extensive clinical trials, involving the treatment of over 35 000 migraine attacks in over 7000 patients, and the drug has demonstrated proven clinical efficacy *via* both the subcutaneous and oral routes of administration.[35] Thus, 86% of patients obtained relief after two hours following a single 6 mg subcutaneous dose and 75% after four hours following a single 100mg oral dose compared with up to 37% in the placebo treated group (Figure 1).

The onset of headache relief with sumatriptan is rapid, occurring 10 minutes after injection and 30 minutes after the tablet. In a comparative study against ergotamine (2 mg, plus caffeine, 200 mg), 66% of sumatriptan-treated patients obtained relief at 2 hours compared with 48% on ergotamine and, although associated migraine symptoms such as nausea, vomiting and photophobia were effectively relieved by sumatriptan, ergotamine treatment actually provoked nausea and vomiting in a number of patients.

A few specific adverse events are associated with the use of sumatriptan but the majority of these are mild, transient, and resolve spontaneously without intervention. Such events include tingling, feelings of warmth, heaviness or pressure, and vertigo. We have also established that the clinical efficacy of sumatriptan is maintained after long-term usage, regardless of the number of migraine attacks treated, and that there is no difference in the nature, severity,

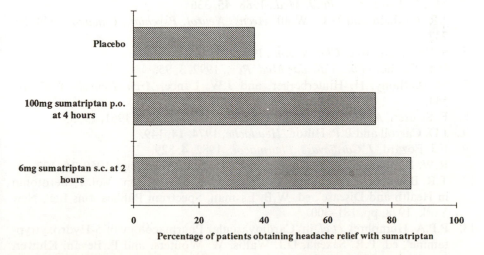

Figure 1: *Headache relief with sumatriptan*

and incidence of adverse events when comparing short-term and long-term usage of the drug.

10 CONCLUSIONS

In this account, which covers over fifteen years of intensive research, we have highlighted the major pharmacological and chemical advances that led to the discovery and development of sumatriptan: the first prescription drug to be marketed exclusively for the acute treatment of migraine. Although there is currently much scientific debate relating to the mode of action of suma-triptan,[36] there is no doubt that the new drug provides a novel, effective treatment for migraine and its associated symptoms. Above all, sumatriptan is highly regarded by many migraine sufferers in the community because it helps them to enjoy a normal existence and, as such, significantly improves their quality of life.

11 ACKNOWLEDGEMENTS

We would like to acknowledge the following chemists and biologists who made a significant contribution to the discovery of sumatriptan: David Bays, Darko Butina, Peter Clark, Ian Coates, Mike Dowle, Brian Evans, Pam Gaskin, Keith Mills, Martin Owen, Marion Perren, and Colin Webb.

12 REFERENCES

1. Headache Classification Committee of the International Headache Society. Classification and diagnostic criteria for headache disorders, cranial neuralgias and facial pain. *Cephalagia*, 1988, **7** (suppl. 8), 1.
2. J.T. Osterhaus and R.J. Townsend, *Cephalagia*, 1991, **11** (11), 103.
3. M.L.E. Espir *et al.*, *Br. J. Med.*, 1988, **45**, 336.
4. J.R. Graham and H.G. Wolff, *Archs. Neurol. Psychiat., Chicago*, 1938, **39**, 737.
5. S. Diamond, *Med. Clin. N. Am.*, 1991, **75**, 545.
6. H.E. Connor *et al.*, *Vascular Med. Rev.*, 1992, **3**, 95.
7. M. Anthony, H. Hinterberger, and J.W. Lance, *Arch. Neurol.*, 1967, **16**, 544.
8. F. Sicuteri, A. Testi, and B. Anselmi, *Int. Arch. Allergy*, 1961, **19**, 55.
9. J.D. Carroll and B.P. Hilton, *Headache*, 1974, **14**, 149.
10. F.J. Fozard, *J. Cardiovasc. Pharmacol.*, 1982, **4**, 829.
11. R.W. Kimball, A.P. Friedman, and E. Valleejo, *Neurology*, 1960, **10**, 107.
12. T.R. Bosin, in 'Availability, Localisation and Disposition'. Vol. 1, 'Serotonin in Health and Disease', ed. W.B. Essman, Spectrum Publications Inc., New York, 1978, pp. 181–300.
13. P.P.A. Humphrey *et al*, in 'Cardiovascular Pharmacology of 5-Hydroxytryp-tamine', ed. P.R. Saxena, D.I. Wallis, W. Wouters, and P. Bevan, Kluwer, Dordrecht, 1990, p. 417.

14. P.R. Saxena, *Eur. J.Pharmacol.*, 1974, **27**, 99.
15. P.R. Saxena, *Headache*, 1972, **12**, 44.
16. J.W. Lance, M. Anthony, and B. Somerville, *Br. Med. J.*, 1970, **2**, 327.
17. P.B. Bradley *et al.*, *Neuropharmacology*, 1986, **25**, 563.
18. E. Apperley, P.P.A. Humphrey, and G.P. Levy, *Br. J. Pharmacol.*, 1976, **58**, 211.
19. W. Feniuk *et al.*, *Br. J. Pharmacol.*, 1985, **86**, 697.
20. E. Apperley and P.P.A. Humphrey, *Br. J. Pharmacol.*, 1986, **87**, 131P.
21. S.J. Gunning, K.T. Bunce, and P.P.A. Humphrey, *Br. J. Pharmacol.*, 1988, **93**, 238P.
22. 'Ergot Alkaloids and Related Compounds', ed. B. Berde and H.O. Schild, Springer-Verlag, Berlin, 1978.
23. H.E. Connor *et al.*, *Br. J. Pharmacol.*, 1986, **87**, 417.
24. M.A. Trevethick, W. Feniuk, and P.P.A. Humphrey, *Life Sci.*, 1986, **38**, 1521.
25. M.J. Sumner, W. Feniuk, and P.P.A. Humphrey, *Br. J. Pharmacol.*, 1989, **97**, 292.
26. P.P.A. Humphrey and W. Feniuk, 'Classification of functional 5-hydroxy-tryptamine receptors', in 'Pharmacology, International Congress Series 750 (Proceedings of Xth International Congress of Pharmacology-I.U.P.H.A.R.), ed. M.J. Rand and D. Raper, Elsevier Science Publishers, Netherlands, 1987, p. 277.
27. P.P.A. Humphrey and W. Feniuk, 'The sub-classification of functional 5-HT-like receptors', in 'Serotonin (Proceedings of the Heron Island Meeting, September 1987)', ed. E.J. Mylecharane, J.A. Angus, I.S. de la Lande, and P.P.A. Humphrey, Macmillan Press Limited, London, 1989.
28. P.P.A. Humphrey, W. Feniuk, and M.J. Perren, '5-HT in migraine: Evidence with 5-HT$_1$-like receptor agonists for a vascular aetiology', in 'Migraine, A Spectrum of Ideas', ed. M. Sandler and G. Collins, Oxford University Press, London, 1989.
29. A. Doenicke *et al.*, *Cephalalgia*, 1987, **7**(6), 438.
30. J. Brand, M. Hadoke, and V.L. Perrin, *Cephalalgia*, 1987, **7**(6), 402.
31. P.A. Fowler *et al.*, *Cephalalgia*, 1989, **9**(9), 57.
32. V.L. Perrin *et al.*, *Cephalalgia*, 1989, **9**(9), 63.
33. A. Doenicke, D. Melchart, and E.M. Bayliss, *Cephalalgia*, 1989, **9**(9), 89.
34. P.P.A. Humphrey *et al.*, *Drugs of the Future*, 1989, **14**(1), 35.
35. M.J.B. Tansey, A.J. Pilgrim, and K. Lloyd, *J. Neuro. Sci.*, 1993, **114**, 109.
36. M.D. Ferrari and P.R. Saxena, *TiPS*, 1993, **14**, 129.

CHAPTER 19

Drug Development

JANE ORMEROD

1 INTRODUCTION

Drug Development is a very complex process requiring a great deal of co-ordination and communication between a wide range of different functional groups. It is expensive, particularly in the later phases of clinical development, where studies involve hundreds of patients. It is currently estimated that the development of a new drug costs about $230 million (1987 dollars)[1] and takes somewhere between 7 and 10 years from initiation of preclinical development to first marketing (excluding regulatory delays). Drug development is a high risk business; although the rate is increasing, only about ONE out of every TEN new chemical entities studied in human beings for the first time will ever become a product.[2] As a drug candidate progresses through development the risks of failure decrease as 'hurdles' are overcome along the way. Typical reasons for failure include unacceptable toxicity, lack of efficacy, or inability to provide advantages over competitive products (Figure 1).

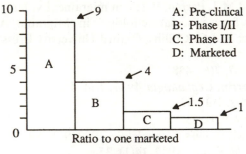

A: Pre-clinical
B: Phase I/II
C: Phase III
D: Marketed

Attrition Rate of New Chemical Entities (NCE's) entering development. On average only about 1 in 400-1,000 compounds synthesized enters development.

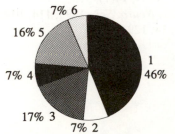

Reasons for termination of development of NCE's (excluding anti-infectives)

1: Lack of efficacy
2: Pharmacokinetics
3: Animal toxicity
4: Miscellaneous
5: Adverse effects in man
6: Commercial reasons

Figure 1: *Attrition rates[3] and reasons for termination[4] of NCEs*

2 PLANNING FOR DEVELOPMENT

Assessment of whether a drug candidate is likely to provide competitive advantages highlights the need first to have in place a set of product 'goals' or target product profile.[5] Particular attention should be paid to the differentiation from competitors. This is becoming more and more critical with the increasing emphasis on limited formularies, healthcare costs, and pharmacoeconomics (discussed later in the chapter).

A target profile will define the indication(s) that a drug candidate will be developed for, along with goals such as once a day dosing, faster onset of action, better side effect profile than a major competitor. The target profile can be refined and revised as a drug candidate moves through development and new data on the drug candidate or competitors become available. The logical next steps are to define the development strategy, for example, which indications to develop first,

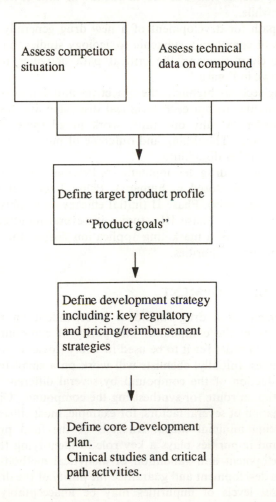

Figure 2:   *Defining a new drug development plan*

which countries to aim to market the drug in and then to define the core clinical studies necessary to achieve regulatory approval and commercial success (see Figure 2)

This chapter will describe the main activities required for successful development of a new drug. All these activities, many of which are interdependent, need to be carefully planned and co-ordinated. Speed to market with collection of high quality data is critical for success. The path of activities which determine the time it will take to get to registration is called, in project management terms, the critical path. It is vital to plan and prepare before studies begin and to monitor and manage problems so as to ensure that the **critical path** remains on schedule. With increased economic pressures and competitive intensity it is important for companies to explore ways to shorten this critical path. Running activities in parallel, or overlapping studies which would usually run sequentially, often involves an increase in risk but the dividends in time-saving can make such strategies worthwhile.

The critical path for development of a new drug generally runs through the initial synthesis of compound, subacute toxicology studies, and then the clinical programme. A chart showing the critical path activities for a typical drug candidate is shown in Figure 3.

The following sections highlight the objectives and activities of drug development work. Activities within each technical discipline are described broadly in chronological order. At any one time, work in all these disciplines may be proceeding in parallel. The timing and outcome of much of the work has direct impact on work in other disciplines.

The major phases of drug development are Preclinical (studies required before the compound can be dosed in humans), Phase I (clinical studies usually in healthy human volunteers), Phase II (initial efficacy and safety and dose finding studies in patients), and Phase III (studies in several hundred patients). There then follows assembly of a marketing application dossier for subsequent review by country regulatory authorities.

3 CHEMICAL DEVELOPMENT

Rapid development of a drug candidate is dependent on the availability of sufficient quantity of the compound. The purity of compound needs to reach certain standards in order for it to be used in safety (toxicology), pharmaceutical, and clinical studies. Initially, chemists will work on a small to medium scale to investigate production of the compound by several different methods so as to identify the optimum route for synthesising the compound. 'Optimum' here may mean a combination of several factors, for example, most efficient, cheapest, safe, or that producing minimal waste. Analysis of the final product as well as intermediates and impurities plays a key role in identifying the best method of synthesis. Development and validation of analytical methods are necessary to support process development and guarantee the purity of the drug substance.

In some cases levels of impurities may be unacceptably high and either improved purification procedures will need to be developed or the synthetic

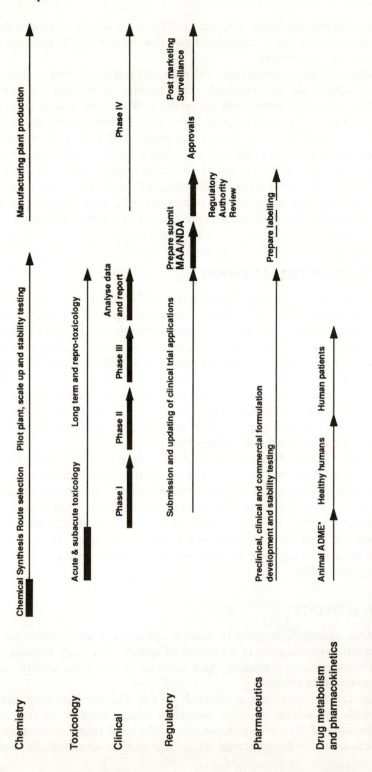

Figure 3: *The major processes in new drug development*

process may require significant alterations. The main aim is to ensure that the composition of compound is understood and that ultimately the material that is prepared is as pure as possible.

As a drug candidate progresses through development, larger and larger amounts of compound are required. The amount of material required for different tests will often depend on the actual potency and dosage form of the compound. A pilot plant can be regarded as a mini-manufacturing set-up. Before transferring to a pilot plant, extensive evaluation and testing of the chemical synthesis is undertaken to ensure that any changes and hazards are minimised. Procedures are optimised, particular attention being paid to developing environmentally acceptable ways of disposing of waste products. Commercial production of bulk drug substance for production of a drug, once approved and marketed, will likely take place on a larger scale or at a registered manufacturing plant.

4 FORMULATION DEVELOPMENT

The dosage form of a drug is the form by which it is administered to the patient. There are a vast array of possible dosage forms ranging from transdermal patches to inhalers to intranasal medicines. The more common dosage forms include oral tablets or capsules, oral liquids, topical ointments or creams, and injectables. The dosage form or forms chosen for a particular drug candidate will be defined in the target profile.

Sometimes a more simple dosage form, for example an oral solution, is chosen for early clinical studies in human beings. This may save time and upfront costs at an early, high-risk stage of the drug development process. Later clinical studies would use the expected marketed dosage form.

Whatever the dosage form, the combination of drug and other materials which constitute it must fulfil certain criteria. One of the most important is that of adequate stability. That means a predetermined potency level must remain after, for example, two or three years. The stability data generated on a dosage form will determine its shelf-life and recommended storage conditions. Early in development the shelf-life may be limited to several months. This will not be a problem provided it is sufficient to cover use of the drug over the duration of the clinical study or studies.

5 PHARMACOLOGY

Before a drug candidate is given to man, its pharmacological effects on major systems are often investigated in a number of species. The body systems studied include cardiovascular, respiratory, and nervous systems; the effects on gross behaviour can also be studied.

Experiments are sometimes conducted to see whether the drug candidate interferes with the actions of other medicines which, because of their specific effects or because of their common use, are likely to be taken concurrently with the drug candidate. Any synergism or antagonism of drug effects should be investigated, and any necessary warning issued to clinical investigators. (It may be judged necessary to investigate such effects further in clinical studies, and any potential or proven drug interactions are likely to be noted in the product labelling for the drug.)

It may also be appropriate to identify a substance for possible use in the management of overdosage, particularly if the therapeutic margin of the drug candidate is small.

6 SAFETY EVALUATION

The objective of animal toxicology testing, carried out prior to the administration of a drug to man, is to reject compounds of unacceptable toxicity and to identify potential target organs and timings for adverse effects of the drug. This means that in early human studies these organs and tissues can be monitored with particular attention. It is important to establish whether toxic effects are reversible or irreversible, whether they can be prevented and, if possible, the mechanism of the toxicological effects. It is also important to interrelate drug response to blood levels in humans and blood levels in various animal species.

The toxicological studies required for the evaluation of a drug candidate in man will be relevant to its proposed clinical use in terms of route of administration and duration of treatment of the clinical studies. The size and frequency of the doses and the duration of the toxicology studies are major determinants of permissible tests in man. Countries, including UK, USA, Australia, and Nordic countries, have regulatory guidelines which relate the duration of treatment allowed in man to the length of toxicity studies required in two species. Points from the guidelines are referenced in the subsequent sections.

Initially, the pharmacological effects of increasing doses of the test substances are established in acute toxicity studies in small numbers of animals, generally using two routes of administration (one being that used in man). Results provide a guide to the maximum tolerated doses in subsequent chronic toxicity tests, aid selection of dose levels, and identify target organs.

The main aim of the subsequent sub-acute toxicity tests is to determine whether or not the drug candidate is adequately tolerated after administration to animals for a prolonged period as a guide to possible adverse reactions in man. Two to four week (daily dosing) studies are required, using the same route of administration as in man, in two species (one non-rodent) prior to administration of the compound to man. Three dose levels are usually necessary: the low daily dose should be a low multiple of the expected therapeutic dose, and the highest dose should demonstrate some toxicity.

A general guide for the evaluation of new chemical entities would be that toxicology studies of a minimum duration of 14 days are required to support single-dose exposure of a new drug candidate in normal volunteers in Phase I. Toxicology studies of 30 days duration are required to support clinical studies of 7 to 10 days duration. Clinical studies of greater than 7 to 10 days up to 30 days duration require the support of at least 90 day toxicology studies. These requirements illustrate the need to plan ahead in drug development. The duration and approximate timings for future clinical trials need to be considered well in advance in order to schedule and conduct the appropriate toxicology studies to support the clinical programme and avoid any delays.

Two types of safety test are used to detect the ability of the drug candidate to produce tumours in man. The first are short-term *in vitro* genotoxicity tests, for example bacterial tests. The second are long-term animal carcinogenicity studies which are conducted in mice and rats; their length of often 2 years covers a large part of the lifespan of the animal. Mice and rats are used because of their relatively short life span, small size, and ready availability. Also, knowledge which has accumulated concerning spontaneous diseases and tumours in particular strains of these species helps greatly in the interpretation of results.

Long-term toxicology and carcinogenicity studies are conducted in order to obtain approval to test and finally to market a product for chronic administration to man. These studies may need to start during the late preclinical/early clinical phase in order to 'support' the subsequent clinical programme. Long-term toxicity studies will normally include toxicity studies of six and twelve months duration in two species (one non-rodent). Any toxicity previously detected may be investigated more closely, for example extra enzymes looked at in blood samples.

Reproductive toxicology is that part of toxicology dealing with the effects of compounds on reproduction – fertility, foetal abnormalities, post-natal development. Prior to clinical studies in women of child-bearing age, regulatory authorities require teratology data from two species (normally rat and rabbit) as well as clinical data from male volunteers. No reproductive data are required prior to clinical studies in male subjects. The effects of compounds on reproduction differ with the period of the reproductive cycle in which exposure takes place and studies are designed to look at these phases. Teratology studies are designed to detect foetal abnormalities, fertility studies to investigate the compounds' effect on reproductive performance, and peri- and post-natal studies to study the development of pups.

7 DRUG METABOLISM AND PHARMACOKINETICS

Drug metabolism and pharmacokinetic (DMPK) studies are required to build a knowledge of metabolism of a compound together with the way in which the levels of the compound and its metabolites vary according to the dose administered and the length of time from when it was administered.

There is rarely a definitive regulatory requirement for metabolism data at the preclinical/early clinical stage of drug development. However, metabolism studies aid interpretation of toxicological results and study design and help in the extrapolation of animal safety and efficacy data to man. Development of assays is required to measure drug and major metabolite levels in biological fluids or tissues. Aims are to develop rapid and reproducible methods. HPLC is normally used for separation although other techniques such as GLC may be used where suitable. Detection may be UV, flurometric, electrochemical, mass spectroscopy, to give some examples. When the activity of the compound is very high and consequently only trace amounts of material will actually be present in body fluids or tissues, detection problems may arise. RIA (radio-immuno assay) may provide greater sensitivity as well as giving the potential to analyse a greater number of compounds in a given time. However, an RIA is likely to take longer to develop and lack of specificity can be a problem.

Information on plasma concentrations of compound and/or metabolites is required in support of toxicology studies and to aid selection of dose levels. There is an initial need to establish the region of pharmacokinetic linearity, *i.e.* range in which dose *vs.* AUC (area under the curve – from concentration–time curves) may be regarded as linear. Identification of causes of non-linearity such as metabolic saturation of absorption/elimination processes will help in the understanding of toxicological or pharmacological events.

8 CLINICAL

Once adequate animal studies have been completed and analysed, the pharmaceutical company will decide whether or not to take the drug into the human phase of research. This step often involves approval from company experts, clinical investigators and their Ethics Committees, and in some countries, for example USA, review by a government agency – in this example, the FDA (US Food and Drugs Administration). A new drug is first reviewed by the FDA when a sponsoring company submits an investigational new drug application (IND) to FDA. Within 30 days the FDA must let the sponsor know whether in its judgement the proposed clinical study is sufficiently safe.[6] If so, the IND is considered to be 'in effect' and the clinical study may proceed. If not, the FDA may place the clinical study 'on hold' until their concerns are satisfactorily addressed.

In planning the clinical programme it is important to refer to the target profile and explore the potential clinical benefits of new drug candidates as early as possible so as to reject drug candidates which fail to meet the desired goals. The phases of clinical development alongside major decision checkpoints are shown in Figure 4.

The main objectives of the initial investigations of a new drug candidate in man are to:

- Determine the safety and tolerance in man.
- Determine the pharmacokinetics and bioavailability for a range of doses.
- Determine the pharmacological profile.

Well designed and well conducted early studies in man are important because results from these enable studies later in development to be better designed in terms of dose range and frequency, and better monitoring of side effects and toxicity. Initial clinical trials should be designed so as to ensure that the maximum information can accrue from studies in minimal numbers of subjects, thus reducing the spread of risk.

To begin with, single, increasing doses of the drug candidate are administered to a small number of subjects, who are monitored intensively. In this way an

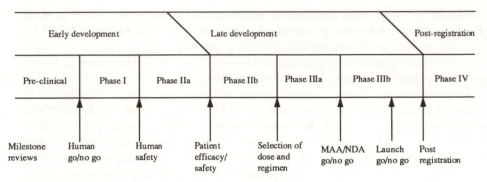

Figure 4: *Drug development phases and decision checkpoints*

indication of the maximum tolerated dose is obtained. The subjects are usually young, healthy male volunteers. One advantage of using healthy volunteers is that it is more easy to define the cause of any adverse reactions. Adverse reactions include both 'toxic effects' (unwanted actions of the substance on organs or tissues of the body sufficient to impair their function or to cause cell death) and 'side effects' (unexpected and unwanted effects caused by known or expected pharmacological actions of the substance at or around the therapeutic dose). Female volunteers of childbearing potential are not used in clinical trials until the results of adequate reproductive toxicology tests are available in animals. Usually these tests are not available prior to Phase I and volunteers studies are invariably conducted in males. Clinical trials can be conducted in males without any reproductive data in animals, in countries including USA and UK. In contrast, in Japan, male fertility studies in animals are required prior to volunteer Phase I studies. Although the majority of initial clinical studies are conducted in normal healthy (male) subjects, there are instances where this is inappropriate, for example, products indicated for cancer chemotherapy or AIDS. In these cases initial clinical studies may be undertaken in patients.

During a Phase I trial, in addition to safety data, pharmacokinetic data can be obtained by sampling body fluids from single-dose and subsequent repeat-dose studies. Half-life, area under the curve, clearance, and accumulation can be determined. Studies using radiolabelled material are often performed to establish the metabolite profile and routes of excretion in man, and to compare with the data obtained in toxicology species. Therapeutic effects can seldom be measured in Phase I, although pharmacological action may be detectable. Such data, if available, can provide valuable indications of clinical usefulness and of therapeutic dose ranges and can help in the planning and design of later clinical trials. In some instances pharmacological activity of potential benefit in disease can be demonstrated in non-patient volunteers by the treatment of induced effects.

The route of administration in man should be the same as that used in the toxicology studies. The formulation used should ideally be the simplest presentation consistent with the objectives of the study. The starting dose in man can be derived in different ways from the animal data: for example, 1% of the dose (unit weight) which has produced any effect on animals, 10–20% of the maximum tolerated dose in animals, or alternatively scrutiny of effective and safe doses in man of closely related compounds .

When satisfactory single-dose human data are available, repeated-dose Phase I studies may be conducted. The number of doses given to volunteers should be the minimum that will yield the required information and will be constrained by the duration of the completed two species animal toxicology studies. In multiple dose studies the interval between doses is usually approximately one half-life – 'rounded-up' to a convenient dosing regimen, for example, once daily or 8 hourly.

Placebo administration acts as a control in Phase I studies and a randomised, controlled study provides a strong design in that it removes bias in allocation of subjects to a control or drug group, provides comparable groups, and allows valid statistical tests.

The cut-off points between the Phases I, II, and III clinical trials are somewhat subjective and arbitrary. Phase II studies are designed to evaluate safety and efficacy in patients for whom the drug is intended. They provide confirmation on the effective dose and the therapeutic ratio. Dosing usually begins with a single dose lower than the expected therapeutic dose, taking into account any differences in the absorption, distribution, and metabolism which might arise from abnormalities resulting from the disease process.

The initial studies are usually small and patients are monitored intensively for therapeutic and adverse effects. Often, the initial studies are conducted on hospital patients, inpatients rather than outpatients. Later Phase II studies entail a more rigorous demonstration of a drug's efficacy. These studies are often controlled against placebo or a competitor compound (the latter to establish the comparative advantages and disadvantages of the new medicinal product). In the first instance, subjects with incompetence of any target organs which are expected to be affected by the pharmacological action of the drug candidate, or of any other important organs (especially the liver and kidney), must be excluded unless this type of abnormality is an integral part of their disease process.

In the UK, clearance for studies in patients is required from the Medicine's Control Agency (Committee for Safety of Medicines – CSM) of the Department of Health. A pharmaceutical company will require a Clinical trial Exemption (CTX) or Certificate (CTC) for which information is required on the chemistry, pharmacy, and preclinical safety of the compound. Permission or refusal of a CTX comes through in 35 days after application, unless an extension is requested by the MCA.

Multiple-dose studies will involve a decision on the dosing frequency or interval between individual doses. The half-life of the compound in the blood and/or the duration of the pharmacological effect will determine the dosing frequency.

There may be some constraint here imposed by the target product profile such that dosing which is more frequent than once a day is not competitive. A decision may have to be made about the viability of the drug candidate if pharmacokinetic/pharmacodynamic data point to a need for bid (twice daily) or tid (three times daily) dosing.

Phase III studies are large studies, in terms of patient numbers. Their aim is to establish the efficacy and safety of a treatment in order to substantiate the best method of treatment for patients. The duration of treatment should be long enough to induce a satisfactory response of the target disease and be related to the probable use by patients. The trials often include direct comparison with other available treatments. Thus the data address not only how efficacious and safe is the drug candidate but what is its relative efficacy and safety *versus* other medicines. Such comparative data are not only useful in marketing the drug but also increasingly in assessing the cost–benefit/pharmacoeconomics of the drug candidate *versus* other treatments. Whether placebo or another drug is used as a comparator will also depend on the disease being treated and the ethics of the trial. In the UK and Europe it is generally considered unethical to use a placebo in a chronic study if an effective therapy is available. The FDA, however, still require at least one well designed placebo-controlled study to gain registration approval. Placebos should 'match' the active drug in all physical respects such that the patient and clinical investigator cannot tell them apart.

Numbers of patients in the Phase III studies are based on the need to demonstrate differences in efficacy and/or safety in the drug candidate group *versus* the active comparator or placebo group. For active comparator trials it is necessary to have a good understanding of the expected safety and efficacy in order to predict the differences expected with the drug candidate and thus the required sample size. Transnational companies will usually carry out Phase III trials on a multi-national basis.

Additional clinical studies are conducted in parallel to the Phase II and III studies. These may include interaction studies with drugs which are likely to be prescribed concurrently, food interactions studies and special populations, for example elderly or renally or hepatically impaired patients. The results from these studies will be reflected in the labelling (prescribing information) for the drug as, for example, contraindications warnings, adverse reactions.

The task in Phases I to III is to try and establish the degree of efficacy and the degree of side effects of a new drug candidate. The purpose of conducting all the preclinical and clinical studies is to enable the placement of new drugs on the market. In each major country there is a Government department (Regulatory Authority) which reviews the data, to determine whether the product should be granted a licence. Although guidelines on the information necessary for approval differ throughout the world, three basic criteria must be met; products must be of proven quality, safety, and efficacy. Each regulatory dossier or marketing approval application (MAA) contains volumes of data. Providing the data in a user friendly manner is very important. To date most MAAs have been provided as hard copy but increasingly some companies are implementing electronic submissions. The regulatory dossier is the culmination of many years work; the quality of the data together with the therapeutic need for the targeted disease will to a significant extent determine the approval times for marketing of the drug.

A point worth highlighting is that pharmacoeconomics data are increasingly needed at the time of product registration and when negotiating product pricing and reimbursement. Data that measure the value of the benefit of a new drug in terms of better health and the value of cost saving, for example, in terms of need for surgical interventions or residential care, need to be collected. In the future, the concern about value for money is unlikely to subside. Cost-containment for healthcare expenditure is a worldwide issue. Pharmaceutical companies now need to provide evidence to decision-makers, regulators, healthcare providers, formulary holders, insurers, doctors, pharmacists, and patients, of the value of new products.

At time of marketing usage of the drug may still be limited to 1000–2000 patients and attention is now being drawn to the limitations of this in terms of rarer side effects. Also, once the drug has been marketed it is available for widespread use and such use is not always in accordance with the manufacturer's recommendations. These aspects often produce reports, sometimes anecdotal, of new effects either advantageous or, more often, disadvantageous.

The aim of post-marketing stage of drug evaluation, in addition to continuing clinical trials, is to conduct long-term surveillance of the efficacy and safety of the drug in general use. Post-marketing clinical trials usually involve collection of a smaller amount of clinical data per patient than for Phase II or III studies. However, the trials must be of adequate scientific standard and sufficiently well documented to be compiled into a report which could be expected to be publishable in a medical journal. All adverse reactions notified to pharmaceutical companies should be kept in an appointed register. Documentation of unusual effects should be extensive enough so that any retrospective analysis of the files would allow consideration of any possible causes or contributory factors.

In summary, drug development requires effective integration and execution of many activities from diverse groups, under demanding cost, schedule, and performance requirements. It is important to set product goals at the start of development and to explore these 'advantages' as early as possible so as to reject drug candidates which fail. The plan for development of a new drug candidate provides an important road-map for organising multi-disciplinary activities towards desired results. It should also indicate a series of checkpoints at which data will be reviewed to assess if the product goals are likely to be met. This will be pivotal to ensuring that any new drug candidate justifies the investment in its development and offers benefits in the healthcare of its target patients.

9 REFERENCES

1. J.A. DiMasi, R.W. Hansen, H.G. Grabowski, and L. Lasagnon, *J. Health Economics*, 1991, **10**, 107.
2. D.L. Azarnoff, and R.L. Hertin, 'Drug Development: Risks and Problems', *Ann. N. Y. Acad. Sci.*, 1984.
3. R.G. Halliday, S.R Walker, and C.H Lumley, *J. Pharm. Med.* 1992, **2**, 139.
4. 'Trends and Changes in Drug Research and Development', B.C. Walker, and S.R. Walker, Kluwer, London, 1987.
5. J. Kranzler, N. Selby, D. Taylor, and F. Weber, *Pharmaceutical Executive*, March 1989.
6. D. Farley, *ASM News*, 1988, **54**, No 12.

Appendix 1: SUMMARY OF RECEPTOR PROPERTIES

Adapted from TiPS Receptor Nomenclature Supplement 1993 {Elsevier Science Publishers Ltd. (UK)}

	Agonists	Antagonists	Radioligands	Effectors
Adenosine	Review: TiPS (1991) 12, 326			
A_1	(2-Cl)-N^6-cyclo-pentyladenosine	DPCPX; 8-cyclo-pentyltheophylline	[^{3}H]DPCPX; [^{125}I]APNEA; [^{3}H]cyclopentyl-adenosine	cAMP↓ K$^+$↑Ca^{2+}↓
A_{2A}	CGS 21680 PAPA-APEC	CP 66713; KF 17837	[^{3}H]CGS 21680; [^{3}H]NECA; [^{3}H]PAPA-APEC	cAMP↑
A_{2B}	-	-	[^{3}H]NECA	cAMP↑
α_1-Adreno-	Review: TiPS (1991) 12, 62			
α_{1A}	Phenylephrine	WB 4101	-	IP$_3$/DG
α_{1B}	Phenylephrine	CEC (irreversible)	-	IP$_3$/DG
α_{1C}	Phenylephrine	WB 4101; CEC(irreversible)	-	IP$_3$/DG
α_{1D}		WB 4101	-	-
α_2-Adreno-	Review: Ann. Rev. Pharmacol. Toxicol. (1993) 33, 263			
α_{2A}	oxymetazoline	yohimbine; fluparoxan	-	cAMP↓ K$^+$ ↑Ca^{2+}↓
α_{2B}	UK14304	prazosin; ARC 239	-	cAMP↓ Ca^{2+}↓
α_{2C}	UK14304	yohimbine	-	cAMP↓
β-Adreno-	Review: Prog. in Med. Chem. (1985) 22, 121			
β_1	xamoterol	CGP 20712A; betaxolol	[^{3}H]bisoprolol	cAMP↑
β_2	procaterol	ICI 118551; α -methylpropranolol	[^{3}H]ICI 118551	cAMP↑
β_3	NA>adrenaline	BRL 37344	-	cAMP↑
Angiotensin	Review: TiPS (1992) 13, 365			
AT_1	AII>AIII	EXP 31274; SKF 108566	[^{3}H]losartan; [^{125}I]EXP 985 [^{3}H] or [^{125}I] AII	IP$_3$/DG; cAMP↓
AT_2	AII=AIII	PD 123177; CGP 42112A	[^{125}I]CGP 42112A; [^{3}H] or [^{125}I] AII	cGMP↓
Atrial natriuretic peptide	Review: TiPS (1990) 11, 245			
ANP_A	ANP>BNP	[L-α-aminosuberic acid]-NP$_{7-28}$	[^{125}I]ANP	cGMP↑
ANP_B	CNP>>ANP~BNP	-	[^{125}I]CNP	cGMP↑
Bombesin	Review: Comprehensive Medicinal Chemistry (1990) 3, 926			
BB_1	NMB	-	[^{125}I]BH-NMB; [^{125}I][Tyr^4]bombesin	IP$_3$/DG
BB_2	GRP~bombesin	[D-Phe^6]bombesin$_{6-13}$OEt; AcGRP$_{20-26}$ OEt	[^{125}I]GRP; [^{125}I][D-Tyr^6]bombesin$_{6-13}$OMe	IP$_3$/DG

	Agonists	Antagonists	Radioligands	Effectors

Bradykinin   Review: TiPS (1990) **11**, 156

B_1	BK_{1-8}; Sar[D-Phe^8]BK$_{1-8}$	[Leu^8]BK$_{1-8}$; [des-Arg^{10}]HOE 140	[^{3}H]BK$_{1-8}$	-
B_2	kallidin ~ BK [Hyp^3,Tyr(Me)^8]BK	HOE 140; NPC 567	[^{125}I]-[Tyr^8]BK; [^{3}H]D-Arg[Pro^2, Hyp^3,Thi^5,D-Tic^7,Tic^8]BK	IP$_3$/DG

CGRP

CGRP$_1$	α- and β-CGRP	CGRP$_{8-37}$	[^{125}I]α- and β-CGRP	cAMP
CGRP$_2$	α- and β-CGRP	[Cys(ACM)^{2,7}]CGRP	[^{125}I]α- and β-CGRP	cAMP

Cannabinoid   Review: TiPS (1990) **11**, 395

	(-)Δ^{9}tetrahydrocannabinol CP55940; WIN 55212-1	-	[^{3}H]CP55940 [^{3}H]WIN55212-2	cAMP

Cholecystokinin   Review: Ann. Rev. Pharmacol. Toxicol. (1991) **31**, 469

CCK$_A$	CCK$_8$; A 71623	devazepide; PD 140548	[^{3}H]devazepide	IP$_3$/DG
CCK$_B$ (gastrin)	CCK$_4$; gastrin	CI 988; L 365260; LY 262691	[^{3}H]L 365260; [^{3}H]PD 140376	IP$_3$/DG

Dopamine   Review: TiPS (1991) **12**, 7.

D$_1$	SKF 38393 fenoldopam	SKF 83566; SCH 39166	[^{3}H]SCH 23390 [^{125}I]SCH 23982	cAMP↑ (IP$_3$/DG?)
D$_2$	N-0437 bromocriptine	(-)sulpiride, YM 091512 BRL 25594, domperidone	[^{125}I]iodosulpiride [^{3}H]YM 091512	cAMP↓ K$^+$↑; Ca^{2+}↓
D$_3$	quinpirole; 7-OH-DPAT	AJ-76	[^{125}I]iodosulpiride	
D$_4$	-	clozapine	[^{3}H]spiperone	cAMP↓
D$_5$	-	SCH 23390	-	cAMP↑

Endothelin   Review: TiPS (1993) **14**, 225

ET$_A$	ET-1~ET-2>ET-3	BQ 123; FR 139317	[^{125}I]ET-1; [^{125}I]ET-2	IP$_3$/DG
ET$_B$	[Ala^{1,3,11,15}]ET-1	[Cys^{11,15}]ET-1$_{11-21}$	[^{125}I]ET-3; [^{125}I]-[Ala^{1,3,11,15}]ET-1	IP$_3$/DG

GABA   Reviews: TiPS (1993) **14**, 259; TiPS (1992) **13**, 446.

GABA$_A$ (competitive)	isoguvacine, muscimol	bicuculline SR 95531	[^{3}H]muscimol; [^{3}H]GABA [^{3}H]SR 95531	GABA$_A$-gated Cl$^-$ channel
GABA$_A$ (BDZ.)	diazepam; (inverse agonists DMCM)	flumazenil, ZK 93426	[^{3}H]flunitrazepam [^{3}H]flumazenil [^{35}S]TBPS	GABA$_A$-gated Cl$^-$ channel
GABA$_B$	L-baclofen; SKF 97541	saclofen; CGP 36742	[^{3}H]L-baclofen; [^{3}H]GABA	cAMP↓; K$^+$↑; Ca^{2+}↓

Galanin   Review: TiPS (1992) **13**, 312

	galanin	galantide	[^{125}I]-[Tyr^3]galanin	cAMP↓; K$^+$↑;Ca^{2+}↓

	Agonists	Antagonists	Radioligands	Effectors
Glutamate (ionotropic)		Review: TiPS (1990) 11, 126		
NMDA (competitive)	NMDA	CGS 19755 CGP 37849	[3H]CGS 19755; [3H]CPP; [3H]dizocilpine	int. Na+/ K+/Ca2+
NMDA (modulatory)	glycine, HA 966	5,7-dichlorokynurenate MNQX; L 689560	[3H]glycine; [3H]MK801; [3H]TCP	-
AMPA	AMPA;	NBQX	[3H]AMPA; [3H]CNQX	int. Na+/K+
kainate	kainate, domoate	NBQX	[3H]kainate	int. Na+/K+
Glutamate (metabotropic)		Review: TiPS (1993) 14, 13		
mGluR₁	ACPD; DHPG	-	-	IP3/DG
mGluR₂	ACPD	-	-	cAMP↓
mGluR₃	ACPD	-	-	cAMP↓
mGluR₄	ACPD	-	-	cAMP↓
mGluR₅	ACPD	-	-	IP3/DG
Glycine	glycine	strychnine	[3H]strychnine	int. Cl⁻
Histamine	Review: Pharmacol. Revs. (1990), 42, 46			
H₁	2-(*m*-F-phenyl)- histamine	mepyramine; triprolidine	[3H]mepyramine [125I]iodobolpyramine	IP3/DG
H₂	dimaprit, impromidine	cimetidine; ranitidine	[3H]tiotidine [125I]iodoaminopotentidine	cAMP↑
H₃	R-α- methylhistamine	thioperamide iodophenpropit	[3H]R-α-methylhistamine [125I]iodophenpropit	-
5-HT	Review: TiPS (1993) *14*, 233			
5-HT₁A	8-OH-DPAT	WAY 100135	[3H]8-OH-DPAT	cAMP↓, K+↑
5-HT₁B	CP 93129	cyanopindolol	[125I]GTI	cAMP↓
5-HT₁D	sumatriptan	GR 127935	[125I]GTI	cAMP↓
5-HT₁E	GR 85548 (+1D)	-	[3H]5-HT	cAMP↓
5-HT₁F	sumatriptan (+1D)	-	[125I]LSD	cAMP↓
5-HT₂A	α-methyl-5-HT	ritanserin; ICI 170809	[3H]ketanserin	IP3/DG
5-HT₂B	α-methyl-5-HT	LY 53857 (non-comp)	[3H]5-HT	IP3/DG
5-HT₂C	mCPP	SB 200646	[3H]mesulergine	IP3/DG
5-HT₃	2-methyl-5-HT	granisetron, tropisetron, ondansetron, BRL 46470	[3H]zacopride; [3H]granisetron	int. cation channel
5-HT₄	5-MeO-tryptamine renzapride, BIMU8	GR 113808 SB 204070	[3H]GR 113808 [125I]SB 207710	cAMP↑

	Agonists	Antagonists	Radioligands	Effectors
Leukotriene	**Review: TiPS (1989) 10, 103**			
LTB_4	LTB_4	LY 255283; ONO-LB 457	$[^3H]LTB_4$	IP_3/DG
LTC_4	N-methyl-LTC_4	-	$[^3H]LTC_4$	-
LTD_4	LTD_4	ICI 198615; MK 571; SKF 104353	$[^3H]LTD_4$; $[^3H]ICI$ 198615	IP_3/DG
Melatonin	melatonin	luzindole	2-$[^{125}I]$iodomelatonin	cAMP↓
Muscarinic	**Review: TiPS (1993) 14, 308**			
M_1	methacholine	pirenzepine; telenzepine	$[^3H]$pirenzepine; $[^3H]$QNB	IP_3/DG
M_2	methacholine	methoctramine; himbacine	$[^3H]$QNB	cAMP↓ K^+↑
M_3	methacholine	hexahydrosiladifenidol	$[^3H]$QNB	IP_3/DG
M_4	methacholine	tropicamide	$[^3H]$QNB	cAMP↓
Neuropeptide Y	**Review: TiPS (1991) 12, 389**			
Y_1	$[Pro^{34}]$NPY	-	$[^{125}I]$ or $[^3H]$NPY	cAMP↓
Y_2	NPY_{18-36}	-	$[^{125}I]$ or $[^3H]$NPY	cAMP↓ Ca^{2+}↓
Neurotensin	NT	SR 48692	$[^3H]$-NT	IP_3/DG
Nicotinic	**Review: Ann. Rev. Pharmacol. Toxicol. (1991) 31, 37**			
muscle	suxamethonium	α-bungarotoxin	$[^{125}I]$ or $[^3H]$α-bungarotoxin	int.Na^+/K^+/Ca^{2+}
		(gallamine, decamethonium - channel blockers)		
neuronal	dimethylphenyl-piperazinium	κ-bungarotoxin methylcaconitine	$[^{125}I]$ or $[^3H]$κ-bungarotoxin $[^3H]$nicotine	int.Na^+/K^+/Ca^{2+}
		(hexamethonium; mecamylamine - channel blockers)		
Opioid	**Review: TiPS (1990) 11, 70**			
μ	DAMGO; PL 017	CTAP; naloxone	$[^3H]$DAMGO; $[^3H]$DAGO	cAMP↓ K^+↑
δ	DPDPE; DSBULET [D-Ala²]deltorphin	ICI 174864; naltrindole	$[^3H]$DPDPE; $[^3H]$naltrindole	cAMP↓ K^+↑
κ	U 69593; CI 977; ICI 197067	norbinaltorphimine	$[^3H]$U 69593; $[^3H]$CI 977	Ca^{2+}↓
PAF	C-PAF	CV 6209; WEB 2086; L 659989	$[^3H]$PAF; $[^3H]$WEB 2086	IP_3/DG
Prostanoid	**Review: TiPS (1990) 11, 301**			
DP	BW 245C; ZK 110841	BWA 868C	$[^3H]PGD_2$	cAMP↑
EP_1	17-phenyl-ω-trinor-PGE_2	SC 19220	$[^3H]PGE_2$	IP_3/DG
EP_2	butaprost; AH 13205	-	$[^3H]PGE_2$	cAMP↑
EP_3	enprostil, GR 63799	-	$[^3H]PGE_2$	IP_3/DG, cAMP↓
FP	fluprostenol	-	$[^3H]PGF_{2\alpha}$	IP_3/DG
IP	cicaprost	-	$[^3H]$iloprost	cAMP↑
TP	U 46619; STA_2; I-BOP	GR 32191; SQ 29548	$[^3H]$SQ 29548; $[^{125}I]$I-BOP	IP_3/DG

	Agonists	Antagonists	Radioligands	Effectors
P$_2$ Purinoreceptors	Review: TiPS (1993) <u>14</u>, 50			
P$_{2X}$	α,β-methyleneATP	ANAPP$_3$	[^{3}H]α,β-methyleneATP	int. cation channel
P$_{2Y}$	ADPβF; homo-ATP 2-MeS-ATP; ADPβS	-	[^{35}S]ADPβS [^{35}S]ADPαS	IP$_3$/DG
P$_{2Z}$	3'-O-(benzoyl-benzoyl)ATP	2-MeS-L-ATP	-	int. cation channel
P$_{2T}$	2-MeS-ADP	2-Cl-ATP ; ATP	β[^{32}P]2-MeS-ADP	int. cation channel; cAMP↓
P$_{2U}$	UTPγS	-	[^{32}P]UTPγS	IP$_3$/DG
Somatostatin	Ann. Rev. Physiol. (1992) <u>54</u>, 455			
SS$_1$	-	-	[^{125}I]-[Tyr^{11}]SS	-
SS$_2$	MK 678	-	[^{125}I]MK 678	K$^+$↑ Ca^{2+}↓
SS$_3$	-	-	[^{125}I]-[Tyr^{11}]SS	cAMP↓
SS$_4$	-	-	[^{125}I]-[Tyr^{11}]SS	cAMP↓
Tachykinin	Review: Ann. Rev. Neurosci. (1991) <u>14</u>, 123			
NK$_1$	SP-OMe; GR 73632 [Pro^9]SP	CP 99994; RP 67580 GR 82334	[^{3}H] [Pro^9]SP; [^{3}H] or [^{125}I]BH-SP	IP$_3$/DG
NK$_2$	[β-Ala^8]NKA$_{4-10}$ GR 64349	SR 48968; GR 94800; L659877	[^{3}H]NKA; [^{125}I]iodohistidyl-NKA	IP$_3$/DG
NK$_3$	senktide; [Pro^7]NKB	[Trp^7,β-Ala^8]NKA$_{4-10}$	[^{3}H]senktide; [^{125}I]-[MePhe^7]NKB	IP$_3$/DG
Oxytocin and Vasopressin	Review: Comprehensive Medicinal Chemistry (1990) <u>3</u>, 881			
OT	[Thr^4,Gly^7]OT	*cyc*(D1-Nal,Ile,DPip, Pip,DHis,Pro)	[^{125}I]d(CH$_2$)$_5$[Tyr(Me)^2, Thr^4,Orn^8,Tyr^9-NH$_2$]OT	IP$_3$/DG
V$_{1A}$	-	OPC 21268	[^{125}I]Phaa,DTyr(Me),Phe,Gln, Asn.Arg-Pro,Arg,TyrNH$_2$	IP$_3$/DG
V$_{1B}$	-	-	-	IP$_3$/DG
V$_2$	δ[DArg^8]VP δ[Val^4]AVP	OPC 31260; δ(CH$_2$)$_5$[DIle^2,Ile^4]AVP	[^{3}H]δ[Val^4]AVP; [^{3}H]δ[DArg^8]VP	cAMP↑
VIP	VIP	-	[^{125}I]VIP; [^{125}I]PHI	cAMP↑
GRF	GRF	-	[^{125}I]GRF	cAMP↑
PACAP	PACAP	PACAP$_{6-27}$	[^{125}I]PACAP	cAMP↑
secretin	secretin	-	[^{125}I]secretin	cAMP↑

Appendix 2: SUMMARY OF ION CHANNEL PROPERTIES

Type	Conductance	Blockers	Properties	Function
Ca^{2+} channels				
L	~25 pS	dihydropyridines phenylalkylamines benzothiazepines	High voltage activated; long lasting current; slow inactivation modulated by protein Kinase A-dependent phosphorylation	Excitation: contraction of cardiac and smooth muscle; secretion coupling in endocrine cells and neurones
N	~12-20 pS	-	High voltage activated moderate inactivation	neurotransmitter release
T	~8 pS	octanol, nickel flunarizine (non- selective)	Low voltage activated slower inactivation	SA pacemaker activity in heart repetitive spike activity in neurones and endocrine cells
P	~10-12 pS	-	Moderate voltage activated non-inactivated	In some CNS neurones (Purkinge cells)
K$^+$ channels (voltage dependent)				
Delayed rectifier I_{KV}	5-60 pS	forskolin, phencyclidine 9-aminoacridine, 4AP, TEA, local anaesthetics	Delayed activation following membrane depolarisation. Inact.in ~ secs. or on repolarization	repolarization of AP in skeletal muscle; slow wave activity in smooth muscle.
A-channel I_A	20 pS	phencyclidine, 4AP, tetra-H-aminoacridine phencyclidine	Fast activation by depolarization after hyperpolarization. Rapid inactivation	prolongs interspike interval in hippocampal, pyramidal cells. regulation of firing frequency
slow delayed rectified $I_{K,S}$	~1 pS	LY 97241	Very slow activation Very slow inactivation	slow component of delayed rectifying current in heart; K$^+$ homeostasis (kidney)
inward rectified I_{IR}	5-30 pS	TEA, Cs$^+$,Ba^{2+}	open at resting potential, current reduced during depolarisation	Resting K$^+$ conductance and plateau phase of cardiac AP in cardiac and skeletal muscle
Sarcoplasmic reticulum $I_{K(SR)}$	150 pS	decamethonium hexamethonium, 4AP	voltage dependent, low K$^+$/Na$^+$ selectivity	Skeletal and cardiac muscle SR membranes:
K$^+$ channels (Ca^{2+}-activated)				
high conductance $I_{BK(Ca)}$	100-250 pS	TEA and Ba^{2+} (<mM); quinine; tubocurarine	opened by high conc. K$^+$ openers; opening increases with Ca↑ and membrane depolarisation	AP repolarization; control of secretion from chromaffin, pituitary, pancreatic β–cells
intermediate conductance $I_{IK(Ca)}$	18-50 pS	TEA; quinine; cetiedil; nitrendipine; calmodulin antagonists	activated by [Ca^{2+}]$_i$; red cell channel opened by metabolic exhaustion	volume regulation
small conductance $I_{SK(Ca)}$	6-14 ps	tubocurarine; quinine; mepacrine; 9-aminoacridine	little or no voltage dependence	long AHPs' intestinal smooth muscle relaxation; hyper-kalaemic response to α agonists
nonspecific cation $I_{K/Na(Ca)}$	25-30 pS	sensitive to 4AP and quinine	[Ca]$_i$ increases open probability; voltage insensitive; no dis-crimination between Na$^+$ and K$^+$	cardiac pacemaker; pacemaker depolarizations; depol. afterpot. and plateau pot. in skeletal muscle

Type	Conductance	Blockers	Properties	Function

Receptor-coupled channels

Type	Conductance	Blockers	Properties	Function
Muscarinic-inactivated $I_{K(M)}$	3-18 pS	W7; Ba^{2+}	time/voltage-dependent K^+, slow activating; non-inactivating; inhib. by PTX -insens. G proteins coupled to IP_3/DG	enhances depolarizing stimuli; hormonal control of neuronal excitability; facilitates AP discharge
Atrial muscarinic-activated $I_{K(ACh)}$	25-50 pS	Cs^{2+}; Ba^{2+}; 4AP; TEA; quinine	low-threshold voltageactivation; muscarinic and adenosine receptors activate directly via G_i-like G protein	vagal slowing of heart; (inhibitory action of $GABA_A$, α_2-adreno- and opioid receptors?)
5-HT-inactivated $I_{K(5-HT)}$	55 pS	Ba^{2+}	weakly voltage-dependent K^+, open at resting potential. 5-HT inactivates via cAMP-dependent phosphoryl-ation. FMRF amide opens channel	presynatic facilitation by 5-HT of transmitter release in *Aplysia* sensory neurones.

Other K^+ channels

Type	Conductance	Blockers	Properties	Function
ATP-sensitive $I_{K(ATP)}$ (several)	5-200 pS	sulfonylureas AZ-DF 265; lidocaine	$[ATP]_i$ inhibits opening; opened by K^+ channel openers; some show voltage dependence	in CNS, skeletal,cardiac and smooth muscle; control resting pot./regulation of GABA release
Na^+-activated $I_{K(Na)}$	220 pS	TEA; 4AP	activated by $Na^+ > 20$ mM; insensitive to voltage, $[ATP]_i$ or $[Ca^{2+}]_i$	repolarization and opposes depolarization
cell-volume-sensitive $I_{K(VOL)}$	16-40 pS	quinidine; lidocaine; cetiedil	opens when cells swell	volume regulation

Na^+ channels

Type	Conductance	Blockers	Properties	Function
I		tetrodotoxin; saxitoxin	-	CNS; spinal cord > brain; also in heart; located in cell bodies
II	20 pS	tetrodotoxin; saxitoxin	$V_{50} \sim -41$ mV; $V_h \sim -64$ mV	CNS brain > spinal cord in un-myelinated axons; conduction of action potential
III	16 pS	tetrodotoxin; saxitoxin	$V_{50} \sim -10$ mV; $V_h \sim -40$ mV	embryonic and neonatal central neurones
μ1	-	μ-conotoxin	-	innervated skeletal muscle
h1	-	tetrodotoxin, saxitoxin (<200)	'tetrodotoxin-resistant' $V_h \sim -67$ mV	heart; embryonic and denervated skeletal muscle

Appendix 3: ENZYME COMMISSION CLASSIFICATION OF ENZYMES

- first number indicates to which of the six classes the enzyme belongs
- second number indicates the subclass
- third figure indicates the sub-subclass
- fourth figure the serial number

1. OXIDOREDUCTASES: catalyse oxidoreduction systems:

1.1 acting on CH-OH: **1.2** acting on C=O: **1.3** acting on CH-CH: **1.4** acting on $CH-NH_2$:
1.5 CH-NH: **1.6** NADH or NADPH: **1.7** other Nitrogen compounds: **1.8** Sulfur compounds:
1.9 HEME: **1.10** Diphenols: **1.11** H_2O_2: **1.12** Hydrogen:
1.13 single donor with incorporation of O_2: **1.14** Paired donor with incorporation of O_2:
1.15 superoxide radicals as acceptor: **1.16** oxidizing metal ions: **1.17** acting on CH_2
1.18 reduced ferredoxin: **1.19** reduced flavodoxin: **1.97** Other oxidoreductases

2. TRANSFERASES: transfers a group from donor to acceptor

2.1 transfers one-carbon groups: **2.2** aldehyde or ketone: **2.3** acyltransferases
2.4 glycosyltransferases: **2.5** alkyl or aryl (not methyl): **2.6** nitrogen containing groups
2.7 phosphorus containing groups: **2.8** sulfur containing groups

3. HYDROLASES: hydrolysis of various bonds

3.1 esters : **3.2** glycosidases: **3.3** ethers: **3.4** peptidases and proteinases: **3.5** carbon-nitrogen
bonds other than peptide: **3.6** acid anhydrides: **3.7** carbon-carbon bonds: **3.8** halide bonds:
3.9 phosphorus-nitrogen bonds: **3.10** sulfur-nitrogen bonds: **3.11** carbon-phosphorus:

4. LYASES: cleave bonds by non-hydrolytic and non-oxidative mechanism

4.1 carbon-carbon cleavage: **4.2** carbon-oxygen cleavage: **4.3** carbon-nitrogen cleavage:
4.4 carbon-sulfur cleavage: **4.5** carbon-halide cleavage: **4.6** phosphorus-oxygen cleavage
4.99 other lyases

5. ISOMERASES: catalyse changes within one molecule.

5.1 racemases and epimerases (**5.1.1**: amino acids; **5.1.2**: hydroxy acids; **5.1.3**:
carbohydrates): **5.2** *cis-trans*-isomerases: **5.3** intramolecular oxidoreductases (including
5.3.1: sugar isomerases; **5.3.2**: keto-enol tautomerases; **5.3.3**: C=C shift; **5.3.4**: S-S
transposition): **5.4** intramolecular transferases (including acyl, phospho-, amino-): **5.5**
intramolecular lyases: **5.99** other isomerases

6. LIGASES: (synthases and synthetases) connect two molecules with hydrolysis of ATP or similar triphosphate

6.1 forming C-O bonds: **6.2** forming C-S bonds: **6.3** forming C-N bonds
6.4 forming C-C bonds: **6.5** forming phosphoric ester bonds

Example of Classification: EC 1.5.1.3 Dihydrofolate reductase:

7,8-dihydrofolate + NADPH → 5,6,7,8-tetrahydrofolate + NADP

No.	Classification
1	Oxidoreductase
5	Acting on C-N bond of donors
1	With NAD or NADP as Acceptor
3	Specific number indicating dihydrofolate reductase

Appendix 4: SCHEMATIC REPRESENTATIONS OF MECHANISMS OF PROTEASES

$$RCONHR' \rightarrow RCOOH + H_2NR'$$

1. Schematic representation of aspartate proteinase catalytic mechanism

2. Schematic representation of serine (X = O) and cysteine (X = S) peptidase catalytic mechanism

3.   Schematic representation of metalloproteinase catalytic mechanism

Appendix 5: TABLE OF SUBSTITUENT CONSTANTS π, MR, F, R AND σ.

Substituent	π	MR	F	R	σ_{meta}	σ_{para}
Br	0.86	8.88	0.44	-0.17	0.39	0.23
Cl	0.71	6.03	0.41	-0.15	0.37	0.23
F	0.14	0.92	0.43	-0.34	0.34	0.06
I	1.12	13.94	0.40	-0.19	0.35	0.18
NO_2	-0.28	7.36	0.67	0.16	0.71	0.78
N_3	0.46	10.20	0.30	-0.13	0.27	0.15
H	0.00	1.03	0.00	0.00	0.00	0.00
OH	-0.67	2.85	0.29	-0.64	0.12	-0.37
SH	0.39	9.22	0.28	-0.11	0.25	0.15
NH_2	-1.23	5.42	0.02	-0.68	-0.16	-0.66
NHOH	-1.34	7.22	0.06	-0.40	-0.04	-0.34
SO_2NH_2	-1.82	12.28	0.41	0.19	0.46	0.57
CF_3	0.88	5.02	0.38	0.19	0.43	0.54
OCF_3	1.04	7.86	0.38	0.00	0.38	0.35
SO_2CF_3	0.55	12.86	0.73	0.26	0.79	0.93
SCF_3	1.44	13.81	0.35	0.18	0.40	0.50
CN	-0.57	6.33	0.51	0.19	0.56	0.66
CO_2^-	-4.36	6.05	-0.15	0.13	-0.10	0.00
1-Tetrazolyl	-1.04	18.33	0.52	0.02	0.52	0.50
CHO	-0.65	6.88	0.31	0.13	0.35	0.42
CO_2H	-0.32	6.93	0.33	0.15	0.37	0.45
NHCHO	-0.98	10.31	0.25	-0.23	0.19	0.00
$CONH_2$	-1.49	9.81	0.24	0.14	0.28	0.36
Me	0.56	5.65	-0.04	-0.13	-0.07	-0.17
$NHCONH_2$	-1.30	13.72	0.04	-0.28	-0.03	-0.24
$NHC=S(NH_2)$	-1.40	22.19	0.23	-0.05	0.22	0.16
OMe	-0.02	7.87	0.26	-0.51	0.12	-0.27
CH_2OH	-1.03	7.19	0.00	0.00	0.00	0.00
SOMe	-1.58	13.70	0.52	0.01	0.52	0.49
SO_2Me	-1.63	13.49	0.54	0.22	0.60	0.72
SMe	0.61	13.82	0.20	-0.18	0.15	0.00
NHMe	-0.47	10.33	-0.11	-0.74	-0.30	-0.84
$NHSO_2Me$	-1.18	18.17	0.25	-0.20	0.20	0.03
CF_2CF_3	1.68	9.23	0.44	0.11	0.47	0.52
$CH=CH_2$	0.82	10.99	0.07	-0.08	0.05	-0.02
COMe	-0.55	11.18	0.32	0.20	0.38	0.50
OCOMe	-0.64	12.47	0.41	-0.07	0.39	0.31
CO_2Me	-0.01	12.87	0.33	0.15	0.37	0.45
NHCOMe	-0.97	14.93	0.28	-0.26	0.21	0.00
$NHCO_2Me$	-0.37	16.53	0.14	-0.28	0.07	-0.15
C=O (NHMe)	-1.27	14.57	0.34	0.05	0.35	0.36
NHC=S (Me)	-0.42	23.40	0.27	-0.13	0.24	0.12
Et	1.02	10.30	-0.05	-0.10	-0.07	-0.15

Substituent	π	MR	F	R	σ_{meta}	σ_{para}
CH$_2$OMe	-0.78	12.07	0.01	0.02	0.02	0.03
OEt	0.38	12.47	0.22	-0.44	0.10	-0.24
SOEt	-1.04	18.35	0.52	0.01	0.52	0.49
SEt	1.07	18.42	0.23	-0.18	0.18	0.03
NHEt	0.08	14.98	-0.11	-0.51	-0.24	-0.61
SO$_2$Et	-1.09	18.14	0.54	0.22	0.60	0.72
N(Me)$_2$	0.18	15.55	0.10	-0.92	-0.15	-0.83
cPr	1.14	13.53	-0.03	-0.19	-0.07	-0.21
CO$_2$Et	0.51	17.47	0.33	0.15	0.37	0.45
iPr	1.53	14.96	-0.05	-0.10	-0.07	-0.15
nPr	1.55	14.96	-0.06	-0.08	-0.07	-0.13
N$^+$(Me)$_3$	-5.96	21.20	0.89	0.00	0.88	0.82
Si(Me)$_3$	2.59	24.96	-0.04	-0.04	-0.04	-0.07
1-Pyrryl	0.95	21.85	0.50	-0.09	0.47	0.37
2-Thienyl	1.61	24.04	0.10	0.04	0.09	0.05
3-Thienyl	1.81	24.04	0.04	-0.06	0.03	-0.02
nBu	2.13	19.61	-0.06	-0.11	-0.08	-0.16
tBu	1.98	19.62	-0.07	-0.13	-0.10	-0.20
OnBu	1.55	21.66	0.25	-0.55	0.10	-0.32
N(Et)$_2$	1.18	24.85	0.01	-0.91	-0.23	-0.90
CH$_2$Si(Me)$_3$	2.00	29.61	-0.15	-0.07	-0.16	-0.21
Pentyl	2.67	24.26	-0.06	-0.08	-0.08	-0.16
Ph	1.96	25.36	0.08	-0.08	0.06	-0.01
OPh	2.08	27.68	0.34	-0.35	0.25	-0.03
SO$_2$Ph	0.27	33.20	0.56	0.18	0.61	0.70
NHPh	1.37	30.04	-0.02	-0.38	-0.12	-0.40
NHSO$_2$Ph	0.45	37.88	0.21	-0.18	0.16	0.01
2,5-diMe-1-pyrryl	1.95	31.15	0.52	-0.10	0.49	0.38
c-Hexyl	2.51	26.69	-0.13	-0.10	-0.15	-0.22
2-Benzthiazolyl	2.13	38.88	0.25	0.06	0.27	0.29
COPh	1.05	30.33	0.30	0.16	0.34	0.43
CO$_2$Ph	1.46	32.31	0.33	0.13	0.37	0.44
OCOPh	1.46	32.33	0.23	-0.08	0.21	0.13
N=CHPh	-0.29	33.01	0.09	-0.63	-0.08	-0.55
NHCOPh	0.49	34.64	0.09	-0.27	0.02	-0.19
CH$_2$Ph	2.01	30.01	-0.08	-0.01	-0.08	-0.09
CH$_2$OPh	1.66	32.19	0.02	0.02	0.03	0.04
C≡CPh	2.65	33.21	0.12	0.05	0.14	0.16
CH=CHPh (trans)	2.68	34.17	0.06	-0.12	0.03	-0.07
N(Ph)$_2$	3.61	54.96	0.07	-0.29	0.00	-0.22

Substituents highlighted are those suggested by David Livingstone (SB) as suitable substituents for investigating π, MR (molar refractivity), F (Field) and R (Resonance)

Compound selection programme called "Paragon" is available from University of Portsmouth Enterprise Ltd (UPEL), U.K.

Appendix 6: AN EXAMPLE OF A CRAIG DIAGRAM PLOT OF σ VS π

(J. Med. Chem. 1970, **14**, 680)

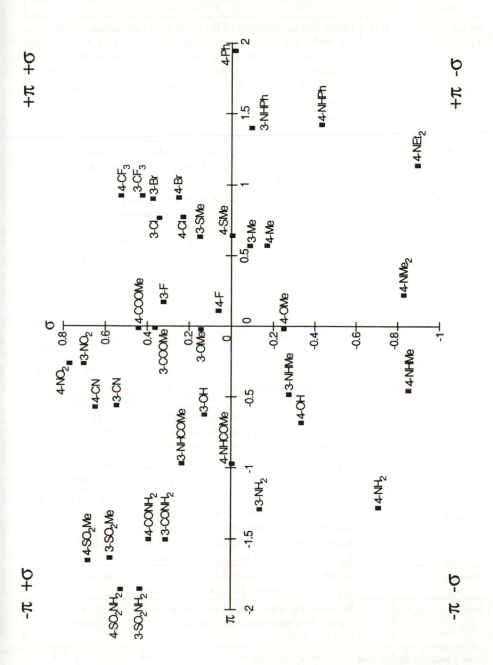

Appendix 7: SUMMARY OF COMMON ROUTES OF ADMINISTRATION*

Route		Comments
Intra-Cerebro Ventricular	ICV	Direct into the ventricle of the brain, rapid immediate effect limited by low surface area, elimination via the CSF and possible local metabolism. Diffusion from ventricles into the brain should be fast, otherwise the drug may leave the ventricles with the CSF. Re-entry to the brain via the blood may be <u>faster</u>.
Intra-Venous	IV	Guaranteed systemic exposure, rapid blood levels/effect limited by protein binding/metabolism/distribution. Central activity limited by brain penetration
Intra-Arterial	IA	Guaranteed systemic exposure, rapid blood levels/effect limited by protein binding/metabolism/distribution. Central activity limited by brain penetration
Sub-Cutaneous	SC	Systemic exposure produced more slowly than IV. Only small dose volume appropriate and there is the possibility of precipitation at the dosing site. Other properties same as IV but slow release may increase effects of metabolism etc.
Intra-Muscular	IM	Systemic exposure produced more slowly than IV. Only small dose volume appropriate and there is the possibility of precipitation at the dosing site. More reproducible route of administration than SC.
Dermal/Topical		Systemic exposure limited by surface area and absorption through epidermal barrier.
Intra-Peritoneal	IP	Absorption into either hepatic portal vein (and in this case first pass metabolism is important) or systemic system. Precipitation may occur in peritoneum. Systemic exposure may be highly variable by this route.
Intra-Duodenal	ID	Systemic exposure limited by absorption from the gut, gut wall metabolism and first pass elimination. Gut transit time/housekeeper waves also important.
Intra-Hepatic Portal Vein	IPV	Systemic exposure limited by first pass elimination. Avoids malabsorption through gut wall and gut wall metabolism.
Per Os (by mouth)	PO	Systemic exposure limited by gastric emptying rate and acid and gastric enzyme stability. Acidic compounds can be directly absorbed. Differences may occur from fed versus starved status. As for ID systemic exposure limited by absorption from the gut, gut wall metabolism and first pass elimination.
Buccal		Systemic exposure limited by low surface area but this route of administration avoids first pass elimination
Rectal		Systemic exposure limited by absorption through gut wall. Avoids first pass elimination in first 6" of gut but absorption may be variable.

*Kindly supplied by Ann Lewis, SmithKline Beecham Pharmaceuticals, Welwyn Garden City, U.K.

Appendix 8: APPROXIMATE CONVERSION FACTORS FOR ΔLOG TO RATIO

ΔLog	0	0.1	0.2	0.3	0.4	0.5	0.6	0.7	0.8	0.9
ratio	1	1.25	1.5	2	2.5	3	4	5	6	8
ΔLog	1.0	1.1	1.2	1.3	1.4	1.5	1.6	1.7	1.8	1.9
ratio	10	12.5	15	20	25	30	40	50	60	80

Appendix 9: CONVERSION FACTORS FOR SOLUTIONS AND DOSAGES; MOLAR VS WEIGHT

Solution; weight to molar: $X\ \mu g/mL = X \div M.Wt.\ mM \equiv 1000X \div M.Wt.\ \mu M$

M.Wt.	100	150	200	250	300	350	400	450	500
1μg/mL =	10μM	6.7μM	5μM	4μM	3.3μM	2.9μM	2.5μM	2.2μM	2μM
1μM =	0.1 μg/mL	0.15 μg/mL	0.2 μg/mL	0.25 μg/mL	0.3 μg/mL	0.35 μg/mL	0.4 μg/mL	0.45 μg/mL	0.5 μg/mL

Dosage; molar to weight: $X\ \mu M/kg = X \times M.Wt.\ \mu g/kg \equiv X \times M.Wt. \div 1000\ mg/kg$

M.Wt.	100	150	200	250	300	350	400	450	500
1mg/kg =	10 μM/kg	6.7 μM/kg	5 μM/kg	4 μM/kg	3.3 μM/kg	2.9 μM/kg	2.5 μM/kg	2.2 μM/kg	2 μM/kg
1μM/kg =	0.1 mg/kg	0.15 mg/kg	0.2 mg/kg	0.25 mg/kg	0.3 mg/kg	0.35 mg/kg	0.4 mg/kg	0.45 mg/kg	0.5 mg/kg

Subject Index